T0137230

Rare Diseases of the Immune System

Series Editors
Lorenzo Emmi
Domenico Prisco

Editorial Board:

Systemic Vasculitis
Lorenzo Emmi
Carlo Salvarani
Renato Alberto Sinico

Autoimmune Disease
Pier Luigi Meroni
Dario Roccatello
Marco Matucci-Cerinic
Lorenzo Emmi

Autoinflammatory Syndromes
Marco Gattorno
Fabrizio de Benedetti
Rolando Cimaz

Primary Immunodeficiency
Alessandro Plebani
Cosima Baldari
Mario Milco D'Elios

Systemic Fibroinflammatory Disorders
Augusto Vaglio

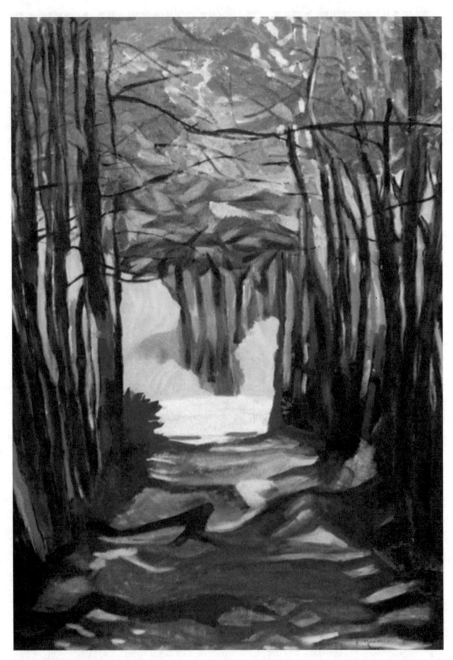

Profondità luminosa
Laura Maddii Emmi (Private collection)

Carlo Salvarani · Luigi Boiardi
Francesco Muratore
Editors

Large and Medium Size Vessel and Single Organ Vasculitis

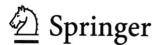

Springer

Editors
Carlo Salvarani
Rheumatology Unit
Azienda Unita' Sanitaria Locale IRCCS
di Reggio Emilia
Reggio Emilia
Italy

Rheumatology Unit
Università di Modena e Reggio Emilia
Modena
Italy

Francesco Muratore
Rheumatology Unit
Azienda Unita' Sanitaria Locale IRCCS
di Reggio Emilia
Reggio Emilia
Italy

Luigi Boiardi
Rheumatology Unit
Azienda Unita' Sanitaria Locale IRCCS
di Reggio Emilia
Reggio Emilia
Italy

ISSN 2282-6505   ISSN 2283-6403   (electronic)
Rare Diseases of the Immune System
ISBN 978-3-030-67177-8   ISBN 978-3-030-67175-4   (eBook)
https://doi.org/10.1007/978-3-030-67175-4

© Springer Nature Switzerland AG 2021, corrected publication 2021
This work is subject to copyright. All rights are reserved by the Publisher, whether the whole or part of the material is concerned, specifically the rights of translation, reprinting, reuse of illustrations, recitation, broadcasting, reproduction on microfilms or in any other physical way, and transmission or information storage and retrieval, electronic adaptation, computer software, or by similar or dissimilar methodology now known or hereafter developed.
The use of general descriptive names, registered names, trademarks, service marks, etc. in this publication does not imply, even in the absence of a specific statement, that such names are exempt from the relevant protective laws and regulations and therefore free for general use.
The publisher, the authors, and the editors are safe to assume that the advice and information in this book are believed to be true and accurate at the date of publication. Neither the publisher nor the authors or the editors give a warranty, expressed or implied, with respect to the material contained herein or for any errors or omissions that may have been made. The publisher remains neutral with regard to jurisdictional claims in published maps and institutional affiliations.

This Springer imprint is published by the registered company Springer Nature Switzerland AG
The registered company address is: Gewerbestrasse 11, 6330 Cham, Switzerland

Preface

The vasculitides are a heterogeneous group of relatively rare conditions that can occur independently by other conditions (primary vasculitis), or they can represent a manifestation of a well-established disease (secondary vasculitis). Vasculitis may be localized to a single organ or vascular bed, or, they are, more commonly, generalized. The most widely accepted classification system, the 2012 Revised Chapel Hill Consensus Conference (2012 CHCC), is based on vessel size predominantly involved (large-, medium-, and small-vessel vasculitis) and association with antineutrophil cytoplasmic antibodies (ANCA). (Jennette JC, Falk RJ, Bacon PA, et al. 2012 revised International Chapel Hill Consensus Conference Nomenclature of Vasculitides. Arthritis Rheum. 2013;65(1):1–11). Furthermore, vasculitis affecting vessels of variable size and single organ vasculitis are included. According to the 2012 CHCC definition, single organ vasculitis is a vasculitis involving arteries or veins of any size in a single organ without evidences indicating the presence of a systemic vasculitis. The involved organ and vessel type should be included in the name (e.g., cutaneous small-vessel vasculitis, testicular arteritis, central nervous system vasculitis). Vasculitis distribution may be unifocal or multifocal (diffuse) within an organ.

This book will provide detailed and updated information on the nosology, pathology, pathogenesis, clinical presentation, diagnosis, and treatment of large- and medium-sized vessel and single organ vasculitis, critically discussed by the most expert physicians and researchers in the field. Among the conditions considered are giant cell arteritis, Takayasu arteritis, polyarteritis nodosa, primary central nervous system vasculitis, isolated aortitis, isolated gastrointestinal vasculitis, cutaneous vasculitis, and isolated genitourinary vasculitis. Finally, arterial and venous involvement in Behcet's disease will be discussed as well.

The role of histopathology in the diagnosis and prognosis of these vasculitides will also be evaluated. The role of imaging studies in diagnosing and monitoring these diseases will be addressed and, in particular, indications and limitations of the available imaging modalities will be discussed to provide better anatomic and functional information to the referring physicians, which would improve patient care. The expanding role of biological agents for the treatment of vasculitides will be addressed, and the current therapeutic approaches to these diseases in clinical practice will be discussed.

We believe that this book, the first ever published on single organ vasculitis, will be a cornerstone for medical practitioners, internists, specialists, researchers, and postgraduate students interested in the fields of vasculitis and rare diseases.

Reggio Emilia, Italy   Carlo Salvarani
                                                                                          Luigi Boiardi
                                                                                      Francesco Muratore

Contents

Part I

Giant Cell Arteritis

Classification Criteria

1

Fabrizio Cantini and Carlotta Nannini

Abstract

GCA is usually classified according to the American College of Rheumatology (ACR) 1990 criteria. This set of criteria were designed to distinguish the different types of vasculitides but not to establish a differential diagnosis. Five criteria were finally selected and a patient shall be classified as having GCA if at least 3 of 5 criteria are satisfied. The presence of any 3 or more of the 5 criteria is related with a sensitivity of 93.5% and a specificity of 91.2%. The use and the application of the criteria set is relatively simple. Biopsy is the only invasive procedure. Limitations of temporal artery biopsy lead to develop noninvasive procedures in order to detect GCA like ultrasound, MRI, and PET CT. Due to numerous uncertainties regarding the optimal GCA diagnosis based on temporal artery biopsy, and the advent of modern vascular imaging techniques prompted different societies to develop recommendations for GCA management.

Keywords

Classification criteria · Giant cell arteritis · Large vessel vasculitis · Specificity Sensitivity · Temporal artery biopsy

Giant cell arteritis (GCA) also known as temporal arteritis is a chronic granulomatous vasculitis of large and medium-sized arteries [1].

GCA is usually classified according to the American College of Rheumatology (ACR) 1990 criteria [2].

F. Cantini (✉) · C. Nannini
Rheumatology Department, Prato Hospital, Prato, Italy

© Springer Nature Switzerland AG 2021
C. Salvarani et al. (eds.), *Large and Medium Size Vessel and Single Organ Vasculitis*, Rare Diseases of the Immune System,
https://doi.org/10.1007/978-3-030-67175-4_1

This set of criteria were designed to **distinguish** the **different** types of vasculitides but not to establish a differential diagnosis from other vasculitis disorders. Therefore, these criteria should be used for classification purposes rather **than for diagnosis**.

The vasculitis study group developed *the traditional format classification* and the *classification tree* comparing 214 patients with GCA with 593 controls with other forms of vasculitis. Thirty-three variables were selected as potentially important discriminators against other forms of vasculitis (Table 1.1). The number of cases and controls, the sensitivity and the specificity are reported in Table 1.1.

A "short list" of criteria was created including 3 single items and 7 combined items selected among the 33 variables reported in Table 1.1. The "short list" with 10 variables would have the potential to discriminate GCA cases from controls (Table 1.2).

Table 1.1 Variables list. Comparison of the sensitivity and specificity of potential criteria variables for giant cell arteritis[a] (adapted from Hunder GG Arthritis and Rheum 1990; 33:1122–1128)

Criterion	No. of pts. (Min-Max n)	No. of controls (Min-Max n)	Sensitivity (Min-Max %)	Specificity (Min-Max %)
History				
[i.e.: age at disease onset ≥50 years[b,c,d]; headache, new, localized[b,c,d]; Claudication, variables[b,d]; Polymyalgia rheumatica[b]...]	210–214	577–593	11.3–98.6	63.8–99.8
Physical				
[i.e.: Ischemic optic neuritis; visual abnormality[b]; amaurosis fugax; TA abnormality[b,c,d]; scalp tenderness or nodules[b,d]...]	209–214	473–588	4.7–57.3	88.8–99.7
Laboratory				
[i.e.: ESR (Wetergren) ≥ 50 mm/h [b,d]; serum alkaline phosphatase or Aspartate aminotransferase >1.5 times normal...]	203–207	439–514	8.4–86.5	47.7–81.1
Arterybiopsy				
[i.e.: predominantly mononuclear cell infiltration with granulomatosus inflammation and giant cells; Abnormal biopsy[b,c,d]]	210–211	320–322	84.3–92.9	73.1–88.2

[a]Values are the number of cases or controls with the variable described or tested. The sensitivity is the proportion of cases positive for the variable tested or described. The specificity is the proportion of controls negative for the variable tested or described. *TA* temporal artery, *ESR* erythrocyte sedimentation rate
[b]Criterion is one of the final "short list" of variables ($n = 10$)
[c]Criterion is used for the traditional format classification
[d]Criterion is used for the tree classification

Table 1.2 Short list

Criterion history	Criterion physical	Criterion laboratory	Criterion artery biopsy
1. Age at disease onset ≥50 years 2. Headache, new, localized (combined items) 3. Claudication (combined item) 4. Polymialgia rheumatica (combined item)	5. Visual abnormality (combined item) 6. TA abnormality (combined item) 7. Scalp tenderness or nodules (combined item)	8. ESR ≥ 50 mm/h 9. Serum alkaline phosphatase >1.5 times normal	10. Abnorml biopsy (combined item)

Table 1.3 1990 criteria for the classification of giant cell (temporal) arteritis (traditional format)[a]

Criterion	Definition
1. Age at disease onset ≥50 years	Development of symptoms or findings beginning at the age 50 or older
2. New headache	New onset or new type of localized pain in the head
3. Temporal artery abnormality	Temporal artery tenderness to palpation or decreased pulsation, unrelated to arteriosclerosis of cervical arteries
4. Elevated erythrocyte sedimentation rate	Elevated erythrocyte sedimentation rate by the Westergren method ≥50 mm/h
5. Abnormal artery biopsy	Biopsy specimen with artery showing vasculitis characterized by a predominance of mononuclear cell infiltration or granulomatous inflammation, usually with mononucleated giant cells

[a]For purpose of classification, a patient shall be said to have giant cell (temporal) arteritis if at least 3 of 5 criteria are present. The presence of any 3 or more criteria yields a sensitivity of 93.5% and a specificity of 91.2%

Traditional format classification. Five criteria were finally selected among the 10 variables in the "short list": age ≥ 50 years at disease onset, new onset of localized headache, temporal artery tenderness or decreased temporal artery pulse, elevated erythrocyte sedimentation rate (according Westergren method) ≥ 50 mm/h, and biopsy sample including an artery with necrotizing arteritis characterized by a predominance of mononuclear cell infiltrates or a granulomatous process with mononucleated giant cells. Table 1.3 records the final sets of criteria with their definition. A patient shall be classified as having GCA if at least 3 of 5 criteria are satisfied. The presence of any 3 or more of the 5 criteria is related with a sensitivity of 93.5% and a specificity of 91.2%.

Tree classification. Six are the criteria used to build the tree classification, selected among the 10 variables in the "short list" (Table 1.2). These criteria are the same as for the *traditional format* except for ESR that is excluded and other two items included: scalp tenderness and claudication of the jaw or tongue or on deglutition.

The best of several tree classifications was obtained using the computer program CART [3]. Criteria used for the *tree classification* are reported with their definitions in Table 1.4.

Table 1.4 Criteria and definitions used for the classification of giant cell (temporal) arteritis (tree format)

Criterion	Definition
1. Age at disease onset ≥50 years	Development of symptoms or findings beginning at the age 50 or older
2. New headache[a]	New onset or new type of localized pain in the head
3. Claudication of jaw, tongue, or on deglutition	Development or worsening of fatigue or discomfort in muscles of mastication, tongue, or swallowing muscle while eating
4. Temporal artery abnormality	Temporal artery tenderness to palpation or decreased pulsation, unrelated to arteriosclerosis of cervical arteries
5. Scalp tenderness or nodules[a]	Development of tender areas or nodules over the scalp, away from the temporal artery or other cranial arteries
6. Abnormal artery biopsy	Biopsy specimen with artery showing vasculitis characterized by a predominance of mononuclear cell infiltration or granulomatous inflammation, usually with mononucleated giant cells

[a]Used as surrogate if artery biopsy is not available (criterion2) or if temporal artery abnormality is not present (criterion5)

Among them, the presence of temporal artery tenderness or decreased pulsation recognized cases from controls better than any other criterion. When these items were not available, scalp tenderness was used as a surrogate. When biopsy was not performed, headache served as a surrogate. The classification tree reached an overall sensitivity of 95.3% and specificity of 90.7%.

The use and the application of either criteria set is relatively simple. Biopsy is the only invasive procedure even if it is performed with local anesthesia, and it has a low morbidity rate. Severe complications can occur occasionally including the facial nerve damage, skin necrosis, brow ptosis, removing a vein or nerve by mistake and stroke [4]. TAB may require also the anticoagulation interruption with possible health issues and organizing challenge [4].

The diagnosis of GCA still continues to require the TAB confirmation since an inflammatory infiltrate in the media with the presence of giant cells and elastophagia can be considered characteristic of GCA [5]. These features are not always found. An isolated, inflammatory infiltrate in the periadventitia [6] or vasculitis (rarely necrotizing) of small vessels surrounding the temporal artery [6] is less common and may be found in other systemic vasculitis [7, 8].

Moreover, the typical skip lesion of GCA (areas of normal artery alternate to inflamed areas) can contribute to the false-negative biopsy in particular in specimens less than 2 cm in length [9, 10].

Bowling and colleagues [11] demonstrated that 80% of the TABs performed at their institute were negative and the glucocorticoid regimen was modified only in 7.8% of the cases.

Therefore, different societies across Europe and the USA suggest to not delay the prompt use of corticosteroids in particular in patients at higher risk of neuro-ophthalmic complications.

TAB can remain positive for 2–6 weeks after treatment initiation [12–14].

Additionally, the sensitivity of TAB is lower in patients with GCA with large vessel involvement who lack temporal arteritis [4].

Limitations of TA biopsy lead to develop noninvasive procedures in order to detect GCA. Schmidt in 1995 reported "hypoechoic halo" as a diagnostic finding of GCA on Doppler ultrasound (US) [15], representing inflammation of the vessel wall. The reported diagnostic accuracy of the halo sign and the other ultrasonographic findings like stenosis and occlusion vary across the study. Schmidt initially reported that all patients with GCA had hypoechoic halo [15], but later the same group found that the halo sign had a sensitivity and specificity of 73% and 100%, respectively [4].

US evaluation was also compared with physical examination and the results were that halo around the temporal artery (any halo or halo 1 mm or greater in thickness) modestly increased the probability of biopsy-proven giant cell arteritis, but did not improve the diagnostic accuracy of a careful physical examination [16].

A recent meta-analysis of 8 studies and 605 patients found that US had a pooled sensitivity and specificity of 77% and 96%, respectively [17].

Due to numerous **uncertainties** regarded the optimal GCA diagnosis based on temporal artery biopsy and the advent of modern vascular imaging techniques, different societies prompted to develop **recommendations** for GCA management [12–14].

The French study group for large vessel vasculitis formulated that GCA should be defined as an arteritis of the aorta and/or its branches in a person with 50 years of age and older with cranial (clinical or histologic evaluation) or ophthalmic involvement. For research purposes, the ACR classification criteria should be used to classify a vasculitis as GCA [12].

Temporal artery biopsy (TAB) still remains the **gold standard** for GCA diagnosis with high certainty. Temporal artery imaging with Doppler **ultrasonography** or MRI cannot replace the TAB as a first choice diagnostic evaluation. Angio CT, angio MRI, or FDG-PET scan support a clinical diagnosis of extracranial GCA with description of arteritis of aorta and its branches, but imaging cannot replace TAB as a first choice examination [12].

The Delphi exercise-based EULAR recommendations [13], developed 7 statements for the management of the large vessel vasculitis. Regarding diagnosis, also Eular Committee underlined the importance of TAB performance when GCA is suspected and as stated before TAB should not **delay** the treatment, and a **contralateral** biopsy is not routinely indicated.

The British society and the British health professionals in Rheumatology **developed recommendations** for GCA diagnosis and management [14]. The British groups pointed out that the early recognition and diagnosis is paramount. Particular attention should be paid to predictive features of ischemic neuro-ophthalmic complications. Urgent **referral** for rheumatologic evaluation is proposed for all patients with GCA. TAB should be considered when a GCA diagnosis is suspected. Imaging techniques **demonstrated promising sensitivity and specificity** for the diagnosis and monitoring **of** GCA, but, **to date, cannot replace TAB.**

References

1. Salvarani C, Cantini F, Hunder GG. Polymyalgia rheumatica and giant cell arteritis. Lancet. 2008;372:234–45.
2. Hunder GG, Bloch DA, Michael BA, Calabrese LH, Fauci AS, Fries JF, et al. The American College of Rheumatology 1990 Criteria for Classification of Giant Cell Arteritis. Arthritis Rheum. 1990;8:1122–8.
3. CART: California Statistical Software. Lafayette, CA; 1984.
4. Halbach C, McClelland CM, Chen J, Li S, et al. Use of noninvasive imaging in giant cell arteritis. Asia-Pac J Ophthalmol. 2018;7:260–4.
5. Lie JT. Illustrated histopathologic classification criteria for selected vasculitis syndrome. American College of Rheumatology subcommittee on Classification of Vasculitis. Arthritis Rheum. 1990;33:1074–87.
6. Cavazza A, Muratore F, Boiardi L, Restuccia G, Pipitone N, Pazzola G, et al. Inflamed temporal artery: histologic findings in 354 biopsies, with clinical correlations. Am J Surg Pathol. 2014;38:1360–70.
7. Esteban MJ, Font C, Hernandez-Rodriguez J, Valls-Solé J, Sanmartì R, Cardellach F, et al. Small vessel vasculitis surrounding a spared temporal artery: clinical and pathological findings in a series of 28 patients. Arthritis Rheum. 2001;44:1387–95.
8. Genereau T, Lortholary O, Pottier MA, Michon-Pasturel U, Ponge T, de Wazières B, et al. Temporal artery biopsy: a diagnostic tool, for systemic necrotizing vasculitis. Arthritis Rheum. 1999;42:2674–81.
9. Reinhard M, Smidth D, Hetzel A. Color-coded sonography in suspected temporal arteritis experience after 83 cases. Rheumatol Int. 2004;24:340–6.
10. Alberts M. Temporal arteritis: improving patient evaluation with a new protocol. Perm J. 2013;17:56–62.
11. Bowling K, Rait J, Atkinson J, Srinivas G. Temporal artery biopsy in the diagnosis of giant cell arteritis: does the end justify the means. Ann Med Surg. 2017;20:1–5.
12. Bienvenu B, Ly KH, Lambert M, André M, Benhamou Y, Bonnotte B, et al. Management of giant cell arteritis: recommendations of French study group for large vessel vasculitis. Rev Med Interne. 2016;37:154–65.
13. Mukhtyar C, Guillevin L, Cid MC, Dasgupta B, de Groot K, Gross W, et al. Eular recommendations for the management of large vessel vasculitis. Ann Rheum Dis. 2009;68:318–23.
14. Dasgupta B, Borg FA, Hassan N, Alexander L, Barraclough K, Bourke B, et al. BSR and BHPR guidelines for the management of giant cell arteritis. Rheumatology. 2010;49:1594–7.
15. Schmidt WA, Kraft HE, Volker L, Vorpahl K, Gromnica-Ihle EJ. Colour doppler sonography to diagnose temporal arteritis. Lancet. 1995;354:866.
16. Salvarani C, Silingardi M, Ghirarduzzi A, Lo Scocco G, Macchioni P, Bajocchi G, et al. Is duplex ultrasonography useful for diagnosis of giant cell arteritis? Ann Int Med. 2002;20(137):232–8.
17. Nielson BD, Gormsen LC, Hansen IT, Keller KK, Therkildsen P, Hauge EM. Three days of high dose glucocorticoid treatment attenuates large vessel v18F-FDG uptake in large vessel giant cell arteritis but with a limited impact on diagnostic accuracy. Eur J Nucl Med Mol Imaging. 2018;45:119–1128.

Epidemiology and Genetics

2

Fabrizio Cantini and Carlotta Nannini

Abstract

Giant cell arteritis (GCA) is the most frequent primary systemic vasculitis among patients ≥50 years of age, peaking in the seventh and eighth decade of life. The annual incidence rate of GCA increases with advancing age up to a maximum in the 70–79 year age group and then decreases slowly. Women are more affected than males with 3:1 ratio. The highest incidence is reported in North European countries and in North American population of the same descent with an incidence that varies between 32.4/100,000 people, older than 50 years of age in Norway and 18.9/100,000 people in Olsted County, Minnesota, USA Prevalence in GCA follows the same latitude distribution of incidence with higher prevalence in the Northern hemisphere compared to the Southern Europe and non-European country.

Prevalence study from Mayo Clinic reported that prevalence rate of GCA between 1950 and 2009 among women was 304 (95% CI 229–375) and among men was 91 (95% CI 46–156) per 100,000 population older than 50 years of age.

Compared with general population, all cause SMR (standardized mortality ratio) was not increased in GCA patients (SMR 1.081, 95% CI 0.963–1.214, $p = 0.184$) and the stratification by regions showed no significant increase in all cause SMR in Europe and the USA. Sex-specific meta-analysis provided by four out of eight studies included revealed the pooled SMR for women was 1.046 (95% CI 0.834–1.314, $p = 0.696$) and for men was 1.051 (95% CI 0.974–1.133, $p = 0.204$).

Female sex is the most important genetic risk factors for GCA as reported above.

Polymorphisms of the HLA II gene in particular the presence of HLA DRB1*04 alleles (both HLA DRB1*0401 and HLA DRB1*0404) are systematically associated with GCA supporting the thesis that GCA is driven by an antigen-based immune response.

F. Cantini (✉) · C. Nannini
Rheumatology Department, Prato Hospital, Prato, Italy

© Springer Nature Switzerland AG 2021
C. Salvarani et al. (eds.), *Large and Medium Size Vessel and Single Organ Vasculitis*, Rare Diseases of the Immune System,
https://doi.org/10.1007/978-3-030-67175-4_2

Keywords

Incidence · Mortality · Prevalence

2.1 Epidemiology

Giant cell arteritis (GCA) is the most frequent primary systemic vasculitis among patients ≥50 years of age [1], peaking in the seventh and eighth decade of life [2, 3]. In Northwestern Spain infact, the annual **incidence** rate of GCA increased with advancing age up to a maximum in the 70–79 year age group and then decreased slowly [4]. Similar results were obtained in the Olmsted County Minnesota USA population-based study, where the annual incidence increased with advanging age, in the 50–59 age groups was 0.6/100,000 population, while in the over 80 age group the annual incidence was 73.9/100,000 [5]. GCA mainly affects white individuals [6], and it is more common in women than in men [7] with a lifetime risk for GCA of 1.0% in female sex and 0.5% in males [1]. In north European countries, 3:1 ratio of women to men was detected [8, 9], comparable results were observed in the Olmsted County, Minnesota, USA, among 74 patients diagnosed between 2000 and 2009, 80% were women and 20% were men [5].

A lower female male ratio was observed in Israel and in Southern Europe [10, 11].

The incidence of GCA has ranged widely across the world depending on the characteristics of population. In Japan, the reported GCA incidence was 1.7/100,000 [12] while in Gothenburg, Sweden reached 22 per 100,000 [13].

In Olmsted County, Minnesota, USA composed by a predominant white population with northern European ancestry, the incidence of GCA is 19.8% per 100,000 [5]. Few case reports and case series demonstrated that GCA can affect people of any racial background such as Indians, Chinese, African, and Latins but the epidemiological data in these areas are insufficient and incidence/prevalence studies are required to a more accurate project of potential global burden of GCA [14]. The most recent epidemiologic studies are from Italy, Norway, and the UK [15–17]. Table 2.1 summarizes the annual incidence of GCA in the different regions of the world.

Most of the studies on GCA published in the last 30 years support the clue of an increase evidence of GCA with **latitude** in the North hemisphere [3]. As Table 2.1 shows the highest incidence is reported in North European countries and in North American population of the same descent with an incidence that varies between 32.4/100,000 people, older than 50 years of age in Norway [18] and 18.9/100,000 people in Olsted County, Minnesota, USA [2]. The incidence is markedly reduced in the Mediterranean countries and in the Southern Europe with an annual incidence that varies between 12.9/100,000 people in Spain [4] and 1.1/100,000 people in Turkey [29]. A lower incidence is reported among black people from Tennessee [30] with an incidence of 0.4/100,000. Similar results were reported in Japan [12].

Table 2.1 Incidence rates for giant cell arteritis

Study, year	Country (Region/city)	Method of diagnosis	Study period	Population incidence >50 years of age (per 100,000 people/year)
Haugeberg et al. (2003) [18]	Norway (North and West)	ACR criteria	1992–1996	32.4
Baldursson et al. (1994) [19]	Iceland (Nationwide)	ACR criteria	1984–1990	27.0
Boesen et al. (1987) [8]	Denmark (Danish county)	Biopsy proven Clinical GCA	1982–1985	23.3
Nordborg et al. (2003) [20]	Sweden (Gothenborg)	Biopsy proven	1976–1995	22.2
Smeeth et al. (2006) [17]	UK (Nationwide)	Clinical criteria	1990–2001	22.0[a]
Elling et al. (1996) [21]	Denmark (Nationwide)	Biopsy proven	1982–1994	20.4
Kermani et al. (2010) [2]	USA (Minnesota)	ACR criteria	2000–2004	18.9
Salvarani et al. (2004) [22]	USA (Minnesota)	ACR criteria	1950–1999	18.8
Brekke et al. (2017) [16]	Norway (West)	ACR criteria	1972–2012	16.7
Gonzalez Gay et al. (2007) [4]	Spain (Lugo)	Biopsy proven	2001–2005	12.9
Abdul-Rahman et al. (2011) [23]	New-Zealand (Otago)	Biopsy proven	1996–2005	12.7
Bas-Lando et al. (2007) [10]	Israel (Jerusalem)	Biopsy proven or ACR criteria	1980–2004	11.3
Ramsted and Patel (2007) [24]	Canada (Saskatoon)	Biopsy proven	1998–2003	9.4
Barrier et al. (1982) [25]	France (Loire-Atlantique)	Biopsy proven or clinical features	1970–1979	9.4[b]
Pucelj et al. (2018) [26]	Slovenia (Ljubljana)	Biopsy proven or ACR criteria or TA CDS	2012–2017	8.7
Salvarani et al. (1991) [27]	Italy (Reggio Emilia)	Biopsy proven or clinical features	1980–1988	6.9
Salvarani et al. (2017) [15]	Italy (North)	Biopsy proven	1986–2012	5.8
Dunstan et al. (2014) [28]	Australia (South)	Biopsy proven	1992–2011	3.2
Pamuk et al. (2009) [29]	Turkey (Northwest)	ACR criteria	2002–2008	1.1

[a]Reported for people over 40 years
[b]Reported for people over 55 years. *ACR* American college of Rheumatology, *TA CDS* temporal artery color Doppler ultrasonography

Several epidemiologic studies reported a progressive increase in incidence of this vasculitis in particular between 1950 and 1980/1990 [4, 11, 24, 31] but more recent reports from Israel and Olmsted County, Minnesota reported the incident rates leveled off and remained steady with minimal fluctuations through 2009 [31, 32].

Fewer are the **prevalence** studies on GCA. Table 2.2 summarized these data from different regions of the world. Prevalence in GCA follows the same latitude distribution of incidence with higher prevalence in the Northern hemisphere compared to the Southern Europe and non-European country. Prevalence study from Mayo Clinic [31] reported that prevalence rate of GCA between 1950 and 2009 among women was 304 (95% CI 229–375) and among men was 91 (95% CI 46–156) per 100,000 population older than 50 years of age. The prevalence rate increased precipitously from age 50–54 to age 90 in both sexes. Moreover, the authors reported that prevalence estimates remained stable over the long period of observation.

Differences in prevalence and incidence reports in these cohorts are most likely related to differences in disease classification and diagnostic criteria, temporal artery biopsy evaluation, as well as genetic and geographic factors.

The population **health burden** of these disease among older people continued to be substantial. The incident GCA cases will increase secondary to an aging population, therfore in projected worldwide disease burden study on GCA was found that by 2050 more than three million people will have been diagnosed with GCA in Europe, North America, and Oceania [14]. If current treatment will not change, over 140,000 patients with GCA in the USA will come up with acute visual symptoms and receive hospital admission for appropriate treatment with consequent important economic impact con sanitary cost. By 2050, in the USA, US$1.3 billion is expected to have been spent on inpatient management of visual impairment-associated GCA. Moreover, since oral and intravenous corticosteroids still remain the cornerstone of GCA treatment, the treatment side effects should be considered in the long-term management of these patients. By 2050, in the USA, around 360,000 patients with GCA are expected to develop a steroid-induced fractures, a total amount of money to manage this side effect is more than US$6.58 billion.

Several studies have addressed the issue about **mortality** in patients with GCA. However, the conclusions are inconsistent due to the small number of studies, their small sample sizes, and the clinical heterogeneity. A recent meta-analysis combined the published data of all cause, sex-specific, region-specific, and cause-specific standardized mortality ratios (SMRs) in patients with GCA [39]. Eight studies were included and seven analyzed all-cause mortality. Compared with general population, all cause SMR was not increased in GCA patients (SMR 1.081, 95% CI 0.963–1.214, $p = 0.184$) and the stratification by regions showed no significant increase in all cause SMR in Europe and the USA. Sex-specific meta-analysis provided by four out of eight studies included revealed the pooled SMR for women was 1.046 (95% CI 0.834–1.314, $p = 0.696$) and for men was 1.051 (95% CI 0.974–1.133, $p = 0.204$); therefore, no sex-specific significant differences in SMR were demonstrated. In contrast, the risk of mortality of cardiovascular disease was significantly increased with an SMR of 1.312 (95% CI 1.136–1.516, $p < 0.001$).

Table 2.2 Prevalence studies on GCA

Study, year	Country	Age, years	Method of diagnosis	GCA prevalence rate per 100,000 (95% CI)		
				Overall	Female	Male
Crowson CS et al. 2015 [31]	USA	≥50	ACR1990	204 (161,254)	304 (229.375)	91 (46,156)
Catanoso M et al. 2012 [15]	Italy	≥50	Positive TAB, ACR1990	87.9 (75.8,101.4)		
Lawrence RC 2000 [33]	USA	≥50	ACR1990	228 (192,268)	344	200
Yates M et al. 2013 [34]	UK	≥55	ACR1990	250 (110,390)	330 (120,550)	160 (0–320)
Kobayashi S et al. 1997 [12]	Japan	≥50	ACR1990	1.5		
Gonzalez Gay MA et al. (1991) [35]	Spain	≥50	Hunder	60		
Herlyn K et al. 2006–1994 [36]	Germany	≥50	ACR1990	44 (2004) (39.9,48.1) 24(1996) (1.64,31.5)	61.2 (54.4,66.0)	21.9 (19.0,25.)
Pamuk ON et al. [29]	Turkey	≥50	ACR1990	20 (16,24)		
Adrianakos A et al. 1996 [37]	Greece	≥50	ACR1990	80 (10,150)		
Mohammad A et al. 2011 [38]	Sweden	≥50	Positive TAB	110 (100,120)		

ACR American College of Rheumatology, *GCA* giant cell arteritis, *TAB* temporal artery biopsy

Chazal and colleagues [40] using the death certificates compiled by French Epidemiological Centre on Medical Causes of Death for the period 2005 and 2014 reported the mean age of death was 86 ($\pm$6.8) years and the overall age of SMR among GCA patients was 7.2 per million people. Throughtout the study period, the mean age of death was significantly increased ($r = 0.17$, $p < 0.0001$). The most frequent associated diseases were cardiovascular (79%) and infectious (35%).

From the same French death certificate database between 1980 and 2011 Aouba and colleagues [41] reported the annual SMR for GCA increased to a peak in 1997 then decreased in the following years (Spearman's correlation test, both $P < 0.0001$). GCA deaths were frequently associated with aortic aneurysm and dissection (1.85% of death certificates), hypertensive disease (20.78% of death certificates), diabetes mellitus (11.27% of death certificates), ischemic disease (16.54% of death certificates), and infectious and parasitic disease (12.12% of death certificates).

UK-based Clinical Practice Research Datalink between 1990 and 2014 was used to identify 9778 newly diagnosed GCA patients [42]. Cases were matched to non-vasculitic patients on age, sex, practice, and years of history before cohort entry. GCA patients compared with controls had increased mortality during the first year following the diagnosis (adjusted HR = 1.51, 95% CI 1.40–1.64) and slighlty increased mortality during the period of 1–5 years after the diagnosis (adjusted HR = 1.06, 95% CI 1.00–1.12). The mortality risk differed by age with a greater increased 1-year mortality in those with a diagnosis at an age less than 65 years, but not by sex or calendar year of the cohort [42].

Survival predictors in giant cell arteritis were evaluated in a recent Italian study [43]. Polymyalgia rheumatica (PMR) at diagnosis and the inflammation limited to the adventia at the temporal artery biopsy appear to be related to a more benign disease, while large vessel involvement at diagnosis is associated with reduced survival [43].

The role of **genetic and environmental factors** (including infectious etiology) on explanation of geographical differences in GCA epidemiologic studies remains unclear [44]. **Geographical variations, seasonal fluctuation, and cyclic pattern** have been observed in the incidence/prevalence of GCA [44].

A **temporal cyclic pattern** of GCA incidence with recurrent peaks and valleys every 7–10 years was demonstrated until 1999 in Mayo Clinic cohort, no peak between 2000 and 2009 [5, 22]. Once the hypothesis is the **theory of sunlight** as a risk factor of GCA. In 1965, Kinmont and McCullum reported 14 patients with GCA who experienced serious vascular complication after sun exposure [45]; moreover, they noticed that the incidence was higher in the summer period. The effect of sun on temporal arteries was demonstrated on histologic specimens; in fact, solar radiation seemed to destroy the essential supportive elastic framework of arteries and since the temporal arteries are superficial on the forehead they resulted vulnerable to sun damage [46]. In a recent study from Mayo Clinic, the impact of **geomagnetic effects and the solar cycle** on GCA incidence was investigated [5].

They reported that GCA rates peaked 0–1 year after strong magnetic activity, possibly suggesting that the effect is cumulative or that the latency between environmental exposure and disease manifestation could be related to complex autoimmune process [47].

However, in the same study [5], they calculated the correlation between solar extreme ultraviolet radiation and GCA incidence but it didn't reach the statistical significance as the geomagnetic impact [47].

Several studies investigated the **seasonality fluctuations** of GCA incidence [48], but this has been a controversial theory. Few studies reported a significant association between the onset of GCA and a specific season or a certain annual fluctuation [10, 13, 21, 28, 32], but the trend is not consistent, some found a peak in summer some other in winter. A Swedish study described a GCA peak in autumn and winter [13] in the UK and Israel studies in spring and summer [10, 32]. There seems to be no overall consensus on seasonality and incidence rate of this disease. A possible explanation could be that the seasonal variation could be associated with peaks of certain infection.

Autoantibodies against various bacterial and/or viral strains (e.g., parainfluenza viruses, adenovirus, respiratory syncytial virus, measles virus, herpes virus type 1 and 2, Epstein–Barr virus and parvovirus B19) have been investigated as possible triggers in susceptible hosts but with inconclusive results [49, 50]. Some studies using advance DNA sequencing techniques revealed abundant quantity of **bacteria and viral DNA** in the arterial wall of patients with GCA [51]. Genetic material from Chlamydia pneumonia [52], from parvovirus B19 [53] as well as Varicella Zoster antigen [54] was detected in temporal artery specimens. However, these results were not confirmed by other authors [55, 56].

In a US retrospective study, data from Medicare and Truven Analytics MarketScan including 16 million individuals reported that previous herpes zoster infection was associated to an increased risk of 2.2 times higher to develop GCA. If patients had been treated with anti-viral therapy, the risk of GCA decreased even below the background risk of the general population (HR0.67 according to Medicare data) [57].

Socioeconomic level as well as **urban** versus **rural living** have been evaluated as possible predictor of GCA development. In a nationwide Swedish study educational level, family income, marital status, and occupation seemed to have only a weak correlation with GCA occurrence [58]. In a British study, a lower socioeconomic status was associated with ischemic symptoms manifestations resulting from GCA. The possible explanation was that individuals living in more deprived areas do not attend medical out-patient clinic as early and therefore are delayed for diagnosis and treatments [59].

Some studies have found a trend, without reaching the statistical significance, that urban lifestyle may predispose individuals to develop GCA [58]. In Northern and Southern Germany, GCA was significantly more prevalent in urban areas compared to rural areas, and it was not clear if it was related to underdiagnosis of GCA in the rural regions due to differences in the healthcare assistance in cities versus rural area [60].

In a recent letter, Brekke LK et al. reported that in the 41-year incidence study conducted in northwestern Norway a mixed urban and rural area, no difference in GCA incidence was detected in urban compared to rural areas [61].

2.2   Genetics

Female sex is the most important **genetic risk factors** for GCA as reported above.

Several studies have outlined the implications of genetic variants on immune and inflammatory pathways in GCA susceptibility since this vasculitis is a **polygenic disease** [62]. Polymorphisms of the HLA II gene in particular the presence of **HLA DRB1*04 alleles** (both HLA DRB1*0401 and HLA DRB1*0404) are systematically associated with GCA supporting the thesis that GCA is driven by an antigen-based immune response [62]. A recent large-scale genetic analysis on GCA was conducted on 1651 case subjects with GCA and 15,306 unrelated control subjects form six different countries of European ancestry using Immunochip array [63]. The study confirmed the involvement of HLA class II region in the pathophysiology of GCA and the association of GCA with HLA DRB1*04 alleles. Moreover, they identified **HLA-DQA1** as an independent novel susceptibility factor, in particular the presence of the classical alleles DQA1*0101, DQA1*0102, and HLA-DQA1*03:01. The level of statistical significance found in the HLA region underlined the importance of **immune system** in the boost of GCA [63]. In the same study, a test on polymorphic amino acid positions revealed DRB1 13, DQ 47, 56, and 76 are relevant for disease occurrence [63].

Mackie SL et al. demonstrated that the susceptibility of HLA DRB1*04 were better explained by amino acids risk residues V, H, and H at positions 11, 13, and 33 [64] in contrast with previous proposal of amino acids in the second hypervariable region [65]. The authors also performed a meta-analysis on geographic distribution of HLA-DRB1*04 and the frequency of GCA. They reported that GCA incidence was independently associated both with the presence of HLA-DRB1*04 and with latitude itself, concluding that different HLA-DRB1*04 frequency in the population can partially explain variations in GCA incidence.

Association between clinical features of GCA patients and the presence of HLA DRB1*04 were reported, in particular higher visual loss and glucocorticoid resistance were documented among GCA patients and the occurrence of HLA DRB1*04 [66, 67].

Among non-HLA genes, polymorphism of genes that encode for **cytokines** (TNF, IFN-g, IL-10, IL-4, IL-6, IL-18, monocyte chemotactic protein-1, IL-12/IL-21, and IL-12 receptor bet2), for molecules involved in endothelial function and genes of innate immune response have been associated with the appearance or the severity of GCA [68].

A recent GWAS analyzed 1,844,133 **genetic variants**, apart from confirming HLA class II as the most important genetic risk factor for GCA, additional genes were identified: plasminogen (PLG) and prolyl 4-hydroxylase subunit alpha 2 (P4HA2) [69]. PLG encodes a secreted blood zymogen involved in angiogenesis and in a wide spectrum of physiological process including wound healing, fibrinolysis, and lymphocites recruitment. The PLG risk alleles seemed to unbalance the metabolism of its encoded proteins leading to the pro-inflammatory features of GCA [69].

P4HA2 encodes a protein critical for collagen biosynthesis, and it is considered an important hypoxia response gene [69].

Genetic variants of the protein tyrosine phosphatase, non-receptor type 22 (PTPN22) are identified as risk factors for GCA [68]. PTPN22 is involved in the negative control of T cell receptor signaling and in the response of Th17 cells that are considered crucial in the pathogenesis of GCA [70].

References

1. Crowson CS, Matteson EL, Myasoedova E, et al. The lifetime risk of adult–onset rheumatoid arthritis and other inflammatory autoimmune rheumatic disease. Arthritis Rheum. 2011;63(3):633–9.
2. Kermani TA, Schafer VS, Crowson CS, et al. Increase in age at onset of giant cell arteritis: a population based study. Ann Rheum Dis. 2010;69:780–1.
3. Gonzalez MA, Vazquez-Rodriguez TR, Lopez-Diaz MJ, et al. Epidemiology of giant cell arteritis and polymyalgia rheumatica. Arthritis Rheum. 2009;61:1454–61.
4. Gonzalez-Gay MA, Miranda-Filloy JA, Lopez-Diaz MJ, et al. Giant cell arteritis in northwestern Spain: a 25 year epidemiologic study. Medicine. 2007;86:61–8.
5. Chandran AK, Udayakumar PD, Crowson CS, et al. The incidence of Giant cell arteritis in Olmsted County Minnesota, over a sixty year period 1950-2009. Scand J Rheumatol. 2015;44:215–8.
6. Levine SM, Hellmann DB. Giant cell arteritis. Curr Opin Rheumatol. 2002;14:3–10.
7. Salvarani C, Cantini F, Boiardi L, Hunder GG. Polymyalgia Rheumatica and giant cell arteritis. N Engl J Med. 2002;347:261–71.
8. Boesen P, Sorensen SF. Giant cell arteritis, temporal arteritis, and polymyalgia rheumatica in a Danish county: a prospective investigation. Arthritis Rheum. 1987;30:294–9.
9. Franzen P, Sutinen S, von Knorring J. Giant cell arteritis and polymyalgia rheumatica in a region of Finland: an epidemiologic, clinical and pathologic study, 1984-1988. J Rheumatol. 1992;19:273–6.
10. Bas-Lando M, Breuer GS, Berkun Y, et al. The incidence of giant cell arteritis in Jerusalem over a 25 years period: annual and seasonal fluctuations. Clin Exp Rheumatol. 2007;25(Suppl 44):S15–7.
11. Gozalez-Gay MA, Garcia-Porrua C, Rivas MJ, et al. Epidemiology of biopsy proven giant cell arteritis in northwestern Spain: trend over a 1 year period. Ann Rheum Dis. 2001;60:367–71.
12. Kobayashi S, Yano T, Matsumoto Y, et al. Clinical and epidemiologic analysis of giant cell (temporal) arteritis from a nationwide survey in 1998 in Japan: the first government-supported nationwide survey. Arthritis Rheum. 2003;49:594–8.
13. Petursdottir V, Johansson H, Nordborg E, et al. The epidemiology of biopsy positive giant cell arteritis: special reference to cyclic fluctuations. Rheumatology. 1999;38:1208–12.
14. De Smit E, Palmer AJ, Hewitt AW. Projected worldwide disease burden from giant cell arteritis by 2050. J Rheumatol. 2015;42:119–25.
15. Catanoso M, Mcchioni P, Boiardi L, et al. Incidence, Prevalence and Survival of biopsy-proven giant cell arteritis in northern Italy during a 26-year period. Arthritis Care Res. 2017;69:430–8.
16. Brekke LK, Diamantopoulos AP, Fevang B-T, et al. Incidence of giant cell arteritis in Western Norway 1972-2012: a retrospective cohort study. Arthritis Res Ther. 2017;19:278–87.
17. Smeeth L, Cook C, Hall AJ. Incidence of polymyalgia rheumatica and temporal arteritis in United Kingdom, 1990-2001. Ann Rheum Dis. 2006;65:1093–8.
18. Haugeberg G, Irgens KA, Thomsen RS. No major differences in incidence of temporal arteritis in northern and western Norway compared with reports from southern Norway. Scan J Rheumatol. 2003;32:318–9.
19. Baldursson O, Steinsson K, Bjornsson J, et al. Giant cell arteritis in Iceland. An epidemiologic and histopathologic analysis. Arthritis Rheum. 1994;37:1007–12.
20. Nordborg C, Johansson H, Petursdottir V, et al. The epidemiology of biopsy positive giant cell arteritis: special reference to changes in the age of population. Rheumatology. 2003;42:549–52.

21. Elling P, Olsson AT, Elling H. Synchronous variations of the incidence of temporal arteritis and polymyalgia rheumatica in different regions of Denmark; association with epidemics of Mycoplasma pneumoniae infection. J Rheumatol. 1996;23:112–9.
22. Salvarani C, Crowson CS, O'Fallon WM, et al. Reappraisal of the epidemiology of giant cell arteritis in Olmstead County, Minnesota, over a fifty-year period. Arthritis Rheum. 2004;15:264–8.
23. Abdul-Rahman AM, Molteno AC, Bevin TH. The epidemiology of giant cell arteritis in Otago, New Zealand: a 9-year analysis. N Z Med J. 2011;124:44–52.
24. Ramstead CL, PAtel AD. Giant cell arteritis in a neuro-ophthalmology clinic in Sasktoon, 1998-2003. Can J Ophthalmol. 2007;42:295–8.
25. Barrier J, Pion P, Massari R, et al. Epidemiologic approach to Horton's disease in the department of Loire-Atlantique. 110 cases in 10 years. Rev Med Interne. 1982;3:13–20.
26. Pucelj NP, Hocevar A, Jese R, et al. The incidence of giant cell arteritis in Slovenia. Clin Rheumatol. 2019;38:285–90.
27. Salvarani C, Macchioni P, Zizzi F, et al. Epidemiologic and immunogenetic aspects of polymyalgia rheumatica and giant cell arteritis in northern Italy. Arthritis Rheum. 1991;34:351–6.
28. Dunstan E, Lester SL, Rischmueller M, Dodd T, et al. Epidemiology of biopsy-proven giant cell arteritis in South Australia. Intern Med J. 2014;44:32–9.
29. Pamuk ON, Donmez S, Karahan B, et al. Giant cell arteritis and polymyalgia rheumatica in northwestern Turkey: clinical features and epidemiological data. Clin Exp Rheumatol. 2009;27:830–3.
30. Smith CA, Fidller WJ, Pinals RS. The epidemiology of giant cell arteritis: report of a ten-year study in Shelby County, Tennessee. Arthritis Rheum. 1983;26:1214–9.
31. Crowson CS, Matteson EL. Contemporary prevalence estimates for giant cell arteritis and polymyalgia rheumatica 2015. Semin Arthritis Rheum. 2017;47:253–6.
32. Sonnenblick M, Nescher G, Friedlander Y, et al. Giant cell arteritis in Jerusalem a 12 year epidemiological study. Br J Rheumatol. 1994;33:938–41.
33. Lawrence RC, Felon DT, Helmick CG, et al. Estimates of prevalence of arthritis and other rheumatic conditions in the United States. Part II. Arthritis Rheum. 2008;58:26–35.
34. Yates M, Grahm K, Watts RA, et al. The prevalence of giant cell arteritis and polymyalgia rheumatica in a UK primary care population. BMC Musculoskelet Disord. 2016;17:285–93.
35. Gonzalez Gay MA, Alonso MD, Aguero JJ, et al. Temporal arteritis in a northwestern area of Spain: study of 57 biopsy proven patients. J Rheumatol. 1992;19:277–80.
36. Herlyb K, Buckert F, Gross WL, et al. Doubled prevalence rates of ANCA-associated vasculitides and giant cell arteritis between 1994 and 2006 in northern Germany. Rheumatology (Oxford). 2014;53:882–9.
37. Andiatikos A, Trontzas P, Christoyannis F, et al. Prevalence of rheumatic diseases in Greece: a cross-sectional population based epidemiological study. The ESORDIG Study. J Rheumatol. 2003;30:1589–601.
38. Mohammad A, Mohammad J, Nilsson JA, et al. Incidence, prevalence and morality rates of biopsy proven giant cell arteritis in Southern Sweden. Arthritis Rheum. 2011;63:1–9.
39. Lee YH, Song GG. Overall and cause-specific mortality in giant cell arteritis. Z Rheumatol. 2018;77:946–51.
40. Chazal T, Lhote R, Rey G, et al. Giant cell arteritis-related mortality in France: a multiple-cause-of-death analysis. Autoimmun Rev. 2018;17:1219–24.
41. Aouba A, Gonzalez Chiappe S, Eb M, et al. Mortality causes and trends associated with giant cell arteritis: analysis of French national death certificate database (1980-2011). Rheumatology (Oxford). 2018;57:1047–55.
42. Li L, Neogi T, Jick S. Mortality in patients with Giant cell arteritis: a cohort study in UK Primary Care. Arthritis Care Res. 2018;70:1251–6.
43. Macchioni P, Boiardi L, Muratore F, et al. Survival predictors in biopsy-proven giant cell arteritis: a northern Italian population-based study. Rheumatology (Oxford). 2019;58(4):609–16.
44. Gabriel SE, Michaud K. Epidemiological studies in incidence, prevalence, mortality and comorbidity of rheumatic diseases. Arthritis Res Ther. 2009;11:229.

45. Kinmont PD, McCallum DI. The aetiology, pathology and course of giant cell arteritis. The possible role of light sensitivity. Br J Dermatol. 1965;77:193–202.
46. O'Brien JP. A concept of diffuse actinic arteritis. The role of actinic damage to elastin in "age change" and arteritis of the temporal artery and polymyalgia rheumatica. Br J Dermatol. 1978;98:1–13.
47. Wing S, Rider LG, Johnson JR, et al. Do solar cycles influence giant cell arteritis and rheumatoid arthritis incidence? BMJ Open. 2015;5:e006636.
48. De Smit E, Clarke L, Sanfilippo PG, et al. Geo-epidemiology of temporal artery biopsy-positive giant cell arteritis in Australia and New Zealand: is there a seasonal influence? RMD Open. 2017;3(2):e000531.
49. Hemauer A, Modrow S, Georgi J, et al. There is no association between polymyalgia rheumatica and parvovirus b19 infection. Ann Rheum Dis. 1999;58:657.
50. Uddhammar A, Boman J, Juto P, et al. Antibodies against chlamydia pneumoniae, cytomegalovirus, enterovirus and respiratory syncytial virus in patients with polymyalgia rheumatica. Clin Exp Rheumatol. 1997;15:299–302.
51. Bahtt AS, Manzo VE, Pedamallu CS, et al. In search of a candidate pathogen for giant cell arteritis: sequencing-based characterization of giant cell arteritis microbiome. Arthritis Rheumatol. 2014;66:1939–44.
52. Wagner AD, Gerard HC, Fresemann T, et al. Detection of chlamydia pneumonia in giant cell vasculitis and correlation with the topographic arrangement of tissue-infiltrating dendritic cells. Arthritis Rheum. 2000;43:1543–51.
53. Gabriel SE, Espy M, Erdam DD, et al. The role of parvovirus B19 in the pathogenesis of giant cell arteritis: a preliminary evaluation. Arthritis Rheum. 1999;42:1255–8.
54. Nagel MA, White T, Khmeleva N, et al. Analysis of varicella zoster virus in temporal arteries biopsy positive and negative for giant cell arteritis. JAMA Neurol. 2015;72:1281–7.
55. Helweg Larsen J, Trap B, Obel N, et al. No evidence of parvovirus B19, chlamydia pneumoniae or human herpes virus infection in temporal artery biopsies in patients with giant cell arteritis. Rheumatology. 2002;41:445–9.
56. Rodriguez-Pla A, Bosch-Gil JA, Echevarria-Mayo JE, et al. No detection of parvovirus b19 or herpesvirus DNA in giant cell arteritis. J Clin Virol. 2004;31:11–5.
57. England BR, Mikuls TR, Xie F, et al. Herpes zoster as a risk for incident giant cell arteritis. Arthritis Rheumatol. 2017;69:2351–8.
58. Zoller B, Li X, Sundquist J, et al. Occupational and socio-economic risk factors for giant cell arteritis: a nationwide study based on hospitalizations in Sweden. Scand J Rheumatol. 2013;42:487–97.
59. Mackie SL, Dasgupta B, Hordon L, et al. Ischemic manifestations in giant cell arteritis are associated with area level socio-economic deprivation, but not cardiovascular risk factors. Rheumatology. 2011;50:2014–22.
60. Reinhold-Keller E, Zeilder A, Gutfleisch J, et al. Giant cell arteritis is more prevalent in urban than in rural populations: results of an epidemiological study of primary systemic vasculitides in Germany. Rheumatology. 2000;39:1396–402.
61. Brekke LK, Fevang BT, Geirmund M. Increased incidence of giant cell arteritis in urban areas? J Rheumatol. 2019;46:327–8.
62. Gonzalez Gay MA, Amoli MM, Garcia-Porrua C, et al. Genetic markers of disease susceptibility and severity in giant cell arteritis and polymyalgia rheumatica. Semin Arthritis Rheum. 2003;33:38–48.
63. Carmona FD, Mackie SL, Martin JE, et al. A large scale genetic analysis reveals a strong contribution of the HLA class II region to giant cell arteritis susceptibility. Am J Hum Genet. 2015;96:565–80.
64. Mackie SL, Taylor JC, Haroon-Rashid L, et al. Association of HLA-DRB1 amino acid residues with giant cell arteritis: genetic association study, meta-analysis and geoepidemiological investigation. Arthritis Res Ther. 2015;17:195–209.
65. Weyand CM, Hicok KC, Hunder GG, et al. The HLA-DRB1 locus as a genetic component in giant cell arteritis. Mapping of a disease-linked sequence motif to the antigen binding site of the HLA-DR molecule. J Clin Invest. 1992;90:2355–61.

66. Gonzalez-Gay MA, Garcia-Porrua C, Llorca J, et al. Visual manifestations of giant cell arteritis. Trend and clinical spectrum in 161 patients. Medicine. 2000;79:283–92.
67. Rauzy O, Fort M, Nourhashemi F, et al. Relation between HLA DRB1 alleles and corticosteroids resistance in giant cell arteritis. Ann Rheum Dis. 1998;57:380–2.
68. Carmona FD, Gonzalez-Gay MA, Martin J. Genetic component of giant cell arteritis. Rheumatology (Oxford). 2014;53:6–18.
69. Carmona FD, Vaglio A, Mackie SL, et al. A genome-wide association study identifies risk alleles in plasminogen and P4HA2 associated with giant cell arteritis. Am J Hum Genet. 2017;5:64–74.
70. Purvis HA, Clarke F, Jordan CK, et al. Protein tyrosine phosphatase ptpn22 regulates il-1 beta-dependent th17 responses by modulating dectin-1 signaling in mice. Eur J Immunol. 2018;48:306–15.

Pathogenesis

3

Stefania Croci, Martina Bonacini, Francesco Muratore,
Luigi Boiardi, Nicolò Pipitone, and Carlo Salvarani

Abstract

Giant cell arteritis (GCA) is an inflammatory disease which mainly affects the extracranial branches of the carotid artery, particularly the temporal arteries. The onset of GCA requires a breakdown of arterial immunoprivilege with the infiltration of immune cells, mainly CD4+ T lymphocytes, macrophages, and dendritic cells (DCs) across the arterial wall. Local production of cytokines, chemokines, growth factors, and enzymes can lead to the amplification of the inflammatory responses and to arterial remodeling. The hyperplasia of the intimal layer can result in luminal stenosis and ischemic events. The etiology of GCA is unknown. However, age-related immune alterations, in genetically predisposed subjects, and environmental triggers seem necessary for the development of the disease. In addition, the existence of a specific GCA-inducing leukocyte repertoire in peripheral blood and the activation of arteries to allow leukocyte entry seem required for the development of GCA. Some immune effectors have been dem-

S. Croci (✉) · M. Bonacini
SSD Autoimmunità, Allergologia e Biotecnologie Innovative, Azienda Unità Sanitaria Locale-IRCCS di Reggio Emilia, Reggio Emilia, Italy
e-mail: stefania.croci@ausl.re.it

F. Muratore · L. Boiardi · N. Pipitone
SC Reumatologia, Azienda Unità Sanitaria Locale-IRCCS di Reggio Emilia, Reggio Emilia, Italy

C. Salvarani
Rheumatology Unit, Azienda Unita' Sanitaria Locale IRCCS di Reggio Emilia, Reggio Emilia, Italy

Rheumatology Unit, Università di Modena e Reggio Emilia, Modena, Italy

© Springer Nature Switzerland AG 2021
C. Salvarani et al. (eds.), *Large and Medium Size Vessel and Single Organ Vasculitis*, Rare Diseases of the Immune System,
https://doi.org/10.1007/978-3-030-67175-4_3

21

onstrated to have a role in GCA pathogenesis: the activation of vascular DCs and T cells, TLR4, TLR5, Janus kinases 1 and 3, CD28 co-stimulation, NOTCH-Jagged pathway, CCR6 expression by T cells, defective PD-1 checkpoint; the production of IL-6, VEGF, MMP-9, IFNγ, ET-1, PDGF, IL-12, IL-23, acute-phase serum amyloid A.

Keywords

Giant cell arteritis · Inflammation · Arterial remodeling · Temporal artery biopsy

3.1   Introduction

Giant cell arteritis (GCA) is characterized by inflammation in the extracranial branches of the carotid artery, particularly the temporal arteries. The gold standard for the diagnosis of GCA is a temporal artery biopsy (TAB) showing infiltration of immune cells mainly CD4+ T lymphocytes, macrophages, and dendritic cells [1, 2]. The causes (etiology) of GCA are currently unknown but the knowledge of the pathways involved in GCA pathogenesis is constantly growing. The onset of GCA requires a breakdown of arterial immunoprivilege. It is associated with ageing because GCA arises in subjects older than 50 years of age. Overall, age-related immune alterations, in genetically predisposed subjects, coupled with environmental triggers seem necessary for the development of the disease [3]. The evidence that identical T cell clones are present in different arteries affected by inflammation and the strong association between GCA and the class II human leukocyte antigen (HLA), particularly with the HLA-DRB1*04 alleles, suggest that GCA is driven by immune responses to specific locally expressed antigens, not yet identified [4, 5].

Experiments performed by Cornelia M. Weyand et al. using human artery-mouse chimeras reconstituted with human peripheral blood mononuclear cells (PBMCs) or alloreactive T lymphocytes have revealed that the activation of arterial dendritic cell (DC) plus a disease-prone repertoire of T cells are both necessary for developing GCA. Arterial DCs could support local T cell triggering once T cells with arteritis potential are present [6–8]. Indeed, normal arteries engrafted in immunodeficient mice can develop arteritis only if they are activated (e.g., with lipopolysaccharide, LPS) and alloreactive T cells or PBMCs from GCA patients but not PBMCs from healthy subjects are injected (Fig. 3.1). Therefore, two conditions must simultaneously occur for the development of GCA: 1) the existence of a GCA-inducing leukocyte repertoire in peripheral blood (systemic component); 2) arterial activation to promote leukocyte entry and expansion in the arterial wall (vascular component).

Immune-mediated alterations in arteries can result in arterial remodeling with intimal hyperplasia which can lead to luminal stenosis and tissue ischemia. In particular, the development and the growing of myofibroblasts represents a critical step in GCA because it can favor arterial occlusion [9, 10].

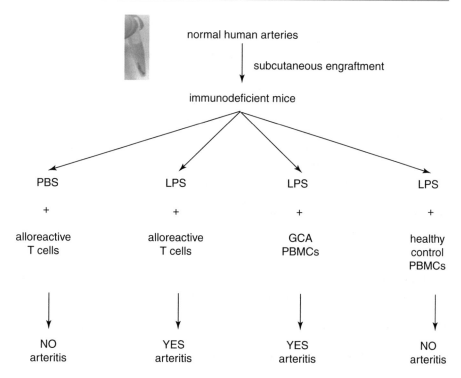

Fig. 3.1 Arterial DC activation plus a GCA-prone repertoire of T cells are necessary for developing GCA. Results of several experiments performed Cornelia M. Weyand et al. from 2004 to 2019 are summarized. Artery-mouse chimeras were obtained by implanting pieces of normal arteries that were free of any inflammation into immunodeficient mice. 6 days after implantation mice were treated with 10 μg lipopolisaccharide (LPS) or control buffer (PBS). 1–2 days later, alloreactive T cells or peripheral blood mononuclear cells (PBMCs) from GCA patients and healthy controls were engrafted in mice. The arterial grafts were recovered 15–18 days after the original implantation and analyzed

3.2 Model of GCA Pathogenesis

A model of GCA immunopathogenesis based on four phases has been recently proposed. Such phases have been depicted in the manuscript by Samson M et al. [10].

Phase 1: Activation of DCs in the adventitia. Resident immature DCs localized in the adventitia act as immune sentinels. After sensing danger signals by means of toll-like receptors (TLRs), particularly TLR-2, TLR-4, and TLR-5, they can produce chemokines and cytokines, present antigens and trigger adaptive immune responses. Activated DCs express CD83 and C-C chemokine receptor type 7 (CCR7), produce T cell-attracting chemokines, such as chemokines (C-C motif) ligand 19 (CCL19) and CCL21 and remain trapped in the arteries initiating and shaping immune responses. Moreover, adventitial microvessels up-regulate Jagged-1 allowing the access to the arterial wall of NOTCH+ leukocytes.

Phase 2: Recruitment, activation, and polarization of CD4+ T lymphocytes. The cytokine milieu recruits CD4+ T lymphocytes in the arterial wall. In case of antigen recognition, CD4+ T lymphocytes are activated, retained in the arterial wall, and polarized toward T helper (Th)1, Th9, Th17, Th21, and Th22 subsets. T lymphocytes show a restricted oligoclonal repertoire.

Phase 3: Recruitment of monocytes/macrophages and CD8+ T lymphocytes. Interleukins produced by CD4+ T lymphocytes, particularly interferon (IFN)γ, induce the production of chemokines and cytokines which attract monocytes and CD8+ T lymphocytes. Monocytes differentiate in macrophages and form granulomas in the media. Macrophages can secrete matrix metalloproteinases (e.g., MMP-2, MMP-9), reactive oxygen species, and nitric oxide leading to lipid peroxidation and the destruction of elastic laminae. Besides, CD8+ T lymphocytes can produce further cytokines and cytotoxic molecules (granzymes and perforin). Loops of amplification of the immune responses occur increasing inflammation.

Phase 4: Vascular remodeling. Feedback mechanisms are induced to restore homeostasis. Several growth factors including platelet-derived growth factor (PDGF), vascular endothelial growth factor (VEGF), fibroblast growth factor (FGF), endothelin (ET)-1 and transforming growth factor (TGF)β are produced, which can promote the transition of vascular smooth muscle cells from a contractile to a secretory phenotype and vascular smooth muscle cell migration to the intima. The formation of a neo-intima made of myofibroblasts and extracellular matrix proteins can result in the occlusion of the arterial lumen.

3.3   Role of Infectious Agents

Incidence of GCA has cyclic fluctuations, with peak incidence rates every 5–7 years, and seasonal fluctuations, with peaks in late winter and autumn suggesting that seasonal infections or solar exposition may be involved in GCA pathogenesis [11]. Different infectious agents such as Parvovirus B19 [12], Chlamydia pneumonia [13], Epstein–Barr Virus [14], Varicella Zoster Virus [15] have been suggested to be involved in the pathogenesis of GCA. Rigorous studies, however, failed in demonstrating a role of these infectious agents. To be noted, according to the data obtained by Weyand CM et al. in human artery-mouse chimeras, any episodes associated to the release of LPS (e.g., bacterial infections) might stimulate arterial DCs, laying the ground for potential arteritis [7]. Up to now, the presence of infectious agents has been searched in the inflamed arteries from GCA patients compared to normal arteries. However, infections might favor arteritis through bystander effects, e.g., activating vascular DCs, or molecular mimicry, which occur when similarities between microbial and self-peptides favor an activation of autoreactive T or B cells in susceptible individuals. If molecular mimicry is involved in GCA pathogenesis has not been investigated yet.

3.4 Genetics

GCA has been associated with MHC class II in many independent studies and particularly with HLA-DRB1*04 alleles [16]. Differently from MHC class II alleles, only a weak association has been detected with MHC class I alleles such as HLA-A*31, HLA-B*8, HLA-B*15, HLA-Cw3, HLA-Cw6, and MHC class I polypeptide-related sequence A (MICA). Outside the HLA region, GCA has been associated with loci which include the protein tyrosine phosphatase non-receptor type 22 (PTPN22), the leucine-rich repeat containing 32 (LRRC32), plasminogen (PLG), and prolyl 4-hydroxylase subunit alpha-2 (P4HA2) [17, 18]. Moreover, polymorphisms in genes encoding a variety of cytokines and growth factors: tumor necrosis factor (TNF)α, interferon (IFN)γ, interleukin (IL)-10, IL-4, IL-6, IL-17, IL-18, IL-21, IL-33, monocyte chemoattractant protein-1 (MCP-1), chemokine (C-C motif) ligand 5 (CCL5), vascular endothelial growth factor (VEGF), intercellular adhesion molecule 1 (ICAM-1), the enzymes metalloproteinase-9 (MMP-9), endothelial nitric oxide synthase (NOS), and myeloperoxidase (MPO), FcγR (Fc fragment of IgG receptor γ), and the pathogen-associated molecular pattern recognition receptor toll-like receptor 4 (TLR4) have been reported to contribute to genetic susceptibility to GCA [9, 10]. However, the results are not always consistent across populations and whether polymorphisms can affect protein activities supporting a causative role in GCA pathogenesis is unknown.

3.5 Immune Effectors of Inflammation in Arteries

The immune infiltrate present in the arteries from patients with GCA is mainly composed of DCs, T lymphocytes (particularly CD4+), macrophages, and multinucleated giant cells (hence, the name). Giant cells are present in about half of the TABs. B lymphocytes and neutrophils are sometimes present in TABs while NK cells have not been reported to date [10]. The classic histologic picture of GCA is a lymphomononuclear inflammatory cell infiltrate crossing all layers (called "transmural"), with or without giant cells. However, inflammation can also be restricted to the adventitia, adventitial vasa vasorum, and/or to the periadventitial small vessels [19, 20].

DCs seem to drive the initiating immunological events in GCA pathogenesis. Adventitial DCs are activated by still unknown triggers, remain in the arteries due to the expression of CCR7 and its ligands, releasing several chemokines and cytokines such as IL-6, IL-18, IL-23, IL-32, IL-33, CCL18, CCL19, CCL20, and CCL21 which attract and activate pathogenic T lymphocytes [10].

The majority of arterial-residing lymphocytes are CD4+, often switched to a memory phenotype (T_{RM}). Compared with TABs from control subjects, TABs from patients with GCA are infiltrated by IFNγ-secreting Th1, IL-9-secreting Th9,

IL-17-secreting Th17, IL-21-secreting Th21, and IL-22-secreting Th22 lymphocytes [21, 22]. To date, two main pathogenic pathways have been characterized in GCA: (i) IL-6/IL-17/Th17 pathway sensitive to the glucocorticoid therapy; (ii) IL-12/IFNγ/Th1 pathway that persists despite treatment with glucocorticoids and likely underlies the chronic phase of the disease [23]. CD8+ T lymphocytes can also infiltrate the arteries. A strong percentage of CD8+ T lymphocyte in TABs is associated with a more severe disease supporting their pathogenic role [24].

B lymphocytes can be detected in TABs from GCA patients but at a lower degree than T lymphocytes. Recently, arterial tertiary lymphoid organs (ATLOs) have been detected in TABs from GCA patients in the adventitial and medial layer of inflamed arteries, not associated with the age of patients, and/or with the occurrence of atherosclerotic lesions, and independent by the degree of arterial inflammation [25]. These ATLOs are formed by B cell aggregates with a follicular dendritic cell network, loosely surrounded by T cells and with high endothelial venules. ATLOs in GCA arteries might have a role in the disruption of the arterial immune privilege, possibly representing the immune sites where immune responses toward unknown arterial wall-derived antigens start.

CD68+ macrophages constitute the major subset of inflammatory cells forming the granulomas and can orchestrate both immune cell functions and tissue remodeling. Moreover, multinucleated giant cells are offspring of macrophages. CD68+ macrophages are heterogeneous in inflamed arteries: some can secrete pro-inflammatory cytokines such as IL-1β and IL-6; others can secrete tissue-degrading metalloproteinases and collagenases [26]. Recently, it has been demonstrated that most macrophages in TABs from GCA patients have the phenotype of non-classical monocytes being CD68+ CD16+ CXCR1+ CCR2^{neg} [27].

Several pro-inflammatory cytokines, chemokines, growth factors, and enzymes have been detected up-regulated in the inflamed arteries from patients with GCA compared to normal arteries: IL-1β, IL-2, IL-6, IL-7, IL-8, IL-9, IL-12p35, IL-12/IL-23p40, IL-23p19, IL-17, IL-18, IL-21, IL-22, IL-27, IL-32, IL-33, IFNγ, TNFα, TGFβ, PTX-3, CCL2, CCL18, CCL19, CCL20, CCL21, CX3CL1, CXCL9, CXCL10, CXCL13, BAFF, APRIL, LT-β, VEGF, FGF, PDGF, NGF, BDNF, ET-1, MMP-2, MMP-12, TIMP-1, TIMP-2. They can promote the recruitment of immune cells, modulate immune cell survival and proliferation, shape the polarization of lymphocyte and monocytes/macrophages, and the phenotype of vascular smooth muscle cells and endothelial cells thus contributing to GCA pathogenesis [9, 10].

3.6   Arterial Remodeling

Arterial resident endothelial cells (ECs) and vascular smooth muscle cells (VSMCs) are key effectors in GCA pathogenesis being the players of tissue remodeling which can lead to lumen occlusion or arterial wall dissection. ECs and VSMCs can respond to the inflammatory mediators acquiring pro-inflammatory properties (e.g., the expression of adhesion molecules and homing chemokines for leukocytes) and new phenotypes (e.g., enhanced proliferation and migratory abilities toward the intima, thus resulting in intimal hyperplasia). ECs of adventitial microvessels and neo-vessels of TAB from GCA patients express high levels of adhesion molecules such as ICAM-1, ICAM-2, PECAM-1, P-selectin, E-selectin, and VCAM-1, all of which are involved in the recruitment of immune cells [10]. In addition, microvascular ECs in the adventitial vasa vasorum but not ECs lining the lumen, express Jagged1, the Notch ligand [28] which can lead to CD4+ T lymphocyte recruitment and lineage differentiation. In particular, VEGF seems involved in such process of activation of adventitial ECs to "open the way" for incoming T cells. Another key growth factor in GCA is platelet-derived growth factor (PDGF) which can be produced by macrophages and giant cells. Multiple arterial stromal cells (e.g., VSMC, fibroblasts) express PDGF receptor and respond with proliferation and enhanced migratory ability. Treatment with the drug imatinib mesylate known to inhibit PDGF signaling, reduced myointimal cell outgrowth from cultured temporal artery sections from patients with GCA [29].

3.7   Epigenetics

Temporal arteries from GCA patients have shown hypo- and hypermethylated loci compared to normal temporal arteries from control subjects based on a high through-put study [30]. Deregulation in mechanisms that control DNA methylation can be thus involved in GCA pathogenesis contributing to up- and down-regulation of gene expression. The most hypomethylated locus was upstream the gene encoding runt-related transcription factor 3 (RUNX3) and the most hypermethylated locus was located in the body of the gene Schlafen family member 12-like (SLFN12L). To be noted, CCR7 was among the most hypomethylated sites in GCA which may reflect the presence of mature DCs in inflamed TABs. Hypomethylation of several genetic risk loci associated with GCA, such as IFNγ, TNF, NLRP1, and PTPN22, has been documented suggesting a possible role for genetic–epigenetic interactions in GCA. Moreover, genes encoding cytokines and proteins which promote T cell activation and differentiation have been found hypomethylated in TABs from patients with GCA (CD3E, CD3G, CD3D, CD3Z, CD28, ZAP70, TNF, IL-6. IL-1β). Finally, hypomethylation of genes of the calcineurin/nuclear factor of activated T cells (NFAT) pathway has suggested that specific inhibitors of this pathway or key downstream molecules, such as IL-21/IL-21R and CD40L, might be exploited for the development of novel therapies for GCA [30].

3.8   MicroRNA

MicroRNA (miRNA, miR) are small non-coding RNAs which can inhibit expression of multiple genes post-transcription. Six miRNA have been detected overexpressed in inflamed TABs from GCA patients compared to non-inflamed TABs: miR146b-5p, −146a, −21, −150, −155, −299- 5p [31]. It is actually unknown whether such miRNAs are biomarkers of specific infiltrating immune cell subsets and activated pathways in inflamed temporal arteries and/or have a functional role in GCA pathogenesis. MiR-146a, −21, −155, and − 150 can be expressed by specific immune cell subsets as well as by arterial cells such as VSMCs, ECs, and fibroblasts. MiR-155 is mainly a pro-inflammatory miRNA. MiR-21 can have both pro- and anti-inflammatory activities. MiR-146a and miR-150 mainly inhibit inflammation by negative feedback circuits. Expression of miR-146b-5p, 146a, −21, and − 155 can be induced by the activation of Nuclear Factor-κB (NF-κB), TLRs, and signal transducer, and activator of transcription 3 (STAT3), suggesting that these pathways might be involved in GCA pathogenesis. Moreover, such miRNAs have been associated to cellular senescence and inflammation thus might be linked to immune ageing in GCA. MiR-21 is the only miRNA overexpressed in GCA that has documented pathogenic effects on VSMCs, endothelial cells, and adventitial fibroblasts, thus emerging as a promising target for the development of novel gene-therapy approaches for GCA. MiR-21 has been detected in spindle-shaped cells of the medial layer and stellate fibroblasts-like cells of the intimal layer in inflamed TABs from GCA patients thus emerging as a potential marker of the phenotypic transition of VSMCs [31].

3.9 Deregulation of the Immune System in Peripheral Blood

GCA is characterized by the hepatic acute-phase response [1, 2]. The laboratory hallmarks of active GCA are increased levels of erythrocyte sedimentation rate (ESR) and/or C-reactive protein (CRP). Some cytokines have been detected at higher concentration in plasma or serum samples from GCA patients compared to healthy subjects: IL-6, sIL-6R, IL-10, IL-18, IL-22, IL-23, VEGF, PTX-3, BAFF, CXCL9, sIL-2R, granzymes A and B, VEGF, CHI3L1, MMP-1, MMP-9, CXCL5, CXCL9, CXCL11, MARCO, M-CSF [32, 33]. GCA patients with very recent optic nerve ischemia have significantly higher PTX3 and VEGF levels compared to other GCA patients and controls suggesting a role for PTX3 and VEGF [34]. Levels of IL-6 and BAFF seem associated with disease activity [35, 36].

In addition, several types of auto-antibodies have been documented in patients with GCA, supporting the activation of B cell responses. In particular, anti-endothelial cell antibodies may induce EC injury [37].

Changes in the percentages and/or absolute numbers of some immune subsets in peripheral blood have also been detected in patients with GCA. The percentages of circulating Th17 and Th21 lymphocytes are increased in GCA patients compared with healthy controls. The percentages of Th22 lymphocytes are similar whereas data on differences in the percentages of Th1 lymphocytes between GCA patients and healthy subjects are controversial [21, 22, 38]. Besides, GCA patients have lower frequencies of circulating anti-inflammatory regulatory CD4+ and CD8+ T cells [38, 39] indicating an imbalance between pathogenic and regulatory T cells which is likely involved in disease pathogenesis. Higher percentages of circulating cytotoxic CD8 T lymphocytes, Tc17, CD63+ CD8+ T cells [24], NKG2D+ CD28+ CD8+ T cells, CD3CD4CD28neg and CD3CD8CD28neg T cells have been detected [40]. Instead decreased numbers of circulating CD19+ B cells (in particular TNFα+ B cells and not IL-10+ B cells) have been found in the peripheral blood of GCA patients [41]. Recently, a reduced expression of the immune checkpoint molecules PD-1 and VISTA have been reported in memory and naïve CD4+ T cells from GCA patients [42]. Reduced PD-1 and VISTA expression may promote an unopposed expansion of Th1 and Th17 responses in GCA patients, strengthening the hypothesis regarding defects of immune checkpoints and regulation in GCA development [42, 43].

Regarding innate immune cells, a higher number of circulating neutrophils with a classically activated phenotype (CD16^{hi}AnxA1^{hi}CD62L^{lo}CD11b^{hi}) has been found in GCA patients, suggesting neutrophil involvement in GCA pathogenesis. Interestingly, therapy with glucocorticoids can dampen neutrophil activation but after 24 weeks of therapy neutrophils can display again an activated phenotype and might thus contribute to GCA flares [44]. Increased number of monocytes particularly CD14+ CD16neg classical monocytes has been reported in peripheral blood from patients with GCA [27]. Moreover, lower percentages of CD80/CD86+ and VISTA+ monocytes have been recently detected in GCA patients compared to healthy controls while the frequencies of PD-L1 and PD-L2-expressing monocytes were similar [42].

3.10 Pathways Proven to be Involved in GCA Pathogenesis

Finding deregulated immune effectors, molecules, and biomarkers associated with a disease does not necessarily mean that they are involved in disease pathogenesis and might be targeted in a therapeutic perspective. Functional studies are needed to demonstrate their role. Indeed, only some of the deregulated immune pathways have been proven to be involved in GCA pathogenesis.

Three preclinical models exist for functional analyses in GCA:

1. A mouse model in which human temporal arteries are engrafted into immunodeficient mice plus/minus transfer of peripheral blood mononuclear cells from GCA patients or alloreactive T cells developed by Cornelia Weyand and collaborators [6, 8, 45];
2. An ex vivo model in which human TAB sections are cultured in matrigel drops for 5 days developed by Maria Cinta Cid and collaborators [46];
3. An ex vivo model in which human TAB sections are cultured for 1 day in serum-supplemented medium developed by Eamonn S Molloy and collaborators [47].

Using the mouse model, it has been demonstrated that the activation of vascular DCs and T cells [6, 7, 45]; the activation of TLR4 (LPS) and TLR5 (flagellin) [48]; the expression of CCR6 by T cells [48]; the activation of NOTCH-Jagged pathway [49]; the inhibition of PD-1 checkpoint [43]; the production of VEGF [28] and MMP9 [50]; the activation of Janus kinases 1 and 3 [8] and CD28 co-stimulation [51] can induce arteritis. Moreover, using the ex vivo models of GCA, a pathogenic role for IFNγ, ET-1, PDGF, IL-12, IL-23, acute-phase serum amyloid A (A-SAA) has been unveiled [29, 47, 52–54]. Table 3.1 summarizes the results of functional

Table 3.1 Functional studies in preclinical models of GCA

Immune intervention	Model	Effects	Reference
T cell depleting antiserum	Artery-mouse chimeras	↓ IFNγ and IL-1β mRNA	[45]
DC depletion with anti-CD83 antibodies	Artery-mouse chimeras	↓ CD3+ T lymphocytes ↓ IFNγ and IL-1β mRNA	[6]
Activation of TLR4 with LPS and TLR5 with flagellin	Artery-mouse chimeras	TLR4 activation: transmural arteritis TLR5 activation: inflammation limited to adventitia	[48]
Depletion of CCR6+ lymphocytes with anti-CCR6 antibodies	Artery-mouse chimeras	↓ Transmural inflammation	[48]
Blocking NOTCH—Jagged1 interaction	Artery-mouse chimeras	↓ CD3+ lymphocytes ↓ TCR mRNA ↓ IFNγ, IL-17, CCR6 mRNA ↑ Smoothelin mRNA	[49]
Treatment with VEGF	Artery-mouse chimeras	↑ Jagged1 by microvascular ECs ↑ CD3+ lymphocytes ↑ IFNγ, IL-17, TNFα, IL-6, T-bet, RORγT, CD68 mRNA Effects reversed by the VEGF inhibitor axitinib	[28]
Blockade of PD-1	Artery-mouse chimeras	↑ CD3+ lymphocytes ↑ TCR, T-bet, RORC, cytokine, and chemokine mRNA ↑ Intima thickness ↑ Microvessels ↑ Endothelial activation ↑ Myofibroblasts	[43]
Inhibition of Janus kinase (JAK)1 and 3 with tofacitinib	Artery-mouse chimeras	↓ CD3+, CD4+, CD8+ lymphocytes ↓ CD4 + CD103+ T_{RM} ↓ CD163, TCR, T-bet, RORC, BCL6, IFNγ, IL-17, IL-21 mRNA ↓ Proliferation ↓ Intima thickness ↓ Microvessels and PDGF, FGF2, VEGF mRNA	[8]
Inhibition of MMP9 with anti-MMP9 antibodies	Artery-mouse chimeras	↓ Migration of T lymphocytes ↓ CD3+ and CD4+ lymphocytes ↓ TCR, CD163, IL-1β, IL-6, IFNγ, IL-21 mRNA ↓ Destruction of the elastic lamina ↓ Intima thickness ↓ Number of microvessels and VEGF, PDGF, FGF2 mRNA Treatment with recombinant MMP9 produced opposite effects	[50]

Table 3.1 (continued)

Immune intervention	Model	Effects	Reference
Blocking CD28 signaling	Artery-mouse chimeras	↓ Tissue-infiltrating T cells ↓ T cell proliferation and cytokine production ↓ T_{RM} ↓ T cell metabolic fitness ↓ Neoangiogenesis and intimal hyperplasia	[51]
Treatment with ET-1	Ex vivo 5-day matrigel culture	↑ αSMA expression ↑ Muscular layer and migration of VSMC toward the intima Opposite effects by treatment with ET-receptor antagonists BQ123 and BQ788	[52]
Inhibition of IFNγ with a neutralizing antibody	Ex vivo 5-day matrigel culture	↓ CXCL9, CXCL10, CXCL11, and STAT-1 ↓ ICAM-1 expression ↓ Number of CD68-expressing cells and giant cells No effects on the number of T cells Treatment with exogenous IFNγ produced opposite effects	[53]
Inhibition of PDGF with imatinib	Ex vivo 5-day matrigel culture	↓ Myofibroblast outgrowth	[29]
Treatment with A-SAA	Ex vivo 1-day culture	↑ IL-6 and IL-8 ↑ Angiogenic tube formation myofibroblast outgrowth ↑ MMP9 activation	[47]
Treatment with IL-12 and IL-23	Ex vivo 1-day culture	↑ Myofibroblast outgrowth	[54]

↑, increase; ↓, decrease

experiments which prove a role of specific immune pathways in the pathogenesis of GCA. These pathways are candidate targets for the development of novel therapies for GCA. Besides, a better understanding of the mechanisms at the basis of GCA can also derive from patient responses to targeted therapies [55, 56]. Treatment of GCA patients with the IL-6 signaling inhibitor tocilizumab and the IL-12/IL-23 signaling inhibitor ustekinumab have proven effective in vivo in patients with GCA, indicating a key role of these cytokines in disease pathogenesis [57, 58].

References

1. Salvarani C, Pipitone N, Versari A, Hunder GG. Clinical features of polymyalgia rheumatica and giant cell arteritis. Nat Rev Rheumatol. 2012;8:509–21.
2. Salvarani C, Cantini F, Hunder GG. Polymyalgia rheumatica and giant-cell arteritis. Lancet. 2008;372:234–45.

3. Mohan SV, Liao YJ, Kim JW, Goronzy JJ, Weyand CM. Giant cell arteritis: immune and vascular aging as disease risk factors. Arthritis Res Ther. 2011;13:231.
4. Weyand CM, Schönberger J, Oppitz U, Hunder NN, Hicok KC, Goronzy JJ. Distinct vascular lesions in giant cell arteritis share identical T cell clonotypes. J Exp Med. 1994;179:951–60.
5. Weyand CM, Goronzy JJ. Giant cell arteritis as an antigen-driven disease. Rheum Dis Clin N Am. 1995;21:1027–39.
6. Ma-Krupa W, Jeon MS, Spoerl S, Tedder TF, Goronzy JJ, Weyand CM. Activation of arterial wall dendritic cells and breakdown of self-tolerance in giant cell arteritis. J Exp Med. 2004;199:173–83.
7. Weyand CM, Ma-Krupa W, Pryshchep O, Gröschel S, Bernardino R, Goronzy JJ. Vascular dendritic cells in giant cell arteritis. Ann N Y Acad Sci. 2005;1062:195–208.
8. Zhang H, Watanabe R, Berry GJ, Tian L, Goronzy JJ, Weyand CM. Inhibition of JAK-STAT signaling suppresses pathogenic immune responses in medium and large vessel vasculitis. Circulation. 2018;137:1934–48.
9. Ciccia F, Rizzo A, Ferrante A, Guggino G, Croci S, Cavazza A, et al. New insights into the pathogenesis of giant cell arteritis. Autoimmun Rev. 2017;16:675–83.
10. Samson M, Corbera-Bellalta M, Audia S, Planas-Rigol E, Martin L, Cid MC, et al. Recent advances in our understanding of giant cell arteritis pathogenesis. Autoimmun Rev. 2017;16:833–44.
11. Petursdottir V, Johansson H, Nordborg E, Nordborg C. The epidemiology of biopsy positive giant cell arteritis: special reference to cyclic fluctuations. Rheumatology. 1999;38:1208–12.
12. Gabriel SE, Espy M, Erdman DD, Bjornsson J, Smith TF, Hunder GG. The role of parvovirus B19 in the pathogenesis of giant cell arteritis: a preliminary evaluation. Arthritis Rheum. 1999;42:1255–8.
13. Wagner AD, Gérard HC, Fresemann T, Schmidt WA, Gromnica-Ihle E, Hudson AP, et al. Detection of Chlamydia pneumoniae in giant cell vasculitis and correlation with the topographic arrangement of tissue-infiltrating dendritic cells. Arthritis Rheumatol. 2000;43:1543–51.
14. Giardina A, Rizzo A, Ferrante A, Capra G, Triolo G, Ciccia F. Giant cell arteritis associated with chronic active Epstein–Barr virus infection. Reumatismo. 2013;65:36–9.
15. Muratore F, Croci S, Tamagnini I, Zerbini A, Bellafiore S, Belloni L, et al. No detection of varicella-zoster virus in temporal arteries of patients with giant cell arteritis. Semin Arthritis Rheum. 2017;47:235–40.
16. Carmona FD, Mackie SL, Martín JE, Taylor JC, Vaglio A, Eyre S, et al. A large-scale genetic analysis reveals a strong contribution of the HLA class II region to giant cell arteritis susceptibility. Am J Hum Genet. 2015;96:565–80.
17. Carmona FD, Vaglio A, Mackie SL, Hernández-Rodríguez J, Monach PA, Castañeda S, et al. A genome-wide association study identifies risk alleles in plasminogen and P4HA2 associated with giant cell arteritis. Am J Hum Genet. 2017;100:64–74.
18. Carmona FD, Coit P, Saruhan-Direskeneli G, Hernández-Rodríguez J, Cid MC, Solans R, et al. Analysis of the common genetic component of large-vessel vasculitides through a meta-immunochip strategy. Sci Rep. 2017;7:43953.
19. Cavazza A, Muratore F, Boiardi L, Restuccia G, Pipitone N, Pazzola G, et al. Inflamed temporal artery: histologic findings in 354 biopsies, with clinical correlations. Am J Surg Pathol. 2014;38:1360–70.
20. Restuccia G, Cavazza A, Boiardi L, Pipitone N, Macchioni P, Bajocchi G, et al. Small-vessel vasculitis surrounding an uninflamed temporal artery and isolated vasa vasorum vasculitis of the temporal artery: two subsets of giant cell arteritis. Arthritis Rheum. 2012;64:549–56.
21. Watanabe R, Hosgur E, Zhang H, Wen Z, Berry G, Goronzy JJ, et al. Pro-inflammatory and anti-inflammatory T cells in giant cell arteritis. Joint Bone Spine. 2017;84:421–6.
22. Zerbini A, Muratore F, Boiardi L, Ciccia F, Bonacini M, Belloni L, et al. Increased expression of interleukin-22 in patients with giant cell arteritis. Rheumatology (Oxford). 2018;57:64–72.
23. Weyand CM, Goronzy JJ. Immune mechanisms in medium and large-vessel vasculitis. Nat Rev Rheumatol. 2013;9:731–40.

24. Samson M, Ly KH, Tournier B, Janikashvili N, Trad M, Ciudad M, et al. Involvement and prognosis value of CD8(+) T cells in giant cell arteritis. J Autoimmun. 2016;72:73–83.
25. Ciccia F, Rizzo A, Maugeri R, Alessandro R, Croci S, Guggino G, et al. Ectopic expression of CXCL13, BAFF, APRIL and LT-β is associated with artery tertiary lymphoid organs in giant cell arteritis. Ann Rheum Dis. 2017;76:235–43.
26. Wagner AD, Goronzy JJ, Weyand CM. Functional profile of tissue-infiltrating and circulating CD68+ cells in giant cell arteritis. Evidence for two components of the disease. J Clin Invest. 1994;94:1134–40.
27. van Sleen Y, Wang Q, van der Geest KSM, Westra J, Abdulahad WH, Heeringa P, et al. Involvement of monocyte subsets in the immunopathology of giant cell arteritis. Sci Rep. 2017;7:6553.
28. Wen Z, Shen Y, Berry G, Shahram F, Li Y, Watanabe R, et al. The microvascular niche instructs T cells in large vessel vasculitis via the VEGF-Jagged1-Notch pathway. Sci Transl Med. 2017;9:399.
29. Lozano E, Segarra M, García-Martínez A, Hernández-Rodríguez J, Cid MC. Imatinib mesylate inhibits in vitro and ex vivo biological responses related to vascular occlusion in giant cell arteritis. Ann Rheum Dis. 2008;67:1581–8.
30. Coit P, De Lott LB, Nan B, Elner VM, Sawalha AH. DNA methylation analysis of the temporal artery microenvironment in giant cell arteritis. Ann Rheum Dis. 2016;75:1196–202.
31. Croci S, Zerbini A, Boiardi L, Muratore F, Bisagni A, Nicoli D, et al. MicroRNA markers of inflammation and remodelling in temporal arteries from patients with giant cell arteritis. Ann Rheum Dis. 2016;75:1527–33.
32. Burja B, Feichtinger J, Lakota K, Thallinger GG, Sodin-Semrl S, Kuret T, et al. Utility of serological biomarkers for giant cell arteritis in a large cohort of treatment-naïve patients. Clin Rheumatol. 2019;38:317–29.
33. Burja B, Kuret T, Sodin-Semrl S, Lakota K, Rotar Ž, Ješe R, et al. A concise review of significantly modified serological biomarkers in giant cell arteritis, as detected by different methods. Autoimmun Rev. 2018;17:188–94.
34. Baldini M, Maugeri N, Ramirez GA, Giacomassi C, Castiglioni A, Prieto-González S, et al. Selective up-regulation of the soluble pattern-recognition receptor pentraxin 3 and of vascular endothelial growth factor in giant cell arteritis: relevance for recent optic nerve ischemia. Arthritis Rheum. 2012;64:854–65.
35. Pulsatelli L, Boiardi L, Assirelli E, Pazzola G, Muratore F, Addimanda O, et al. Interleukin-6 and soluble interleukin-6 receptor are elevated in large-vessel vasculitis: a cross-sectional and longitudinal study. Clin Exp Rheumatol. 2017;35(Suppl 103):102–10.
36. van der Geest KS, Abdulahad WH, Rutgers A, Horst G, Bijzet J, Arends S, Roffel MP, et al. Serum markers associated with disease activity in giant cell arteritis and polymyalgia rheumatica. Rheumatology (Oxford). 2015;54:1397–402.
37. Legendre P, Régent A, Thiebault M, Mouthon L. Anti-endothelial cell antibodies in vasculitis: a systematic review. Autoimmun Rev. 2017;16:146–53.
38. Samson M, Audia S, Fraszczak J, Trad M, Ornetti P, Lakomy D, et al. Th1 and Th17 lymphocytes expressing CD161 are implicated in giant cell arteritis and polymyalgia rheumatica pathogenesis. Arthritis Rheum. 2012;64(11):3788–98.
39. Wen Z, Shimojima Y, Shirai T, Li Y, Ju J, Yang Z, et al. NADPH oxidase deficiency underlies dysfunction of aged CD8+ Tregs. J Clin Invest. 2016;126:1953–67.
40. Dejaco C, Duftner C, Al-Massad J, Wagner AD, Park JK, Fessler J, et al. NKG2D stimulated T-cell autoreactivity in giant cell arteritis and polymyalgia rheumatica. Ann Rheum Dis. 2013;72:1852–9.
41. van der Geest KS, Abdulahad WH, Chalan P, Rutgers A, Horst G, Huitema MG, et al. Disturbed B cell homeostasis in newly diagnosed giant cell arteritis and polymyalgia rheumatica. Arthritis Rheumatol. 2014;66:1927–38.
42. Hid Cadena R, Reitsema RD, Huitema MG, van Sleen Y, van der Geest KSM, Heeringa P, et al. Decreased expression of negative immune checkpoint VISTA by CD4+ T cells facilitates T

helper 1, T helper 17, and T follicular helper lineage differentiation in GCA. Front Immunol. 2019;10:1638.

43. Zhang H, Watanabe R, Berry GJ, Vaglio A, Liao YJ, Warrington KJ, et al. Immunoinhibitory checkpoint deficiency in medium and large vessel vasculitis. Proc Natl Acad Sci U S A. 2017;114:E970–9.

44. Nadkarni S, Dalli J, Hollywood J, Mason JC, Dasgupta B, Perretti M. Investigational analysis reveals a potential role for neutrophils in giant-cell arteritis disease progression. Circ Res. 2014;114:242–8.

45. Brack A, Geisler A, Martinez-Taboada VM, Younge BR, Goronzy JJ, Weyand CM. Giant cell vasculitis is a T cell-dependent disease. Mol Med. 1997;3:530–43.

46. Corbera-Bellalta M, García-Martínez A, Lozano E, Planas-Rigol E, Tavera-Bahillo I, Alba MA, Prieto-González S, et al. Changes in biomarkers after therapeutic intervention in temporal arteries cultured in Matrigel: a new model for preclinical studies in giant-cell arteritis. Ann Rheum Dis. 2014;73:616–23.

47. O'Neill L, Rooney P, Molloy D, Connolly M, McCormick J, McCarthy G, et al. Regulation of inflammation and angiogenesis in giant cell arteritis by acute-phase serum amyloid A. Arthritis Rheumatol. 2015;67:2447–56.

48. Deng J, Ma-Krupa W, Gewirtz AT, Younge BR, Goronzy JJ, Weyand CM. Toll-like receptors 4 and 5 induce distinct types of vasculitis. Circ Res. 2009;104:488–95.

49. Piggott K, Deng J, Warrington K, Younge B, Kubo JT, Desai M, et al. Blocking the NOTCH pathway inhibits vascular inflammation in large-vessel vasculitis. Circulation. 2011;123:309–18.

50. Watanabe R, Maeda T, Zhang H, Berry GJ, Zeisbrich M, Brockett R, et al. MMP (matrix metalloprotease)-9-producing monocytes enable T cells to invade the vessel wall and cause vasculitis. Circ Res. 2018;123:700–15.

51. Zhang H, Watanabe R, Berry GJ, Nadler SG, Goronzy JJ, Weyand CM. CD28 signaling controls metabolic fitness of pathogenic T cells in medium and large vessel vasculitis. J Am Coll Cardiol. 2019;73:1811–23.

52. Planas-Rigol E, Terrades-Garcia N, Corbera-Bellalta M, Lozano E, Alba MA, Segarra M, et al. Endothelin-1 promotes vascular smooth muscle cell migration across the artery wall: a mechanism contributing to vascular remodelling and intimal hyperplasia in giant-cell arteritis. Ann Rheum Dis. 2017;76:1624–34.

53. Corbera-Bellalta M, Planas-Rigol E, Lozano E, Terrades-García N, Alba MA, Prieto-González S, et al. Blocking interferon γ reduces expression of chemokines CXCL9, CXCL10 and CXCL11 and decreases macrophage infiltration in ex vivo cultured arteries from patients with giant cell arteritis. Ann Rheum Dis. 2016;75:1177–86.

54. Conway R, O'Neill L, McCarthy GM, Murphy CC, Fabre A, Kennedy S, et al. Interleukin 12 and interleukin 23 play key pathogenic roles in inflammatory and proliferative pathways in giant cell arteritis. Ann Rheum Dis. 2018;77:1815–24.

55. Terrades-Garcia N, Cid MC. Pathogenesis of giant-cell arteritis: how targeted therapies are influencing our understanding of the mechanisms involved. Rheumatology (Oxford). 2018;57(suppl_2):ii51–62.

56. Watanabe R, Goronzy JJ, Berry G, Liao YJ, Weyand CM. Giant cell arteritis: from pathogenesis to therapeutic management. Curr Treatm Opt Rheumatol. 2016;2:126–37.

57. Stone JH, Tuckwell K, Dimonaco S, Klearman M, Aringer M, Blockmans D, et al. Trial of tocilizumab in giant-cell arteritis. N Engl J Med. 2017;377:317–28.

58. Conway R, O'Neill L, O'Flynn E, Gallagher P, McCarthy GM, Murphy CC, et al. Ustekinumab for the treatment of refractory giant cell arteritis. Ann Rheum Dis. 2016;75:1578–9.

Clinical Manifestations, Differential Diagnosis, and Laboratory Markers

4

Nicolò Pipitone

Abstract

Giant cell arteritis is a large-vessel vasculitis. It is exceptional before 50 years of age, while its incidence increases with advancing age. There is a female predominance, with females being two to three times more frequently affected than males. The hallmark clinical feature of giant cell arteritis is headache. Visual loss, related to vasculitis of the posterior ciliary or, less commonly, the retinal arteries occurs in about one-sixth of patients with giant cell arteritis, usually before treatment with glucocorticoids is started, while jaw claudication is described by half of patients. In some patients, systemic symptoms predominate and may be the only manifestation.

Blood tests typically reveal an inflammatory status, including an elevated erythrocyte sedimentation rate and C-reactive protein; less than 5% of patients with giant cell arteritis have normal inflammatory markers. Autoimmune serology is typically negative; positive anticardiolipin antibodies can occur, but normalize following treatment.

Keywords

Giant cell arteritis · Temporal artery biopsy · Ultrasonography

N. Pipitone (✉)
Arcispedale Santa Maria Nuova, Reggio Emilia, Italy
e-mail: pipitone.nicolo@ausl.re.it, nicolo.pipitone@ausl.re.it

© Springer Nature Switzerland AG 2021
C. Salvarani et al. (eds.), *Large and Medium Size Vessel and Single Organ Vasculitis*, Rare Diseases of the Immune System,
https://doi.org/10.1007/978-3-030-67175-4_4

4.1   Clinical Manifestations of Giant Cell Arteritis

Giant cell arteritis (GCA) affects patients aged 50 years or older; the onset of the disease before such age is exceptional [1], while its incidence progressively increases with advancing age [2]. There is a female predominance, with females being two to three times more frequently affected than males [2]. GCA is typical of Caucasians, especially of Northern European ancestry, and is rare in other ethnicities [2]. GCA is usually classified according to the American College of Rheumatology (ACR) criteria [3]. However, these criteria are not meant to be used for the purpose of making a diagnosis of GCA in the individual patient.

The hallmark clinical feature of GCA is headache, which is described by two-thirds of patients. While typically temporal, headache can also affect other areas of the scalp; it is often persistent and poorly responsive to common analgesic drugs [4, 5]. In patients with pre-existing headache, worsening of pain can be the heralding symptom of GCA. Even when not reported by patients with a suspicion of GCA, direct questioning should always address whether they have headache. Physical examination usually shows tenderness of the temporal arteries and decreased (or sometimes) absent pulse. Less frequently, there may be an erythema overlying the arteries or nodules [4, 5]. A meta-analysis performed to identify the clinical features conducive to a diagnosis of GCA showed that absence of any temporal artery abnormality was the only clinical factor that modestly reduced the likelihood of disease with a likelihood ratio of 0.53. In contrast, predictive physical findings included temporal artery beading (positive likelihood ratio of 4.6), prominence (positive likelihood ratio of 4.3), and tenderness (positive likelihood ratio of 2.6) [1].

In about half of patients, scalp dysesthesia, aggravated by brushing or combing the hair, are associated. Pain on chewing (jaw claudication) is another frequent symptom, described by 50% of patients [5]. Jaw claudication is thought to be due to ischemia of the masseter muscles, and its presence increases the risk for other ischemic manifestations, including visual loss [6]. In contrast, a strong clinical and laboratory inflammatory response protects against ischemic events [7, 8]. Visual loss occurs in about one-sixth of patients with GCA, usually before treatment with glucocorticoids is started [9]. It is typically sudden and painless and can involve one or both eyes. Transient visual loss, also termed amaurosis fugax, is less common (10–15% of cases), but is an ominous sign, since it portends persistent loss of vision in around half of the patients if therapy is not promptly commenced. Likewise, unilateral visual loss is a strong risk factor for visual loss in the contralateral eye in untreated patients [9, 10]. Other risk factors for visual loss include older age at diagnosis and an elevated platelet count at diagnosis [8]. Rarely, visual loss can be the only clinical manifestation of GCA, at least at onset of the disease [11]. In most cases, visual loss is due to anterior ischemic optic neuropathy (AION) related to vasculitis of the posterior ciliary or, less commonly, the retinal arteries. Fundoscopy typically shows a chalky white edematous optic disc [12]. Rarely, visual loss may be due to posterior ischemic optic neuropathy, caused by ischemia of the retrobulbar portion of the optic nerve [9]. Unlike in AION, in posterior ischemic optic neuropathy the appearance of the optic disc on fundoscopy is initially normal, but temporal optic disc pallor develops after a few weeks [9]. Exceptionally, blindness can be result of cortical ischemia; in such cases, the optic disc is unremarkable on fundoscopy [9].

Cranial ischemic events (transient ischemic attacks and stroke) may present early on in the disease course like visual loss, but are less common [13]. Cranial ischemic events are underscored by carotid or vertebral artery involvement [4, 5], whereas intracranial GCA is exceptionally rare [14].

Scalp or lip necrosis are other manifestations attributable to ischemia, but they occur only occasionally [15].

Nearly half of patients describe constitutional features such as fever, fatigue, and weight loss [4]. The fever is usually modest, but can reach up to 40° [13]. Systemic symptoms can be the sole manifestations in about 15% of patients [16].

Musculoskeletal manifestations are frequent in GCA. Polymyalgia rheumatica affects 40% of GCA patients, while another quarter of patients may have a benign, non-erosive peripheral arthritis, tenosynovitis, and carpal tunnel syndrome [4, 5, 17].

GCA may present in some patients with uncommon manifestations. Cough, usually non-productive in nature, occurs in about 10% of patients, possibly due to ischemia of the cough receptors [18]. Atypical, but possible manifestations include peripheral neuropathy [4, 5], audiovestibular dysfunction [19], (usually transient) diplopia [20], dysarthria [21], Charles–Bonnet syndrome (visual hallucinations) [22], facial swelling [23], serosal effusion [24], and myocardial infarction [25]. In some cases, histological findings of GCA are the first clue to the disease; they are usually found in the breast [26] and in the female genital tract [27].

Manifestations due to large-vessel involvement are usually late complications of GCA. Arterial aneurysms (usually of the thoracic, but also of the abdominal aorta), or stenoses (often affecting the upper limb arteries) occur in 9%, 7%, and 14% of patients, respectively [28]. Arm claudication is a symptom of arterial stenosis or occlusion in the upper limbs, whereas thoracic or abdominal pain develops if dissection of the involved arteries occurs. Physical examination may reveal arterial bruits and heart murmurs. An earlier population-based study estimated that patients with GCA have a 17-fold and a 2.4-fold increased risk of developing thoracic and abdominal aortic aneurysms, respectively [29]. In contrast, a more recent study based on a large database in the United Kingdom found that the relative risk of developing aortic aneurysms in GCA was only twofold increased compared to matched controls [30].

Life expectancy is not [31] or only marginally [32] reduced in GCA, except in the subset with large-vessel complications [32].

4.2 Differential Diagnosis of Giant Cell Arteritis

GCA and Takayasu arteritis share a number of features, but GCA occurs almost exclusively in subjects aged 50 or older, whether Takayasu arteritis affects younger patients. Temporal artery involvement and polymyalgia rheumatica point to GCA;

in addition, compared to patients with Takayasu arteritis, patients with GCA have a greater prevalence of jaw claudication (GCA 33%, Takayasu arteritis 5%), blurred vision (GCA 29%, Takayasu arteritis 8%), diplopia (GCA 9%, Takayasu arteritis 0%), and blindness (GCA 14%, Takayasu arteritis 0%) [33]. In terms of large-vessel involvement, there is more left carotid (37% vs 21%) and mesenteric (36% vs 18%) artery disease in Takayasu arteritis and more left and right axillary artery (40% vs 10%) disease in GCA [34]. At ^{18}F-Fluorodeoxyglucose positron emission tomography, ^{18}F-Fluorodeoxyglucose standard uptake max values measured in the arteries are significantly higher in GCA compared to Takayasu arteritis, except for the axillary arteries [35].

Other vasculitides, such as eosinophilic granulomatosis with polyangiitis, granulomatosis with polyangiitis may occasionally affect the temporal arteries; the clinical picture, ANCA status, and the presence of marked fibrinoid necrosis in ANCA-associated vasculitis at temporal artery biopsy suggest the correct diagnosis [36, 37]. Rarely, amyloidosis may present as GCA/polymyalgia rheumatica; the histological features are helpful in clinching the correct diagnosis [38].

Visual loss may be due to GCA (AION, anterior ischemic optic neuropathy), but is more often non-arteritic in nature (NAION, non-arteritic anterior ischemic optic neuropathy). NAION is thought to be related to a lesion to the head of the optic nerve caused by hypotension and is more frequent (90% versus 10%) and less severe than AION. Fundoscopy can aid in the differential diagnosis by showing in NAION a hyperemic edema of the optic disc with a small cap size unlike the "chalky white" appearance of the optic disc in GCA. Normal inflammatory markers point also to a diagnosis of NAION over that of AION [39].

4.3 Laboratory Markers

The laboratory features of giant cell arteritis (GCA) reflect the systemic inflammatory response. An erythrocyte sedimentation rate (ESR) of 50 mm/1st hour or greater is incorporated in the classification criteria of GCA stipulated by the American College of Rheumatology (ACR) [3]. However, ESR values lower than 50 mm/1st hour can also be found in clinical practice [40]. Because the ESR may be nonspecifically elevated for causes unrelated to inflammation (e.g., in the presence of anemia) [41], it is preferable to rely on the C-reactive protein (CRP), which has a higher sensitivity and specificity for active GCA [42]. Both the ESR and CRP reflect ongoing inflammation, but they are not per se specific to GCA, so their role is more important to rule out GCA when they are normal than to point to GCA when they are elevated. In fact, only 4% of patients with GCA have both ESR and CRP in the normal range [43]. When the ESR and CRP are discordant, the non-concordance is usually due to an association of a normal ESR with a raised CRP, but the finding of an elevated ESR with a normal CRP can also be consistent with GCA in the appropriate clinical setting [42]. Serum interleukin-6 (IL-6) is a key molecule that drives the inflammatory status, including the elevation of ESR and CRP, and is a very sensitive measure of inflammation [4], but is not tested in routine clinical practice. Other laboratory indices that reflect systemic inflammation are normochromic normocytic anemia [44], thrombocytosis [45], as well as an reduced albumin [44] and elevated alpha2 fraction at serum protein electrophoresis [46] and a raised fibrinogen [47].

A weak inflammatory response with only modestly elevated ESR and CRP before the institution of glucocorticoid therapy is considered a risk factor for the development of ischemic complications related to GCA [48], but ischemic complications may also occur in the presence of high inflammatory markers [49].

Patients with GCA may also present with other laboratory changes of various types. Liver function tests can be abnormal in one-third to one-fourth of patients, with the alkaline phosphatase being affected in most cases [44]. Isoenzyme studies confirm the hepatic origin of the alkaline phosphatase. The elevation of alkaline phosphatase is usually modest and returns to normal after glucocorticoid treatment [44]. Renal parameters are usually within the normal range [44]. Very occasionally, microscopic hematuria, minimal proteinuria, or both, have been reported. Marked proteinuria is exceptional and warrants investigation for secondary amyloidosis [50]. Thyroid function tests are not routinely performed, and changes in such tests have rarely been described [51]. Autoimmune serology is typically negative [52], whereas positive anticardiolipin antibodies have be found in up to one-half of patients. However, positive anticardiolipin antibodies have not been linked to an increased thrombotic risk in patients with GCA; moreover, they usually normalize following the onset of treatment [53, 54].

Inflammatory indices typically decrease after starting glucocorticoids and are used in clinical practice to monitor response to therapy [44]. Disease flares and relapses are often preceded by a rise in markers of inflammation [55], but their elevation does not inevitably predict clinical worsening [5]. In active disease, ultrasound often shows a hypoechoic halo in the inflamed arteries ("halo sign"), while PET shows increased FDG uptake in the inflamed arteries (Figs. 4.1 and 4.2).

Fig. 4.1 Ultrasound of an inflamed artery showing a hypoechoic halo

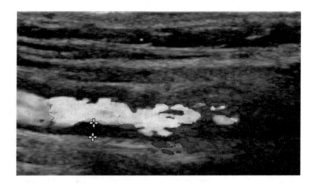

Fig. 4.2 PET showing increased FDG uptake in the thoracic aorta, abdominal aorta, axillary arteries and left carotid artery

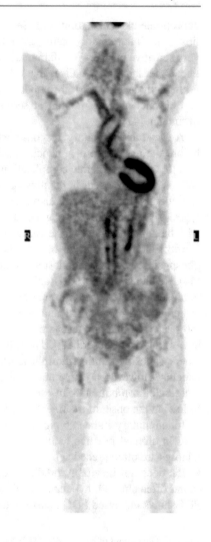

References

1. Smetana GW, Shmerling RH. Does this patient have temporal arteritis? JAMA. 2002;287:92–101.
2. Gonzalez-Gay MA, Vazquez-Rodriguez TR, Lopez-Diaz MJ, et al. Epidemiology of giant cell arteritis and polymyalgia rheumatica. Arthritis Rheum. 2009;61:1454–61.
3. Hunder GG, Bloch DA, Michel BA, et al. The American College of Rheumatology 1990 criteria for the classification of giant cell arteritis. Arthritis Rheum. 1990;33:1122–8.
4. Salvarani C, Cantini F, Hunder GG. Polymyalgia rheumatica and giant-cell arteritis. Lancet. 2008;372:234–45.
5. Salvarani C, Cantini F, Boiardi L, Hunder GG. Polymyalgia rheumatica and giant-cell arteritis. N Engl J Med. 2002;347:261–71.

6. Liozon E, Dalmay F, Lalloue F, et al. Risk factors for permanent visual loss in biopsy-proven giant cell arteritis: a study of 339 patients. J Rheumatol. 2016;43:1393–9.
7. Cid MC, Font C, Oristrell J, et al. Association between strong inflammatory response and low risk of developing visual loss and other cranial ischemic complications in giant cell (temporal) arteritis. Arthritis Rheum. 1998;41:26–32.
8. Salvarani C, Cimino L, Macchioni P, et al. Risk factors for visual loss in an Italian population-based cohort of patients with giant cell arteritis. Arthritis Rheum. 2005;53:293–7.
9. Soriano A, Muratore F, Pipitone N, Boiardi L, Cimino L, Salvarani C. Visual loss and other cranial ischaemic complications in giant cell arteritis. Nat Rev Rheumatol. 2017;13:476–84.
10. Gordon LK, Levin LA. Visual loss in giant cell arteritis. JAMA. 1998;280:385–6.
11. Hayreh SS, Podhajsky PA, Zimmerman B. Occult giant cell arteritis: ocular manifestations. Am J Ophthalmol. 1998;125:521–6.
12. Hayreh SS. Ophthalmic features of giant cell arteritis. Baillieres Clin Rheumatol. 1991;5:431–59.
13. de Boysson H, Liozon E, Lariviere D, et al. Giant cell arteritis-related stroke: a retrospective multicenter case-control study. J Rheumatol. 2017;44:297–303.
14. Salvarani C, Giannini C, Miller DV, Hunder G. Giant cell arteritis: involvement of intracranial arteries. Arthritis Rheum. 2006;55:985–9.
15. Kumar R, Gupta H, Jadhav A, Khadilkar S. Bitemporal scalp, lip and tongue necrosis in giant cell arteritis: a rare presentation. Indian J Dermatol. 2013;58:328.
16. Calamia KT, Hunder GG. Giant cell arteritis (temporal arteritis) presenting as fever of undetermined origin. Arthritis Rheum. 1981;24:1414–8.
17. Salvarani C, Hunder GG. Musculoskeletal manifestations in a population-based cohort of patients with giant cell arteritis. Arthritis Rheum. 1999;42:1259–66.
18. Olopade CO, Sekosan M, Schraufnagel DE. Giant cell arteritis manifesting as chronic cough and fever of unknown origin. Mayo Clin Proc. 1997;72:1048–50.
19. Amor-Dorado JC, Llorca J, Garcia-Porrua C, Costa C, Perez-Fernandez N, Gonzalez-Gay MA. Audiovestibular manifestations in giant cell arteritis: a prospective study. Medicine (Baltimore). 2003;82:13–26.
20. Killer HE, Holtz DJ, Kaiser HJ, Laeng RH. Diplopia, ptosis, and hepatitis as presenting signs and symptoms of giant cell arteritis. Br J Ophthalmol. 2000;84:1319–20.
21. Lee CC, Su WW, Hunder GG. Dysarthria associated with giant cell arteritis. J Rheumatol. 1999;26:931–2.
22. Sonnenblick M, Nesher R, Rozenman Y, Nesher G. Charles Bonnet syndrome in temporal arteritis. J Rheumatol. 1995;22:1596–7.
23. Liozon E, Ouattara B, Portal MF, Soria P, Loustaud-Ratti V, Vidal E. Head-and-neck swelling: an under-recognized feature of giant cell arteritis. A report of 37 patients. Clin Exp Rheumatol. 2006;24:S20–5.
24. Valstar MH, Terpstra WF, de Jong RS. Pericardial and pleural effusion in giant cell arteritis. Am J Med. 2003;114:708–9.
25. Lin LW, Wang SS, Shun CT. Myocardial infarction due to giant cell arteritis: a case report and literature review. Kaohsiung J Med Sci. 2007;23:195–8.
26. McKendry RJ, Guindi M, Hill DP. Giant cell arteritis (temporal arteritis) affecting the breast: report of two cases and review of published reports. Ann Rheum Dis. 1990;49:1001–4.
27. Bajocchi G, Zamorani G, Cavazza A, et al. Giant-cell arteritis of the female genital tract associated with occult temporal arteritis and FDG-PET evidence of large-vessel vasculitis. Clin Exp Rheumatol. 2007;25:S36–9.
28. Bongartz T, Matteson EL. Large-vessel involvement in giant cell arteritis. Curr Opin Rheumatol. 2006;18:10–7.
29. Evans JM, O'Fallon WM, Hunder GG. Increased incidence of aortic aneurysm and dissection in giant cell (temporal) arteritis. A population-based study. Ann Intern Med. 1995;122:502–7.

30. Robson JC, Kiran A, Maskell J, et al. The relative risk of aortic aneurysm in patients with giant cell arteritis compared with the general population of the UK. Ann Rheum Dis. 2015;74:129–35.
31. Matteson EL, Gold KN, Bloch DA, Hunder GG. Long-term survival of patients with giant cell arteritis in the American College of Rheumatology giant cell arteritis classification criteria cohort. Am J Med. 1996;100:193–6.
32. Aouba A, Gonzalez CS, Eb M, et al. Mortality causes and trends associated with giant cell arteritis: analysis of the French national death certificate database (1980-2011). Rheumatology (Oxford). 2018;57:1047–55.
33. Maksimowicz-McKinnon K, Clark TM, Hoffman GS. Takayasu arteritis and giant cell arteritis: a spectrum within the same disease? Medicine (Baltimore). 2009;88:221–6.
34. Grayson PC, Maksimowicz-McKinnon K, Clark TM, et al. Distribution of arterial lesions in Takayasu's arteritis and giant cell arteritis. Ann Rheum Dis. 2012;71:1329–34.
35. Soriano A, Pazzola G, Boiardi L, et al. Distribution patterns of 18F-fluorodeoxyglucose in large vessels of Takayasu's and giant cell arteritis using positron emission tomography. Clin Exp Rheumatol. 2018;36(Suppl 111):99–106.
36. Albreiki D, Al Belushi F, Patel V, Farmer J. When a temporal artery biopsy reveals a diagnosis other than temporal arteritis: eosinophilic granulomatosis with polyangiitis. Can J Ophthalmol. 2016;51:e108–9.
37. Hamidou MA, Moreau A, Toquet C, El Kouri D, de Faucal P, Grolleau JY. Temporal arteritis associated with systemic necrotizing vasculitis. J Rheumatol. 2003;30:2165–9.
38. Salvarani C, Gabriel SE, Gertz MA, Bjornsson J, Li CY, Hunder GG. Primary systemic amyloidosis presenting as giant cell arteritis and polymyalgia rheumatica. Arthritis Rheum. 1994;37:1621–6.
39. Rucker JC, Biousse V, Newman NJ. Ischemic optic neuropathies. Curr Opin Neurol. 2004;17:27–35.
40. Salvarani C, Hunder GG. Giant cell arteritis with low erythrocyte sedimentation rate: frequency of occurrence in a population-based study. Arthritis Rheum. 2001;45:140–5.
41. Salvarani C, Cantini F, Boiardi L, Hunder GG. Laboratory investigations useful in giant cell arteritis and Takayasu's arteritis. Clin Exp Rheumatol. 2003;21:S23–8.
42. Parikh M, Miller NR, Lee AG, et al. Prevalence of a normal C-reactive protein with an elevated erythrocyte sedimentation rate in biopsy-proven giant cell arteritis. Ophthalmology. 2006;113:1842–5.
43. Kermani TA, Schmidt J, Crowson CS, et al. Utility of erythrocyte sedimentation rate and C-reactive protein for the diagnosis of giant cell arteritis. Semin Arthritis Rheum. 2012;41:866–71.
44. Kyle V. Laboratory investigations including liver in polymyalgia rheumatica/giant cell arteritis. Baillieres Clin Rheumatol. 1991;5:475–84.
45. Foroozan R, Danesh-Meyer H, Savino PJ, Gamble G, Mekari-Sabbagh ON, Sergott RC. Thrombocytosis in patients with biopsy-proven giant cell arteritis. Ophthalmology. 2002;109:1267–71.
46. Michael Small J, Gavrilescu K. The serum protein changes in giant cell arteritis. J Neurol Neurosurg Psychiatry. 1963;26:257–61.
47. Gudmundsson M, Nordborg E, Bengtsson BA, Bjelle A. Plasma viscosity in giant cell arteritis as a predictor of disease activity. Ann Rheum Dis. 1993;52:104–9.
48. Salvarani C, Della BC, Cimino L, et al. Risk factors for severe cranial ischaemic events in an Italian population-based cohort of patients with giant cell arteritis. Rheumatology (Oxford). 2009;48:250–3.
49. Schmidt D, Vaith P. Acute-phase response and the risk of developing ischemic complications in giant cell arteritis: comment on the article by Cid et al. Arthritis Rheum. 2000;43:234–6.
50. Monteagudo M, Vidal G, Andreu J, et al. Giant cell (temporal) arteritis and secondary renal amyloidosis: report of 2 cases. J Rheumatol. 1997;24:605–7.

51. Weyand CM, Goronzy JJ. Medium- and large-vessel vasculitis. N Engl J Med. 2003;349:160–9.
52. Hunder GG. Giant cell arteritis and polymyalgia rheumatica. Med Clin North Am. 1997;81:195–219.
53. Liozon E, Roblot P, Paire D, et al. Anticardiolipin antibody levels predict flares and relapses in patients with giant-cell (temporal) arteritis. A longitudinal study of 58 biopsy-proven cases. Rheumatology (Oxford). 2000;39:1089–94.
54. Manna R, Latteri M, Cristiano G, Todaro L, Scuderi F, Gasbarrini G. Anticardiolipin antibodies in giant cell arteritis and polymyalgia rheumatica: a study of 40 cases. Br J Rheumatol. 1998;37:208–10.
55. Kyle V, Cawston TE, Hazleman BL. Erythrocyte sedimentation rate and C reactive protein in the assessment of polymyalgia rheumatica/giant cell arteritis on presentation and during follow up. Ann Rheum Dis. 1989;48:667–71.

Histopathology and Imaging

Histological Features of Giant Cell Arteritis

Nicolò Pipitone

Abstract

The gold standard to diagnose giant cell arteritis is temporal artery biopsy. The classical histologic picture of GCA is a transmural inflammatory infiltrate comprising lymphocytes, macrophages and, in about 50% of cases, giant cells. However, in some patients the inflammation may be restricted to the adventitial layer, to the vasa vasorum, or to the small vessels that surround the temporal artery.

Imaging techniques play a pivotal role both in the diagnosis and in the follow-up of patients with giant cell arteritis. According to the recommendations by the European League Against Rheumatism, imaging procedures should be the first diagnostic test, while temporal artery biopsy should be performed when imaging findings are not contributory. Color Doppler sonography is the modality of choice to image the temporal arteries: inflamed arteries typically show a positive "halo sign," i.e., a hypoechoic (dark) halo around the temporal artery lumen. Color Doppler sonography can also be used to examine the superficial large vessels and to define whether there are lumen changes such as stenoses or aneurysms. Deep, large vessels such as the aorta are best imaged by computerized tomography or magnetic resonance imaging: signs of vasculitis are increased thickness of the vessel wall with enhancement. ^{18}F-Fluorodeoxyglucose positron emission tomography can also be used to demonstrate arterial inflammation. ^{18}F-Fluorodeoxyglucose positron emission tomography can visualize all large vessels and is very sensitive: a vascular smooth, linear pattern with Fluorodeoxyglucose uptake that affects long segments of the arteries is consistent with vasculitis. Imaging changes tend to improve or resolve the following treatment.

N. Pipitone (✉)

Arcispedale Santa Maria Nuova, Reggio Emilia, Italy

e-mail: pipitone.nicolo@ausl.re.it, nicolo.pipitone@ausl.re.it

© Springer Nature Switzerland AG 2021

C. Salvarani et al. (eds.), *Large and Medium Size Vessel and Single Organ Vasculitis*, Rare Diseases of the Immune System,

https://doi.org/10.1007/978-3-030-67175-4_5

Keywords

Giant cell arteritis · Temporal artery biopsy · Ultrasonography

The gold standard to diagnose GCA is temporal artery biopsy. In clinical practice, temporal artery biopsy may be required when the diagnosis of GCA cannot be secured on the basis of clinical and imaging findings alone. The procedure is safe in experienced hands, carrying a very low rate of complications [1, 2]. It is recommended that an adequate sample of artery be excised in order to avoid to incur in false-negative results. In particular, temporal artery biopsies with post-fixation length shorter than 5 mm carry an increased biopsy-negative rate. In a review, the rate of positive biopsies was only 19% with TAB length of 5 mm or less, but increased to 71–79% with TAB lengths of 6–20 mm, and to 89% when TAB length was longer than 20 mm [3]. Temporal artery biopsy can also be affected by glucocorticoid therapy. In newly diagnosed GCA patients treated with high-dose glucocorticoids, temporal artery biopsy is positive in 78% of patients treated for less than 2 weeks, in 65% of those treated for 2–4 weeks, but only in 40% of those treated for longer than 4 weeks [4]. Therefore, while glucocorticoid therapy should not be delayed if there is a strong clinical suspicion of GCA, temporal artery biopsy may safely be performed up to 2 weeks following the institution of treatment. Temporal artery biopsy may also be falsely negative because of sampling error, when an unaffected segment of the artery is excised, because the arteritic lesions of GCA are segmental [5]. This risk may be circumvented by obtaining an arterial sample of adequate length and performing multiple cuts of the histologic specimen. Finally, in some patients with GCA, the temporal arteries may be truly spared; this holds especially for patients with involvement of the aorta and its major branches and accounts for the lower positivity rate of temporal artery biopsy in this patients' group [6].

In an attempt to increase the sensitivity of temporal artery biopsy, Color Doppler sonography-guided biopsy has been investigated in a study on 112 patients with suspected GCA. Fifty patients were randomized to undergo Color Doppler sonography-guided temporal artery biopsy and 55 patients to standard biopsy. No differences in the rate of positive biopsies were found between the two groups, suggesting that Color Doppler sonography-guided temporal artery biopsy does not increase the positive yield of biopsy [7].

The classical histologic picture of GCA is a transmural inflammatory infiltrate comprising lymphocytes, macrophages and, in about 50% of cases, giant cells [8] (Fig. 5.1). The lesion is often characterized by a thicker inflammatory band that surrounds the external elastic lamina and a thinner band along the internal elastic lamina [8]. The media is often relatively spared, but in particularly severe cases it may be damaged by the inflammatory process. Neoangiogenesis is a frequent accompanying feature. Another frequent feature is thickening of the intimal layer, which shows a proliferation of myofibroblasts that lead to stenosis or sometimes occlusion of the vessel lumen; however, intraluminal thrombosis is rare [8].

While transmural inflammatory infiltrate is the most common pattern observed at temporal artery biopsy, in some patients the inflammation may be restricted to the

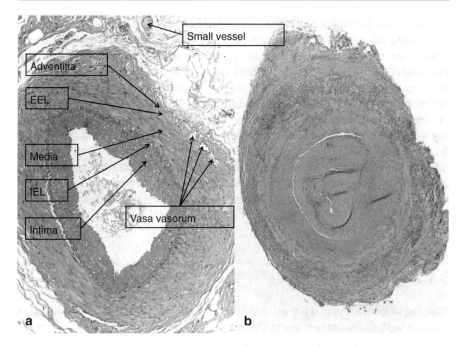

Fig. 5.1 (a) Uninflamed temporal artery. An internal elastic lamina (IEL) and a less-evident external elastic lamina (EEL) separate intima from media and media from adventitia, respectively. Vasa vasorum are localized within adventitia, whereas in the periadventitial tissues there are small vessels devoid of muscular coat. Hematoxylin-Eosin, 40×. (b) A classical example of transmural inflammation, with two concentric bands of inflammation, the thickest along the external elastic lamina and the thinner along the internal elastic lamina, with a relative sparing of the interposed media ("concentric rings" appearance). Hematoxylin-Eosin, 20×. Images courtesy of Dr. Alberto Cavazza, Pathology Department, Arcispedale S. M. Nuova, Reggio Emilia

adventitial layer (7% of all cases), to the vasa vasorum (6.5% of all cases), or to the small vessels that surround the temporal artery (9% of all cases) [8]. Purely adventitial inflammation is characterized by a perivascular inflammatory infiltrate with sparing of the media, while vasculitis of the vasa vasorum shows inflammation limited to the adventitial vessels and small vessel vasculitis shows inflammatory changes restricted to the small periadventitial vessels, which have no muscular coat [8].

The histological patterns of temporal artery biopsy in GCA have also clinical correlates. Specifically, patients with small vessel and vasa vasorum vasculitis, compared to those with transmural inflammation, have a significantly lower frequency of cranial manifestations, including headache, jaw claudication, and abnormalities of the temporal arteries at physical examination; they are also less likely to have a positive ultrasonography (i.e., a positive "halo sign") at ultrasonography [8]. However, polymyalgia rheumatic and visual loss are equally represented in the different subsets, suggesting that limited inflammation does not portend per se a more benign prognosis [8].

When no inflammatory infiltrate is detectable at temporal artery biopsy, there are no histological features that are specific to GCA, including focal mediointimal scar, medial attenuation, intimal hyperplasia, fragmentation of inner elastic lamina, calcification, adventitial fibrosis, and neoangiogenesis [9]. In contrast, a high temporal artery expression of phosphorylated ezrin/radixin/moesin (pERM), a downstream target and surrogate of rho kinase (an intracellular GTPase that regulates several cell processes activated in GCA) has been found in 86% of patients with GCA (including 94% of those with a negative temporal artery biopsy), but only 44% of unaffected controls, suggesting that rho kinase activity is increased in the temporal arteries of GCA patients irrespective of the presence of standard inflammatory changes [10]. Therefore, an increased rho kinase activity at temporal artery biopsy could be useful as a diagnostic marker of GCA. However, this test had also a high frequency of false-positive findings; in addition, it is not available in clinical practice.

5.1　Imaging

Imaging techniques play a pivotal role both in the diagnosis and in the follow-up of patients with GCA. According to the recommendations by the European League Against Rheumatism, imaging procedures should be the first diagnostic "pit stop," while temporal artery biopsy should be performed when imaging findings are not contributory to a diagnosis of GCA [11]. Imaging is the preferred first test because is more cost-effective than temporal artery biopsy and can probe more arteries than biopsy. Since glucocorticoids can cause false-negative imaging findings, it is recommended that imaging be performed as early as possible, within 1 week from symptoms' onset [11]. Both the temporal arteries and the large vessels (the aorta and its major branches) can be imaged [12].

5.2　Temporal Artery Imaging

Color Doppler sonography is the modality of choice to image the temporal arteries in GCA because of its widespread availability, its good visualization of the temporal arteries (with a tenfold higher resolution compared to magnetic resonance) and lack of exposure to ionizing radiation. High-frequency linear probes (18–22 MHz) are best suited to assess the temporal arteries [13]. The classic sign of Color Doppler sonography inflammation of the temporal arteries is the "halo sign," a hypoechoic (dark) halo around the temporal artery lumen, which is visible on both transverse and longitudinal views. In contrast, stenoses and occlusions are less specific to GCA [14] (Fig. 5.2). According to a recent meta-analysis, the "halo sign" has a sensitivity of 68% and a specificity of 81% for the diagnosis of GCA [15]; its specificity approaches 100% when the halo is bilateral [16]. A positive halo sign can be confirmed by a positive "compression test" (pressing with the sonographic probe against an inflamed temporal artery does not collapse it, unlike what happens in a

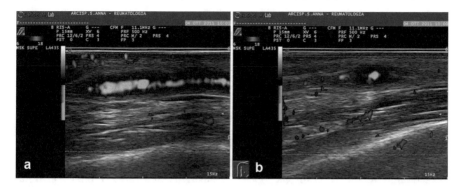

Fig. 5.2 (**a**) Longitudinal view of an inflamed common superficial temporal artery with the hypoechoic wall swelling. (**b**) Transverse view of an inflamed common superficial temporal artery with the hypoechoic wall swelling. Images courtesy of Dr. Giuseppe Germanò, Rheumatology Department, Arcispedale S. M. Nuova, Reggio Emilia

normal artery) [17]. The compression test is very easy to perform, even in the absence of a specific expertise in vascular ultrasonography, and shows an excellent inter-observer agreement [18].

The halo sign usually disappears fairly quickly following the institution of glucocorticoid therapy. In a study, temporal artery Color Doppler sonography performed 0–1 days after onset of glucocorticoid therapy demonstrated 92% sensitivity and 57% specificity for GCA, whereas when Color Doppler sonography was performed over 4 days after onset of GC therapy sensitivity and specificity dropped to 50% and 25%, respectively [19].

1.5 T to 3 T-enhanced magnetic resonance imaging (MRI) is also able to visualize the inflammation in the temporal arteries with roughly the same sensitivity and specificity as Color Doppler sonography [20]. The typical MRI sign of temporal artery inflammation is edema of the vessel wall around the lumen [20]. In contrast, 1 T MRI, although equally specific, is much less sensitive (only 28%) to detect temporal artery inflammation [21]. Similarly to Color Doppler sonography, MRI findings can be affected by glucocorticoid therapy, which leads over time to an attenuation of the mural inflammatory signal and eventually to its disappearance [22].

Neither computerized tomography nor 18F-Fluorodeoxyglucose positron emission tomography have a role in assessing temporal artery inflammation [12].

5.3 Large-Vessel Imaging

There are several imaging modalities that are able to visualize the large arteries. Traditionally, digital subtraction angiography was used to detect large-vessel changes such as stenoses, occlusions, dilation, and aneurysms. However, digital subtraction angiography is unable to depict the arterial wall inflammatory thickening that occurs early on in GCA, before lumen changes occur. For this reason, digital subtraction angiography is not suited to make an early diagnosis of large-vessel arteritis although it may still have a role in guiding interventional procedures such as stenting [12].

Color Doppler sonography can show arterial wall thickening with a halo sign in the inflamed arteries [13]. Color Doppler sonography lends itself particularly well to depict the superficial epiaortic vessels, where its power of resolution is ten times higher than that of MRI. In contrast, Color-Doppler sonography is unable to visualize the thoracic aorta, which is covered by the breast bone, and performs also unsatisfactorily in showing inflammatory changes of the abdominal aorta [12]. Color Doppler sonography has a role as a first-line screening test in patients with suspected large-vessel GCA. In this contest, a sensitivity of 30% [21] to 54% [23] has been reported. However, Color Doppler sonography is less sensitive than 18F-Fluorodeoxyglucose positron emission tomography for the diagnosis of large-vessel GCA. In a study comparing Color Doppler sonography with 18F-Fluorodeoxyglucose positron emission tomography, Color Doppler sonography was able to detect large-vessel involvement in 80% of patients who had large-vessel vasculitis diagnosed according to 18F-Fluorodeoxyglucose positron emission tomography, which was the gold standard [24]. Especially, aortic involvement was often missed by Color Doppler sonography compared with 18F-Fluorodeoxyglucose positron emission tomography.

To study the deep, large vessels such as the thoracic and abdominal aorta computerized tomography (Fig. 5.3) and MRI (or ^{18}F-Fluorodeoxyglucose positron emission tomography) (Fig. 5.4) should be used. Early signs of arterial inflammation are vessel wall thickening and edema, which are best appreciated on contrast-enhanced sequences [12]. T2-weighted MRI sequences may also show arterial wall edema, but they are less sensitive than post-contrast T1 views, which should thus preferentially be used [25]. Computerized tomography angiography and magnetic resonance angiography can be performed together with computerized tomography

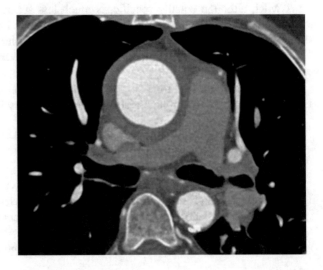

Fig. 5.3 CTA, axial view of the ascending aorta with arterial wall thickening. Image courtesy of Dr. Lucia Spaggiari, Radiology Department, Arcispedale S. M. Nuova, Reggio Emilia

Fig. 5.4 PET coronal view showing increased (grade 3 on a 0–3 scale) 18F-FDG uptake by the thoracic and abdominal aorta as well as by the subclavian and the right common carotid and axillary arteries in a patient with GCA involving large vessels. Image courtesy of Dr. Massimiliano Casali, Nuclear Medicine Department, Arcispedale S. M. Nuova, Reggio Emilia

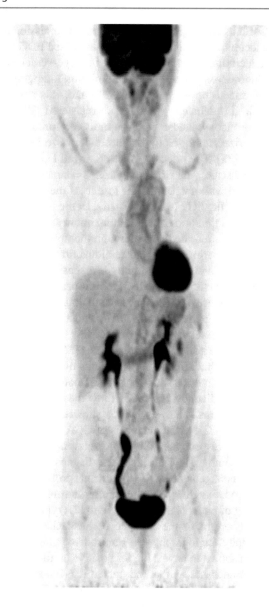

and MRI, respectively, to gain information on vessel lumen changes [12, 26]. The usefulness of computerized tomography angiography in diagnosing large-vessel GCA has been demonstrated by a study in which CTA was able to detect large-vessel involvement in 27 out of 40 patients, with the aorta (65% of patients), the brachiocephalic trunk (48%), the carotid arteries (35%), and the subclavian arteries (43%) being mainly involved [27]. Treatment-naïve patients had a higher frequency of large-vessel vasculitis (77% versus 29%), well in keeping with the notion that glucocorticoids significantly affect the sensitivity of imaging techniques.

[18]F-Fluorodeoxyglucose (FDG) positron emission tomography is a nuclear medicine technique that is able to reveal increased FDG uptake by metabolically active cells, including arterial wall cells in large-vessel vasculitis [12, 28]. Currently, ^{18}F-Fluorodeoxyglucose positron emission tomography is often co-registered with computerized tomography (PET/CT) and, less commonly, with MRI (PET/MRI) [29]. It is debated whether co-registered PET may have an edge over ^{18}F-Fluorodeoxyglucose positron emission tomography alone [30]; in this regard, computerized tomography has been shown to be useful in determining the aortic diameter [31]. The intensity of arterial wall FGD uptake is often expressed using a 0–3 visual scale, where 0 = no uptake, 1 = some uptake but less than that of the liver, 2 = arterial wall uptake similar to that of the liver, and 3 = arterial uptake greater than that of the liver [32]. Alternatively, the intensity of arterial wall uptake can be expressed as the ratio of arterial maximum standard uptake value to that of a reference organ (often the liver) although the optimal cut-off remains debated [33–35]. A study comparing visual and semiquantitative scoring methods demonstrated that visual methods were only slightly less sensitive and more specific than semiquantitative methods [35]. Currently, the European Association of Nuclear Medicine recommends the use of the visual scale to diagnose large-vessel vasculitis. In untreated patients, PET grades 2 and 3 are considered consistent with possibly positive and active large-vessel vasculitis, respectively [34], whereas grade 1 uptake in untreated patients can be a sign of atherosclerosis [36]. A vascular smooth, linear pattern with FDG uptake that affects long segments of the arteries is consistent with vasculitis [37]. A meta-analysis showed that PET had a sensitivity of 90% and a specificity of 98% for the diagnosis of GCA [38]; these results were basically replicated by a more recent meta-analysis, which showed a pooled sensitivity and specificity of PET or PET/CT for the diagnosis of GCA of 83% (95% CI 72–91) and 90% (95% CI 80–96), respectively [39]. The relevance of ^{18}F-Fluorodeoxyglucose positron emission tomography increases the diagnostic accuracy and has an impact on the clinical management in a significant proportion of patients with GCA [40]. ^{18}F-Fluorodeoxyglucose positron emission tomography is particularly valuable in the subset of patients that present with less typical clinical features, such as fever of unknown origin in the absence of headache [6]. Compared with computerized tomography angiography, ^{18}F-Fluorodeoxyglucose positron emission tomography has been shown to have a higher positive predictive value for the diagnosis of GCA [41]; another study that compared ^{18}F-Fluorodeoxyglucose positron emission tomography with magnetic resonance angiography demonstrated that 18F-Fluorodeoxyglucose positron emission tomography was better suited to assess disease activity, while magnetic resonance angiography better captured disease extent [42].

Both false-positive and false-negative findings may occur with imaging techniques. Atherosclerosis is the most common cause of false-positive findings (vessel wall thickening on morphological imaging and increased ^{18}F-Fluorodeoxyglucose vascular uptake with ^{18}F-Fluorodeoxyglucose positron emission tomography). However, changes due to atherosclerosis can usually be distinguished from those due to vasculitis because the former are characterized by eccentric, asymmetrical vessel wall thickening, compared to the smooth involvement of long arterial segments observed in vasculitis [12].

False-negative imaging findings are often observed in patients who are on glucocorticoid therapy. Sometimes even a few days of treatment, a marked drop in sensitivity is observed; this holds for virtually any imaging technique [19, 40].

Imaging techniques have only a limited predictive role for the development of new arterial lesions. In a study on 24 patients with large-vessel vasculitis investigated by MRI, six of sixteen patients had no disease progression despite persistent vessel wall edema, while three patients developed new lesions at sites without vessel wall edema [43]. Regarding ^{18}F-Fluorodeoxyglucose positron emission tomography, in a study baseline vascular 18F-Fluorodeoxyglucose uptake did not correlate with the risk of subsequent relapses [44], whereas uptake in the thoracic aortic was only weakly associated with the risk of developing thoracic aortic aneurysms compared to patients without uptake [45]. Another study confirmed that increased vascular 18F-Fluorodeoxyglucose uptake was a risk factor for the subsequent development of aortic complications [46].

Inconsistent correlations have been reported between imaging findings and laboratory and clinical indices of disease activity [37, 42].

Serial imaging studies are indicated in patients with arterial lesions at baseline. A recent study on 187 patients with GCA demonstrated arterial changes on imaging in 66% patients at the first exam. New abnormalities were observed in 33% patients by year 2; clinical features of active disease were present at only 50% of these cases, suggesting that imaging procedures should be performed even in patients with apparently clinically quiescent disease [47]. On morphological imaging, arterial wall thickening regresses to a variable degree, but such regression is significantly less common in the large vessels than in the temporal arteries [48].

References

1. Salvarani C, Cantini F, Hunder GG. Polymyalgia rheumatica and giant-cell arteritis. Lancet. 2008;372:234–45.
2. Salvarani C, Cantini F, Boiardi L, Hunder GG. Polymyalgia rheumatica and giant-cell arteritis. N Engl J Med. 2002;347:261–71.
3. Breuer GS, Nesher R, Nesher G. Effect of biopsy length on the rate of positive temporal artery biopsies. Clin Exp Rheumatol. 2009;27:S10–3.
4. Narvaez J, Bernad B, Roig-Vilaseca D, et al. Influence of previous corticosteroid therapy on temporal artery biopsy yield in giant cell arteritis. Semin Arthritis Rheum. 2007;37:13–9.
5. Klein RG, Campbell RJ, Hunder GG, Carney JA. Skip lesions in temporal arteritis. Mayo Clin Proc. 1976;51:504–10.
6. Brack A, Martinez-Taboada V, Stanson A, Goronzy JJ, Weyand CM. Disease pattern in cranial and large-vessel giant cell arteritis. Arthritis Rheum. 1999;42:311–7.
7. Giuseppe G, Francesco M, Luca C, et al. Is colour duplex sonography-guided temporal artery biopsy useful in the diagnosis of giant cell arteritis? A randomized study. Rheumatol. (Oxford). 2015;54(3):400–4.
8. Cavazza A, Muratore F, Boiardi L, et al. Inflamed temporal artery: histologic findings in 354 biopsies, with clinical correlations. Am J Surg Pathol. 2014;38:1360–70.

9. Muratore F, Cavazza A, Boiardi L, et al. Histopathologic findings of patients with biopsy-negative giant cell arteritis compared to those without arteritis: a population-based study. Arthritis Care Res (Hoboken). 2016;68:865–70.

10. Lally L, Pernis A, Narula N, Huang WT, Spiera R. Increased rho kinase activity in temporal artery biopsies from patients with giant cell arteritis. Rheumatology (Oxford). 2015;54:554–8.

11. Dejaco C, Ramiro S, Duftner C, et al. EULAR recommendations for the use of imaging in large vessel vasculitis in clinical practice. Ann Rheum Dis. 2018;77:636–43.

12. Pipitone N, Versari A, Salvarani C. Role of imaging studies in the diagnosis and follow-up of large-vessel vasculitis: an update. Rheumatology (Oxford). 2008;47:403–8.

13. Germano G, Monti S, Ponte C, et al. The role of ultrasound in the diagnosis and follow-up of large-vessel vasculitis: an update. Clin Exp Rheumatol. 2017;35(Suppl 103):194–8.

14. Schmidt WA, Kraft HE, Vorpahl K, Volker L, Gromnica-Ihle EJ. Color duplex ultrasonography in the diagnosis of temporal arteritis. N Engl J Med. 1997;337:1336–42.

15. Rinagel M, Chatelus E, Jousse-Joulin S, et al. Diagnostic performance of temporal artery ultrasound for the diagnosis of giant cell arteritis: a systematic review and meta-analysis of the literature. Autoimmun Rev. 2019;18:56–61.

16. Arida A, Kyprianou M, Kanakis M, Sfikakis PP. The diagnostic value of ultrasonography-derived edema of the temporal artery wall in giant cell arteritis: a second meta-analysis. BMC Musculoskelet Disord. 2010;11:44.

17. Aschwanden M, Daikeler T, Kesten F, et al. Temporal artery compression sign—a novel ultrasound finding for the diagnosis of giant cell arteritis. Ultraschall Med. 2013;34:47–50.

18. Aschwanden M, Imfeld S, Staub D, et al. The ultrasound compression sign to diagnose temporal giant cell arteritis shows an excellent interobserver agreement. Clin Exp Rheumatol. 2015;33:S113–5.

19. Hauenstein C, Reinhard M, Geiger J, et al. Effects of early corticosteroid treatment on magnetic resonance imaging and ultrasonography findings in giant cell arteritis. Rheumatology (Oxford). 2012;51:1999–2003.

20. Bley TA, Uhl M, Carew J, et al. Diagnostic value of high-resolution MR imaging in giant cell arteritis. AJNR Am J Neuroradiol. 2007;28:1722–7.

21. Ghinoi A, Zuccoli G, Nicolini A, et al. 1T magnetic resonance imaging in the diagnosis of giant cell arteritis: comparison with ultrasonography and physical examination of temporal arteries. Clin Exp Rheumatol. 2008;26:S76–80.

22. Bley TA, Ness T, Warnatz K, et al. Influence of corticosteroid treatment on MRI findings in giant cell arteritis. Clin Rheumatol. 2007;26:1541–3.

23. Czihal M, Zanker S, Rademacher A, et al. Sonographic and clinical pattern of extracranial and cranial giant cell arteritis. Scand J Rheumatol. 2012;41:231–6.

24. Loffler C, Hoffend J, Benck U, Kramer BK, Bergner R. The value of ultrasound in diagnosing extracranial large-vessel vasculitis compared to FDG-PET/CT: a retrospective study. Clin Rheumatol. 2017;36:2079–86.

25. Geiger J, Bley T, Uhl M, Frydrychowicz A, Langer M, Markl M. Diagnostic value of T2-weighted imaging for the detection of superficial cranial artery inflammation in giant cell arteritis. J Magn Reson Imaging. 2010;31:470–4.

26. Gotway MB, Araoz PA, Macedo TA, et al. Imaging findings in Takayasu's arteritis. AJR Am J Roentgenol. 2005;184:1945–50.

27. Prieto-Gonzalez S, Arguis P, Garcia-Martinez A, et al. Large vessel involvement in biopsy-proven giant cell arteritis: prospective study in 40 newly diagnosed patients using CT angiography. Ann Rheum Dis. 2012;71:1170–6.

28. Pipitone NAM, Versari A, Salvarani C. Usefulness of PET in recognizing and managing vasculitides. Curr Opin Rheumatol. 2018;30:24–9.

29. Einspieler I, Thurmel K, Pyka T, et al. Imaging large vessel vasculitis with fully integrated PET/MRI: a pilot study. Eur J Nucl Med Mol Imaging. 2015;42:1012–24.

30. Balink H, Houtman PM, Collins J. 18F-FDG PET versus PET/CT as a diagnostic procedure for clinical suspicion of large vessel vasculitis. Clin Rheumatol. 2011;30:1139–41.

31. Muratore F, Crescentini F, Spaggiari L, et al. Aortic dilatation in patients with large vessel vasculitis: a longitudinal case control study using PET/CT. Semin Arthritis Rheum. 2019;48:1074–82.
32. Meller J, Strutz F, Siefker U, et al. Early diagnosis and follow-up of aortitis with [(18)F]FDG PET and MRI. Eur J Nucl Med Mol Imaging. 2003;30:730–6.
33. Hautzel H, Sander O, Heinzel A, Schneider M, Muller HW. Assessment of large-vessel involvement in giant cell arteritis with 18F-FDG PET: introducing an ROC-analysis-based cutoff ratio. J Nucl Med. 2008;49:1107–13.
34. Slart RHJA. FDG-PET/CT(A) imaging in large vessel vasculitis and polymyalgia rheumatica: joint procedural recommendation of the EANM, SNMMI, and the PET Interest Group (PIG), and endorsed by the ASNC. Eur J Nucl Med Mol Imaging. 2018;45:1250–69.
35. Castellani M, Vadrucci M, Florimonte L, Caronni M, Benti R, Bonara P. 18F-FDG uptake in main arterial branches of patients with large vessel vasculitis: visual and semiquantitative analysis. Ann Nucl Med. 2016;30:409–20.
36. Belhocine T, Blockmans D, Hustinx R, Vandevivere J, Mortelmans L. Imaging of large vessel vasculitis with (18)FDG PET: illusion or reality? A critical review of the literature data. Eur J Nucl Med Mol Imaging. 2003;30:1305–13.
37. Besson FL, Parienti JJ, Bienvenu B, et al. Diagnostic performance of (1)(8) F-fluorodeoxyglucose positron emission tomography in giant cell arteritis: a systematic review and meta-analysis. Eur J Nucl Med Mol Imaging. 2011;38:1764–72.
38. Soussan M, Nicolas P, Schramm C, et al. Management of large-vessel vasculitis with FDG-PET: a systematic literature review and meta-analysis. Medicine (Baltimore). 2015;94:e622.
39. Lee YH, Choi SJ, Ji JD, Song GG. Diagnostic accuracy of 18F-FDG PET or PET/CT for large vessel vasculitis: a meta-analysis. Z Rheumatol. 2016;75:924–31.
40. Fuchs M, Briel M, Daikeler T, et al. The impact of 18F-FDG PET on the management of patients with suspected large vessel vasculitis. Eur J Nucl Med Mol Imaging. 2012;39:344–53.
41. Lariviere D, Benali K, Coustet B, et al. Positron emission tomography and computed tomography angiography for the diagnosis of giant cell arteritis: a real-life prospective study. Medicine (Baltimore). 2016;95:e4146.
42. Quinn KA, Ahlman MA, Malayeri AA, et al. Comparison of magnetic resonance angiography and (18)F-fluorodeoxyglucose positron emission tomography in large-vessel vasculitis. Ann Rheum Dis. 2018;77:1165–71.
43. Tso E, Flamm SD, White RD, Schvartzman PR, Mascha E, Hoffman GS. Takayasu arteritis: utility and limitations of magnetic resonance imaging in diagnosis and treatment. Arthritis Rheum. 2002;46:1634–42.
44. Blockmans D, De Ceuninck L, Vanderschueren S, Knockaert D, Mortelmans L, Bobbaers H. Repetitive 18F-fluorodeoxyglucose positron emission tomography in giant cell arteritis: a prospective study of 35 patients. Arthritis Rheum. 2006;55:131–7.
45. Blockmans D, Coudyzer W, Vanderschueren S, et al. Relationship between fluorodeoxyglucose uptake in the large vessels and late aortic diameter in giant cell arteritis. Rheumatology (Oxford). 2008;47:1179–84.
46. de Boysson H, Liozon E, Lambert M, et al. 18F-fluorodeoxyglucose positron emission tomography and the risk of subsequent aortic complications in giant-cell arteritis: a multicenter cohort of 130 patients. Medicine (Baltimore). 2016;95:e3851.
47. Kermani TA, Diab S, Sreih AG, et al. Arterial lesions in giant cell arteritis: a longitudinal study. Semin Arthritis Rheum. 2019;48:707–13.
48. Aschwanden M, Schegk E, Imfeld S, et al. Vessel wall plasticity in large vessel giant cell arteritis: an ultrasound follow-up study. Rheumatology (Oxford). 2019;58(5):792–7.

Prognosis and Disease Activity

6

Michael Schirmer and Rick McCutchan

Abstract

Current evidence suggests that overall mortality is not increased in giant cell arteritis (GCA) although cardiovascular complications and comorbidities are more frequent than in the general population. This chapter gives an overview on current evidence of prognostic risks and biomarkers in GCA, including clinical, laboratory, and imaging markers, together with some future perspectives.

Keywords

Biomarker · Comorbidities · Mortality · Prognosis · Vasculitis

Current evidence suggests that overall mortality is not increased in giant cell arteritis (GCA) [1] although cardiovascular (CV) complications and comorbidities are more frequent than in the general population (Tables 6.1 and 6.2).

This chapter gives an overview on current evidence of prognostic risks and biomarkers in GCA, including clinical, laboratory, and imaging markers, together with some future perspectives.

6.1 Risk for Complications and Comorbidities During Disease Course

Overviews on the risk of CV complications and other comorbidities are given in Tables 6.1 and 6.2. In summary, GCA implies an about twofold increased risk for CV disease [2–4], especially for aortic aneurysm, stroke, myocardial infarction, and

M. Schirmer (✉) · R. McCutchan
Medical University of Innsbruck, Internal Medicine II, Innsbruck, Austria
e-mail: michael.schirmer@i-med.ac.at

© Springer Nature Switzerland AG 2021
C. Salvarani et al. (eds.), *Large and Medium Size Vessel and Single Organ Vasculitis*, Rare Diseases of the Immune System,
https://doi.org/10.1007/978-3-030-67175-4_6

Table 6.1 Risks of increased cardiovascular complications in GCA patients compared to general population (Ranges given in brackets indicate 95% confidence intervals). Studies were excluded if not significant or already included in meta-analyses (marked as MA). *CerV* cerebrovascular, *CI* 95% confidence interval, *CIC* cranial ischemic complication, *HR* hazard ratio, *RaR* rate ratio, *MA* meta-analysis, *RiR* risk ratio, *RR* relative risk, *SHR* subhazard ratio

CV complications and comorbidities	Risk vs. general population	Ref.
CV disease	HR 1.49 (1.37–1.62)	[2]
	HR 2.01 (1.62–2.48)[a]	[3]
	HR 3.00 (1.78–5.13)	[4]
Arterial hypertension	RaR 1.31 (1.17–1.46)	[7]
	OR 1.12 (1.03–1.21)	[8]
	HR 1.24 (1.17–1.32)	[9]
Atherosclerosis	RR 1.44 (1.00–2.07)	[9]
	HR 3.70 (1.49–9.44)	[4]
• Aortic aneurysm	HR 1.98 (1.50–2.62)	[9]
	SHR 1.92 (1.52–2.41)	[10]
• CerV accident: Stroke, CIC	HR 1.40 (1.27–1.56)	MA [11]
	RaR 1.40 (1.12–1.74)	[7]
	HR stroke + TIA 1.41 (1.29–1.55)	[9]
• Coronary artery disease	RiR 1.51 (0.88–2.61)	MA [12]
	HR 4.9 (1.52–15.77)	[4]
	OR 1.25 (1.15–1.36)	[8]
	HR 1.37 (1.18–1.59)	[9]
• Pericarditis	OR 1.69 (1.16–2.14)	[13]
• Myocardial infarction	HR 1.57 (1.36–1.82)	[9]
• Angina pectoris	HR 1.77 (1.29–2.43)	[14]
• Heart failure	HR 1.94 (1.39–2.70)[a]	[3]
• Atrial fibrillation	HR 1.36 (1.17–1.58)	[9]
	RR 2.40 (1.74–3.32)	[15]
	HR 1.46 (1.29–1.65)	[9]
	HR 1.29 (1.19–1.39)	[9]
• Peripheral vascular disease	HR 1.88 (1.04–3.41)	MA [16]
	HR 1.75 (1.49–2.06)	[9]
Venous thromboembolic events		
• Venous thromboembolism	HR 2.26 (1.38–3.71)	MA [17]
	HR 2.49 (1.45–4.30)	[18]
	HR 2.03 (1.77–2.33)	[9]
	RR 2.06 (1.75–2.44)	[19]
• Deep venous thrombosis	HR 2.70 (1.39–5.54)	[18]
	HR 1.96 (1.57–2.46)	[19]
	HR 2.50 (1.62–3.85)	[15]
• Pulmonary embolism	HR 2.71 (1.32–5.56)	[18]
	RR 2.25 (1.78–2.85)	[19]

[a]Adjusted for age and sex

peripheral vascular disease (Table 6.1). Similarly, the prevalence of venous thromboembolic events is increased in GCA patients by about twofold (Table 6.1) although antiphospholipid syndrome and GCA appear to be different and independent diseases [5]. The use of an immunosuppressant can be considered as a protective factor

Table 6.2 Summary on risks for non-cardiovascular comorbidities in GCA (ordered according to amount of risk compared to general population, with highest risk rated on top). The risk of diabetes was excluded, as recent data are contradictive [9, 15, 20]. Ranges in brackets indicate 95% confidence interval; *HR* hazard ratio, *MA* meta-analysis, *OR* odds ratio, *RaR* rate ratio, *RiR* risk ratio, *RR* relative risk, *SHR* subhazard ratio

Complication and comorbidity	Risk vs. general population	Ref.
Osteoporosis	RR 2.90 (2.35–3.66)	[15]
• Fractures	RaR 2.81 (2.33–3.37)	[7]
	RaR 1.56 (1.31–1.85)	[7]
Gastritis and duodenitis	RR 2.40 (1.39–4.29)	[15]
Thyroid disease	RaR 1.55 (1.25–1.91)	[7]
• Hypothyroidism	OR 1.30 (1.19–1.42)	[21]
Renal disease, moderate to severe	HR 1.32 (1.25–1.39)	[9]
Psychiatric disease	RaR 1.28 (1.12–1.46)	[7]
• Depression	HR 1.37 (1.26–1.49)	[9]
Dyslipidemia	HR 1.26 (1.15–1.37)	[9]
Obesity	HR 1.23 (1.14–1.32)	[9]
Malignancy	RiR overall 1.14 (1.05–1.22)	MA [22]

against new cardiovascular events, suggesting an effect against vascular inflammation that may favor the new vascular events in GCA [6].

Out of the other non-CV comorbidities, osteoporosis and gastritis are the most important risks of GCA patients (Table 6.2). Both these diseases depend on the use of glucocorticoids (GCs), which is still the first-line treatment for GCA. As a consequence, these diseases have to be routinely considered for monitoring and possible adjunctive treatment during follow-up.

In conclusion, GCA is not only affecting the risk for arterial but also for venous events, and both of them have to be monitored during disease course. Also, non-CV comorbidities should be monitored, especially for osteoporosis and gastritis. As all of the risks for CV and other morbidities mentioned above maybe clinically relevant, they should be included into the information for GCA patients and their carers, both at diagnosis and regularly during follow-up.

6.2 Risk Factors and Biomarkers for Disease Activity in Giant Cell Arteritis

Until today, a single sensitive prognostic clinical parameter or (composite) score to assess disease activity during the course of both cranial GCA and the extracranial large vessel type of GCA is not available. Prognostic risk factors, both the risk factors with increased and those with reduced risk for disease activity and CV complications are separately listed in Tables 6.3 and 6.4. The aim of these tables is to increase the awareness for improved patients' information especially for the factors with increased prognostic risk.

Table 6.3 Summary of prognostic factors for increased disease activity and cardiovascular complications in GCA (with 95% confidence intervals given in brackets). *Aaneurysm* aortic aneurysm, *Adilatation* aortic dilatation, *CHADS2* score of congestive heart failure, age > 75 years, diabetes, stroke, *CIC* cranial ischemic complication, *CRP* C-reactive protein, *CV* cardiovascular, *CEV* cerebrovascular, *DAA* dissection of AA, *ESR* erythrocyte sedimentation rate, *Hb* hemoglobin, *IHD* ischemic heart disease, *Ievent* ischemic event, *RF* risk factor, *LVI* large vessel involvement, *OR* Odds ratio, *pts.* patients, *vs.* versus, *SHR* subhazard ratio

Prognostic factors	Effect on course of GCA	Ref.
Patients' characteristics		
Age	HR malignancy 2.68 (1.87–3.84)	[29]
• <85 years	HR CV event (hospitalization) 5.0	[30]
• >77 years	(1.40–17.54)	[4]
Male gender	OR IHD 2.546 (2.316–2.799)	[8]
	SHR Aaneurysm 2.10 (1.38–3.19)	[10]
Body mass index (1 kg/m² increment)	OR IHD 1.011 (1.003–1.018)	[8]
Disease characteristics		
Large vessel involvement		
• Symptomatic limb involvement	HR CV complication 5.73 (2.94–11.28)	[31]
• Jaw claudication	OR permanent vision loss 2.11 (1.09–4.10)	[30]
CHADS2-score [32]	OR permanent vision loss 10.72 (1.23–93.8)	[33]
• =1	OR permanent vision loss 24.78	[33]
• ≥2	(2.87–213.86)	
Laboratory parameters	OR permanent vision loss 3.1 (1.02–10.14)	[33]
• Thrombocytosis	HR Aaneurysm 3.71 (1.50–9.19)	[34]
• ESR >100 mm/h, Hb <11 g/dL or platelet count >450,000/mm³		
Imaging findings		
• Inflammation of aorta ± branches	HR CV event 3.42 (2.09–5.83)	[6]
• Large-artery stenosis at diagnosis	HR Adilatation 9.30 (3.74–31.05)	[6]
	HR new IE 1.86 (1.01–3.59)	[6]
	HR CV event 2.75 (1.80–4.15)	[6]
	HR new Ievent 6.08 (3.44–10.87)	[6]
Exposition and other risk factors		
Smoking status:	SHR Aaneurysm 2.20 (1.22–3.98)	[10]
• Ex-smoker	OR pericarditis: 1.55 (1.05–2.27)	[13]
• Current smoker	SHR Aaneurysm 3.79 (2.20–6.53)	[10]
	OR IHD 1.493 (1.363–1.635)	[8]
Prior antihypertensive treatment	SHR Aaneurysm 1.62 (1.00–2.61)	[10]
Use of beta blockers	OR CEV Ievent 4.35 (CI, 1.33–14.2)	[35]
Comorbidities	OR IHD 1.665 (CI 1.530–1.812)	[8]
• Diabetes mellitus	HR CV event 2.03 (CI 1.14–3.41)	[6]
• Arterial hypertension	HR new Ievent 3.61 (1.70–7.17)	[6]
• Hyperlipidemia	HR eye symptoms 1.29 (1.10–1.53)	[36]
• CV comorbidities	OR IHD 3.025 (2.700–3.394)	[8]
	HR eye symptoms 1.17 (1.03–1.32)	[34]
	HR Aaneurysm 4.73 (1.87–11.9)	[36]
	OR IHD 3.830 (3.291–4.478)	[8]
	HR CV event 6.20 (2.00–19.24)	[4]
• Previous coronary artery disease	HR new Ievent 5.10 (2.02–11.21)	[6]

Table 6.4 Summary of positive prognostic factors, indicative for a decreased disease activity and cardiovascular complications in GCA (with 95% confidence intervals given in brackets). *Aaneurysm* aortic aneurysm, *CI* 95% confidence interval, *CIC* cranial ischemic complication, *CV* cardiovascular, *CEV* cerebrovascular, *DAA* dissection of Aaneurysm, *HR* hazard ratio, *Ievent* ischemic event, *OR* Odds ratio, *SHR* subhazard ratio

Prognostic factors	Effect on course of GCA	Ref.
Patients' demographics		
Age	HR DAA 0.27 (0.09–0.86)	[29]
Female gender	HR eye symptoms 0.71 (0.64–0.79)	[36]
Disease characteristics		
• Axillary artery vasculitis	OR permanent vision loss 0.08 (0.03–0.27)	[33]
• Cranial signs	HR CV event 0.64 (0.42–0.98)	[6]
• Fever ≥38 °C	OR permanent vision loss 0.30 (0.14–0.64)	[30]
• Constitutional symptoms	OR permanent vision loss 0.28 (0.09–0.81)	[33]
Low ESR	OR CEV Ievent (0.94–0.99)	[35]
Comorbidities and treatment		
Prior diabetes mellitus	SHR Aaneurysm 0.19 (0.05–0.77)	[10]
Low-dose aspirin at follow-up	OR CIC 0.2 (0.03–0.7)	[37]
Statin use	HR CV event 0.993 (0.986–0.999)	[4]

More biomarkers for assessing disease activity in GCA are under ongoing investigation. Only a few studies applied scores. The Birmingham Vasculitis Activity Score (BVAS), which had been developed for different types of vasculitis, has been prospectively evaluated in the follow-up of GCA patients, but showed only limited utility in GCA [23]: Patients with active GCA disease could have a BVAS of 0, and many important ischemic symptoms attributable to active vasculitis were not included in the composite score.

As an important consequence for the clinic, each single sign and symptom has to be separately considered as possible marker for disease deterioration or relapse. Laboratory and imaging biomarkers may then be helpful to provide additional information and support the clinical suspicion or exclusion of GCA disease activity.

From the laboratory perspective, GCA lacks disease-specific serum biomarkers for prognostic purposes. Although multiple parameters have been proposed, these are all unspecific for GCA and have not been validated for monitoring disease activity and estimating disease prognosis [24]. It appears that the most promising biomarkers are serum amyloid A (SAA, 83× > control median values), interleukin-23 (IL-23, 58×), and interleukin-6 (IL-6, 11×), with changed levels of SAA, C-reactive protein (CRP), haptoglobin, erythrocyte sedimentation rate (ESR), MMP-1, MMP-2, and TNF-alpha associated with relapse and visual disturbances [24]. In patients without cranial involvement, antibodies against ferritin maybe useful activity markers [25]. For patients treated with tocilizumab (TCZ), CRP is not valid. As an alternative, osteopontin was proposed for monitoring of these patients under current treatment with tocilizumab [26].

Concerning prognostic imaging biomarkers, the use of sonography, FDG-PET, MR, and CT-angiograms has not been studied sufficiently. Although not yet established, new imaging scores may become helpful for the future [27]. For assessing changes in arterial wall inflammation in response to GCs and methotrexate (MTX), the results are mixed and represent only small patient cohorts. In a prospective study by Blockmans et al., no difference in the predictive value of FDG uptake was found between relapsing and non-relapsing patients [28].

6.3   Additional Biomarkers for Assessment of Prognosis-Relevant Comorbidities

Prognosis-relevant comorbidities maybe age-, disease-, and treatment related. For clinical follow-up of prognosis-relevant comorbidities, selected parameters routinely available and usually applied are listed in Table 6.5.

For immune aging with increased risk of infection and malignancies, but also with increased risk for CV events, no specific laboratory test has been established so far. For experimental purposes, FACS analysis can be performed to evaluate the percentage of proinflammatory CD4$^+$CD28$^-$ T cells out of the CD3$^+$CD4$^+$ T cells [38, 39].

Table 6.5 Summary of prognosis-relevant comorbidities and possible clinical use of biomarkers before and during treatment of GCA (including data from [40], modified). *GC* glucocorticoid, *CT(A)* CT with angiogram, *CV* cardiovascular, *ECG* electrocardiogram, *GC* glucocorticoids, *IL6R* interleukin6-receptor (e.g., with tocilizumab), *MR(A)* MR with angiogram, *MTX* methotrexate

Prognosis-relevant comorbidities	Biomarkers used in clinical practice
Age-related	
• CV-diseases (e.g., atherosclerosis, myocardial infarction)	Sonography, echocardiography, ECG, Trop T/Trop I, Myoglobin
• Immune aging with increased risk of infection and malignances	CRP, procalcitonin
• Renal dysfunction (e.g., with hyperuricemia)	Creatinine
GCA-related	
• Visual deterioration and visual loss	Ophthalmological exam
• GCA-specific CV-diseases (e.g., aortic dilatation/aneurysm, arterial stenosis/occlusion)	Chest radiograph, echocardiography, sonography, MR(A), CT(A), FDG-PET
Treatment-related	
• Under GCs (e.g., weight gain, arterial hypertension, diabetes mellitus, renal dysfunction, osteoporosis, peptic ulcer disease, glaucoma)	Body weight, blood pressure, HbA1c, creatinine, bone density, gastroscopy, gonioscopy/tonometry
• Under IL6R-blockade (e.g., hyperlipidemia, neutropenia, elevation of liver enzymes)	Lipids, neutrophils, liver enzymes
• Under MTX (e.g., leucopenia, elevation of liver enzymes)	Blood count, liver enzymes

References

1. Kermani TA, Warrington KJ. Prognosis and monitoring of giant cell arteritis and associated complications. Expert Rev Clin Immunol. 2018;14:379–88.
2. Robson JC, Kiran A, Maskell J, Hutchings A, Arden N, Dasgupta B, Hamilton W, Emin A, Culliford D, Luqmani R. Which patients with giant cell arteritis will develop cardiovascular or cerebrovascular disease? A clinical practice research datalink study. J Rheumatol. 2016;43:1085–92.
3. Tomasson G, Peloquin C, Mohammad A, Love TJ, Zhang Y, Choi HK, Merkel PA. Risk for cardiovascular disease early and late after a diagnosis of giant-cell arteritis: a cohort study. Ann Intern Med. 2014;160:73–80.
4. Pugnet G, Sailler L, Fournier JP, Bourrel R, Montastruc JL, Lapeyre-Mestre M. Predictors of cardiovascular hospitalization in giant cell arteritis: effect of statin exposure. A French population-based study. J Rheumatol. 2016;43:2162–70.
5. Ruffatti A. Antiphospholipid antibody syndrome and polymyalgia rheumatica/giant cell arteritis. Rheumatology. 2000;39:565–7.
6. de Boysson H, Liozon E, Espitia O, et al. Different patterns and specific outcomes of large-vessel involvements in giant cell arteritis. J Autoimmun. 2019;103:102283. https://doi.org/10.1016/j.jaut.2019.05.011.
7. Mohammad AJ, Englund M, Turesson C, Tomasson G, Merkel PA. Rate of comorbidities in giant cell arteritis: a population-based study. J Rheumatol. 2017;44:84–90.
8. Dagan A, Mahroum N, Segal G, Tiosano S, Watad A, Comaneshter D, Cohen AD, Amital H. The association between giant cell arteritis and ischemic heart disease: a population-based cross-sectional study. Isr Med Assoc J. 2017;19:411–4.
9. Li L, Neogi T, Jick S. Giant cell arteritis and vascular disease-risk factors and outcomes: a cohort study using UK Clinical Practice Research Datalink. Rheumatology (United Kingdom). 2017;56:753–62.
10. Robson JC, Kiran A, Maskell J, Hutchings A, Arden N, Dasgupta B, Hamilton W, Emin A, Culliford D, Luqmani RA. The relative risk of aortic aneurysm in patients with giant cell arteritis compared with the general population of the UK. Ann Rheum Dis. 2015;74:129–35.
11. Ungprasert P, Wijarnpreecha K, Koster MJ, Thongprayoon C, Warrington KJ. Cerebrovascular accident in patients with giant cell arteritis: a systematic review and meta-analysis of cohort studies. Semin Arthritis Rheum. 2016;46:361–6.
12. Ungprasert P, Koster MJ, Warrington KJ. Coronary artery disease in giant cell arteritis: a systematic review and meta-analysis. Semin Arthritis Rheum. 2015;44:586–91.
13. Tiosano S, Adler Y, Azrielant S, Yavne Y, Gendelman O, Ben-Ami Shor D, Comaneshter D, Shalom G, Cohen AD, Amital H. Pericarditis among giant cell arteritis patients: from myth to reality. Clin Cardiol. 2018;41:623–7.
14. Amiri N, De Vera M, Choi HK, Sayre EC, Avina-Zubieta JA. Increased risk of cardiovascular disease in giant cell arteritis: a general population-based study. Rheumatology (United Kingdom). 2016;55:33–40.
15. Petri H, Nevitt A, Sarsour K, Napalkov P, Collinson N. Incidence of giant cell arteritis and characteristics of patients: data-driven analysis of comorbidities. Arthritis Care Res. 2015;67:390. https://doi.org/10.1002/acr.22429.
16. Ungprasert P, Thongprayoon C, Kittanamongkolchai W, Srivali N, Cheungpasitporn W. Peripheral arterial disease in patients with giant cell arteritis: a meta-analysis. Int J Rheum Dis. 2016;19:819–25.
17. Ungprasert P, Koster MJ, Thongprayoon C, Warrington KJ. Risk of venous thromboembolism among patients with vasculitis: a systematic review and meta-analysis. Clin Rheumatol. 2016;35:2741–7.
18. Aviña-Zubieta JA, Jansz M, Sayre EC, Choi HK. The risk of deep venous thrombosis and pulmonary embolism in giant cell arteritis: a general population-based study. J Rheumatol. 2017;44:1184–9.

19. Unizony S, Lu N, Tomasson G, Zhang Y, Merkel PA, Stone JH, Antonio Aviña-Zubieta J, Choi HK. Temporal trends of venous thromboembolism risk before and after diagnosis of giant cell arteritis. Arthritis Rheumatol. 2017;69:176–84.

20. Ungprasert P, Upala S, Sanguankeo A, Warrington KJ. Patients with giant cell arteritis have a lower prevalence of diabetes mellitus: a systematic review and meta-analysis. Mod Rheumatol. 2016;26:410–4.

21. Yavne Y, Tiosano S, Watad A, Comaneshter D, Shoenfeld Y, Cohen AD, Amital H. Association between giant cell arteritis and thyroid dysfunction in a "real life" population. Endocrine. 2017;57:241–6.

22. Ungprasert P, Sanguankeo A, Upala S, Knight EL. Risk of malignancy in patients with giant cell arteritis and polymyalgia rheumatica: a systematic review and meta-analysis. Semin Arthritis Rheum. 2014;44:366–70.

23. Kermani TA, Cuthbertson D, Carette S, et al. The Birmingham vasculitis activity score as a measure of disease activity in patients with giant cell arteritis. J Rheumatol. 2016;43:1078–84.

24. Burja B, Feichtinger J, Lakota K, et al. Utility of serological biomarkers for giant cell arteritis in a large cohort of treatment-naïve patients. Clin Rheumatol. 2018;38:317–29.

25. Baerlecken NT, Linnemann A, Gross WL, et al. Association of ferritin autoantibodies with giant cell arteritis/polymyalgia rheumatica. Ann Rheum Dis. 2012;71:943–7.

26. Prieto-González S, Terrades-García N, Corbera-Bellalta M, et al. Serum osteopontin: a biomarker of disease activity and predictor of relapsing course in patients with giant cell arteritis. Potential clinical usefulness in tocilizumab-treated patients. RMD Open. 2017;3:e000570.

27. Tombetti E, Godi C, Ambrosi A, et al. Novel angiographic scores for evaluation of large vessel vasculitis. Sci Rep. 2018;8:15979.

28. Salvarani C, Soriano A, Muratore F, Shoenfeld Y, Blockmans D. Is PET/CT essential in the diagnosis and follow-up of temporal arteritis? Autoimmun Rev. 2017;16:1125–30.

29. Kermani TA, Warrington KJ, Crowson CS, Hunder GG, Ytterberg SR, Gabriel SE, Matteson EL. Predictors of dissection in aortic aneurysms from giant cell arteritis. J Clin Rheumatol. 2016;22:184–7.

30. Liozon E, Dalmay F, Lalloue F, Gondran G, Bezanahary H, Fauchais AL, Ly KH. Risk factors for permanent visual loss in biopsy-proven giant cell arteritis: a study of 339 patients. J Rheumatol. 2016;43:1393–9.

31. de Boysson H, Espitia O, Liozon E, et al. Vascular presentation and outcomes of patients with giant cell arteritis and isolated symptomatic limb involvement. J Clin Rheumatol. 2020;26(6):248–54.

32. Zhu W-G, Xiong Q-M, Hong K. Meta-analysis of CHADS 2 versus CHA 2 DS 2 -VASc for predicting stroke and thromboembolism in atrial fibrillation patients independent of anticoagulation. Texas Hear Inst J. 2015;42:6–15.

33. Czihal M, Tschaidse J, Bernau C, et al. Ocular ischaemic complications in giant cell arteritis: CHADS 2-score predicts risk of permanent visual impairment. Clin Exp Rheumatol. 2019;37:61–4.

34. Gonzalez-Gay MA, Garcia-Porrua C, Piñeiro A, Pego-Reigosa R, Llorca J, Hunder GG. Aortic aneurysm and dissection in patients with biopsy-proven giant cell arteritis from northwestern Spain: a population-based study. Medicine (Baltimore). 2004;83:335–41.

35. Grossman C, Barshack I, Koren-Morag N, Ben-Zvi I, Bornstein G. Risk factors for severe cranial ischaemic events in patients with giant cell arteritis. Clin Exp Rheumatol. 2017;35:88–93.

36. Ji J, Dimitrijevic I, Sundquist J, Sundquist K, Zöller B. Risk of ocular manifestations in patients with giant cell arteritis: a nationwide study in Sweden. Scand J Rheumatol. 2017;46:484–9.

37. Nesher G, Berkun Y, Mates M, Baras M, Nesher R, Rubinow A, Sonnenblick M. Risk factors for cranial ischemic complications in giant cell arteritis. Medicine (Baltimore). 2004;83:114–22.

38. Mohan SV, Liao YJ, Kim JW, Goronzy JJ, Weyand CM. Giant cell arteritis: immune and vascular aging as disease risk factors. Arthritis Res Ther. 2011;13:231.

39. Maly K, Schirmer M. The story of CD4+ CD28- T cells revisited: solved or still ongoing? J Immunol Res. 2015;2015:348746.

40. Duru N, van der Goes MC, Jacobs JWG, et al. EULAR evidence-based and consensus-based recommendations on the management of medium to high-dose glucocorticoid therapy in rheumatic diseases. Ann Rheum Dis. 2013;72:1905–13.

Treatment and Management

7

Michael Schirmer and Rick McCutchan

Abstract

Treatment and management guidelines for GCA slightly vary between international and national task forces. Therefore, this chapter provides an overview on currently available recommendations of the EULAR task force last updated in 2018, the BSR and BHPR guidelines from 2010, the recommendations of the French Study Group for Large Vessel Vasculitis from 2016 and the guidelines of the Swedish Society of Rheumatology from 2019, which were identified in the literature and reviewed for this book chapter. Besides, the relevant EULAR recommendations for the use of glucocorticoids in rheumatic diseases from 2013 and for imaging from 2018 together with the interdisciplinary recommendations for FDG-PET/CT(A) imaging of the Cardiovascular and Inflammation and Infection Committees of the European Association of Nuclear Medicine (EANM), the Cardiovascular Council of the Society of Nuclear Medicine and Molecular Imaging (SNMMI), and the PET Interest Group (PIG), endorsed by the American Society of Nuclear Cardiology (ASNC) from 2018 were assessed to summarize current evidence necessary for monitoring of GCA and its comorbidities.

Keywords

Guidelines · Management · Recommendations · Review

M. Schirmer (✉) · R. McCutchan
Medical University of Innsbruck, Internal Medicine II, Innsbruck, Austria
e-mail: michael.schirmer@i-med.ac.at

© Springer Nature Switzerland AG 2021
C. Salvarani et al. (eds.), *Large and Medium Size Vessel and Single Organ Vasculitis*, Rare Diseases of the Immune System,
https://doi.org/10.1007/978-3-030-67175-4_7

Treatment and management guidelines for GCA slightly vary between international and national task forces. Therefore, this chapter provides an overview on currently available recommendations of the EULAR task force last updated in 2018 [1], the BSR and BHPR guidelines from 2010 [2], the recommendations of the French Study Group for Large Vessel Vasculitis from 2016 [3] and the guidelines of the Swedish Society of Rheumatology from 2019 [4] were identified in the literature and reviewed for this book chapter. Besides, the relevant EULAR recommendations for the use of glucocorticoids in rheumatic diseases from 2013 [5] and for imaging from 2018 [6] together with the interdisciplinary recommendations for FDG-PET/CT(A) imaging of the Cardiovascular and Inflammation and Infection Committees of the European Association of Nuclear Medicine (EANM), the Cardiovascular Council of the Society of Nuclear Medicine and Molecular Imaging (SNMMI), and the PET Interest Group (PIG), endorsed by the American Society of Nuclear Cardiology (ASNC) from 2018 [7] were assessed to summarize current evidence necessary for monitoring of GCA and its comorbidities.

7.1   General Aspects

General recommendations can be divided into those for time of diagnosis, for monitoring of GCA and those concerning adverse events and comorbidities. Details from the above-mentioned recommendations and guidelines for each of these situations are summarized in Table 7.1. Although not specified in these recommendations, the aim of treat-to-target is important for GCA as for other chronic rheumatic diseases, too, with remission being defined as lack of disease activity as the principal target of disease management. However, an aortic aneurysm may develop even without detectable clinical activity, and even years after disease outset [8]. Such caveats have to be kept in mind as peculiar issues in the management of GCA, arguing for prolonged monitoring even without detectable disease activity over years.

First, treatment is recommended to be initiated as soon as diagnosis is made to prevent further complications. Comorbidities predisposing to an increased risk for worse course of the disease or adverse events to medications have to be considered before start of treatment (see Chap. 6). Patients and their carers should be fully informed about management and risks of treatment.

For monitoring, the EULAR task force recommends assessment of symptoms, clinical findings, and erythrocyte sedimentation rate (ESR) and C-reactive protein (CRP) levels for monitoring of disease activity ([1] recommendation 10). For clinical examination, monitoring is primarily based on symptoms (like jaw and tongue claudication, visual symptoms, vascular claudication of limbs), clinical findings (like bruits and asymmetrical pulses, polymyalgic symptoms, osteoporotic risk factors and fractures). The UK guidelines add a specific recommendation to pay particular attention to the predictive features of ischemic neuro-ophthalmic complications [2]. Concerning laboratory biomarkers, also the French guidelines do explicitly not recommend measuring biomarkers other than C-reactive protein,

Table 7.1 Summary of general recommendations concerning situation at diagnosis, monitoring of GCA for the purpose to optimize treatment, adverse events, and comorbidities. *AE* adverse event, *CRP* C-reactive protein, *CV* cardiovascular, *ESR* erythrocyte sedimentation rate, *GC* glucocorticoid, *LoE* level of evidence, *LoA* (0–10), level of agreement

Year	Recommendation	LoE	LoA (0–10)	Ref.
	At time of diagnosis			
2019/R2	It is vital not to delay treatment, for example while waiting for a temporal artery biopsy			[4]
2019/R1	GCs remain first line for the treatment			[4]
2013/R6	Before starting medium-/high-dose GC treatment consider comorbidities predisposing to AEs. These include diabetes, glucose intolerance, CV disease, peptic ulcer disease, recurrent infections, immune-suppression, (risk factors of) glaucoma, and osteoporosis. Patients with these comorbidities require tight control to manage the risk/benefit ratio	IV		[5]
2013/R1	Explain to patients (and their family and/or carers, including healthcare professionals) the aim of medium-/high-dose GC treatment, and the potential risks associated with such therapy	III		[5]
2013/R2	Discuss measures to mitigate such risks, including diet, regular exercise, and appropriate wound care	III/ IV		[5]
2013/R4	Patients and the patients' treatment teams should receive appropriate, practical advice on how to manage with GC-induced hypothalamic-pituitary-adrenal axis suppression	IV		[5]
2016/9b	The systematic initiation of treatment with intravenous methylprednisolone pulse(s) is not recommended		100	[3]
	Monitoring during follow-up			
2018/ R10	Regular follow-up and monitoring of disease activity is recommended, primarily based on symptoms, clinical findings and ESR/CRP levels	3b	9.6 ± 0.6	[1]
2013/R5	Provide an accessible resource to promote best practice in the management of patients using medium-/high-dose GCs to general practitioners	IV		[5]

(continued)

Table 7.1 (continued)

Year	Recommendation	LoE	LoA (0–10)	Ref.
UK2010/ R7a	Monitoring of therapy should be clinical and supported by the measurement of inflammatory markers. Patients should be monitored for evidence of relapse, disease-related complications, and GC-related complications. In particular, the following features should be sought: Jaw and tongue claudication, visual symptoms, vascular claudication of limbs, bruits and asymmetrical pulses, polymyalgic symptoms, osteoporotic risk factors and fractures, other GC-related complications, other symptoms that may suggest an alternative diagnosis The following investigations should be performed: At each visit: full blood count, ESR/CRP, urea and electrolytes, glucose. Every 2 years: chest radiograph to monitor for aortic aneurysm (echocardiography, PET and MRI may also be appropriate). Bone mineral density may be required Routine follow-up should be planned at: Weeks 0, 1, 3, 6, then Months 3, 6, 9, 12 in the first year. Later (Month 3 onwards) follow-up can be undertaken under shared care *Relapse:* Disease relapse should be suspected in patients with return of symptoms of GCA, ischemic complications, unexplained fever, or polymyalgic symptoms. All patients in whom relapse is suspected should be treated as below, and discussed or referred for specialist assessment. Return of headache should be treated with the previous higher dose of GC. Symptoms of large-vessel disease should prompt further investigation with MRI or PET and use of systemic vasculitis treatment protocols	C		[2]
2016/8a	CT or MRI screening for complications of aortitis is recommended at GCA diagnosis, then every 2–5 years, provided the patient has no contraindications to a potential aorta repair		93.8	[3]
2013/R8	Keep the requirement for continuing GC treatment under constant review, and titrate the dose against therapeutic response, risk of undertreatment, and development of AEs	IV		[5]
2016/15c	A purely biological "relapse" or "recurrence" does not necessarily require GC dose intensification or the initiation of adjunctive therapy but should prompt closer monitoring		96.8	[3]
2018/ R10	In patients in whom a flare is suspected, imaging might be helpful to confirm or exclude it. Imaging is not routinely recommended for patients in clinical and biochemical remission	5	9.4 ± 0.8	[6]
2016/15a	For a first relapse or recurrence, treatment with GCs is recommended at a dose that depends on symptom severity and by at least returning to the previously effective dose		100	[3]

Table 7.1 (continued)

Year	Recommendation	LoE	LoA (0–10)	Ref.
2018/ R7a	In case of major relapse (either with signs or symptoms of ischemia or progressive vascular inflammation), we recommend reinstitution or dose escalation of GC therapy as recommended for new onset disease. For minor relapses, we recommend an increase in GC dose at least to the last effective dose	2b	9.5 ± 1.0	[1]
	Adverse events and comorbidities			
2013/R3	Patients with, or at risk of, GC-induced osteoporosis should receive appropriate preventive/therapeutic interventions	IA		[5]
2013/ R10	All patients should have appropriate monitoring for clinically significant AEs. The treating physician should be aware of the possible occurrence of diabetes, hypertension, weight gain, infections, osteoporotic fractures, osteonecrosis, myopathy, eye problems, skin problems, and neuropsychological AEs	IV		[5]
2016/11a	GCA with uncomplicated and asymptomatic involvement of the aorta or its branches can be treated with the GC regimen recommended for uncomplicated GCA		90.3	[3]
2016/10b	The tapering schedule and duration of glucocorticoid treatment for GCA with ophthalmic involvement should follow the same regimen as that recommended for uncomplicated GCA		96.8	[3]

erythrocyte sedimentation rate, and fibrinogen for monitoring disease activity [3]. Additional laboratory biomarkers maybe necessary for monitoring of GCA complications, comorbidities, and adverse events of GCA-related treatment.

Concerning the imaging biomarkers, the EULAR recommendation for imaging states that imaging "might be helpful in patients with suspected flare, especially when clinical and laboratory parameters are inconclusive" and that "MRA, CTA and/or US may be used for long-term monitoring of structural damage, particularly to detect stenosis, occlusion, dilatation and/or aneurysms, on an individual basis" ([6] recommendation 10 and 11), while the other international consensus on imaging does definitely not support a value of FDG-PET/CT(A) for evaluating response to treatment [7]. It is argued that a positive ^{18}F-FDG-PET persists in up to 60% of patients in full clinical remission, and using sonography, residual changes often remain visible for several months in extracranial arteries.

Important to note, that—if necessary—times of stable remission should be selected for elective surgical interventions or reconstructive surgery (recommendation 9, [1]), while for emergency situations repair of an aortic lesion should be scheduled once the systemic inflammatory response has subsided [3].

7.2　Glucocorticoids as First-Line Treatment

Glucocorticoid (GC) therapy is still considered as first-line therapy in GCA, despite their multiple adverse events. GCs should be started immediately after diagnosis and information of the patient. If the symptoms of GCA do not respond rapidly to high-dose GC treatment, followed by resolution of the inflammatory response, the question of an alternative diagnosis should be raised.

Recommendations for optimal dosage and dose reduction of GCs differ between EULAR and national guidelines (Tables 7.2 and 7.3). EULAR experts start with 40–60 mg/day prednisone-equivalent for induction of remission in active GCA and recommend tapering the GC dose to a target dose of 15–20 mg/day within 2–3 months and after 1 year to ≤5 mg/day. In case of signs and symptoms of reactivated disease, the dosage of GCs should be increased to the latest effective dose and GC-sparing agents be considered (see Sect. 7.3). Specific recommendations with higher dosage regimens apply to ocular and aortic aneurysmatic involvement (Table 7.3).

Monitoring is considered essential for treatment adaptions in GCA and includes: clinical signs and symptoms of GCA-activity and GCA complications,

Table 7.2 Recommendations concerning dosage of GCs, with specific recommendation for eye involvement. Important aspects are marked in bold letters. *GC* glucocorticoids

Year	Recommendation	LoE	LoA (0–10)	Ref.
EULAR 2018/R4	High-dose GC therapy (40–60 mg/day prednisone-equivalent) should be initiated immediately for induction of remission in active GCA. Once disease is controlled, we recommend tapering the GC dose to a target dose of 15–20 mg/day within 2–3 months and after 1 year to ≤5 mg/day	4 5	9.8 ± 0.6 9.5 ± 0.9	[1]
2019/R3	The recommended initial dose of prednisolone is 40–60 mg for 4 weeks, thereafter gradually tapered (until ESR and CRP have been normalized, and signs and symptoms have improved). Thereafter, reduction of the dose by 10 mg every other week to 20 mg daily. Thereafter, reductions of 2.5 mg with 2–4 week intervals to 10 mg daily. If there are no signs of relapse, the dose may be reduced by 1 mg every 1–2 months. After every dose reduction, the patient's ESR and CRP are checked and the return of signs and symptoms is also checked. If signs and symptoms of active disease return, the dose of prednisolone should be increased to the latest effective dose			[4]

Table 7.2 (continued)

Year	Recommendation	LoE	LoA (0–10)	Ref.
UK 2010/R4a	High-dose GC therapy should be initiated immediately when clinical suspicion of GCA is raised. Recommended starting dosages of GC are for uncomplicated GCA (no jaw claudication or visual disturbance): 40–60 mg prednisolone daily. The symptoms of GCA should respond rapidly to high-dose GC treatment, followed by resolution of the inflammatory response. Failure to do so should raise the question of an alternative diagnosis	C		[2]
2016/9a	We recommend treating uncomplicated GCA with oral prednisone at a starting dose of 0.7 mg/kg/day, then gradually tapering to reach 15–20 mg/day at 3 months, 7.5–10 mg/day at 6 months, 5 mg/day at 12 months and weaning off GCs within 18–24 months		100	[3]
UK 2010/R4b	GC reduction should be considered only in the absence of clinical symptoms, signs, and laboratory abnormalities suggestive of active disease. This should be balanced against the need to use the lowest effective dose, patient wishes, and GC side effects. Steroid reduction may also be appropriate if the acute-phase response is deemed to be due to another cause. Suggested tapering regimen: • 40–60 mg prednisolone continued until symptoms and laboratory abnormalities resolve (at least 3–4 weeks) • then dose is reduced by 10 mg every 2 weeks to 20 mg • then by 2.5 mg every 2–4 weeks to 10 mg • then by 1 mg every 1–2 months provided there is no relapse The dose may need adjustment for disease severity, comorbid factors, fracture risk, patient wishes, and adverse events. There are also some patients who will require long-term low-dose GC therapy	C		[2]
2016/11b	For complicated (dilatation, aortic aneurysm, or dissection) or symptomatic (limb claudication or ischemia) aortoarteritis at GCA onset, oral prednisone at 1 mg/kg/day can be prescribed as a starting dose		87.1	[3]
UK 2010/R7b	Relapse: • Jaw claudication requires 60 mg prednisolone	C		[2]
2018/3	Withdraw or delay GC therapy until after PET, unless there is risk of ischemic complications, as in the case of GCA with temporal artery involvement. FDG-PET within 3 days after start of GC is optional as a possible alternative	III	B	[7]

Table 7.3 Recommendations concerning dosage of GCs, with specific recommendation for eye involvement. Important aspects are marked in bold letters. *GC* glucocorticoids

Year	Recommendation	LoE	LoA (0–10)	Ref.
	Eye involvement			
Sweden 2019/R4	If vision is impaired or there are other signs of serious vascular involvement, intravenous methylprednisolone 1000 mg once daily for 3 days may be considered, followed by oral treatment as above			[4]
UK 2010/R4a	Recommended starting dosages of GC are: • Evolving visual loss or amaurosis fugax (complicated GCA): 500 mg to 1 g of i.v. methylprednisolone for 3 days before oral GCs • Established visual loss: 60 mg prednisolone daily to protect the contralateral eye	C		[2]
2016/10a	Suspected GCA with transient or permanent ophthalmic involvement should be treated immediately with 1 mg/kg/day of oral prednisone or 500–1000 mg/day of intravenous methylprednisolone for 1–3 days (followed by oral prednisone at 1 mg/kg/day), according to regimen that can be most rapidly initiated		100	[3]
UK 2010/R7b	Relapse: • Eye symptoms need the use of either 60 mg prednisolone or i.v. methylprednisolone	C		[2]

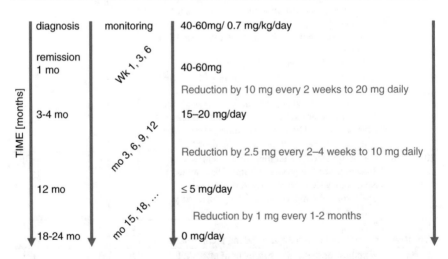

Fig. 7.1 Summary of GC schemes in recommendations and guidelines together with UK proposal for monitoring from 2010 (from Table 7.1). Dosages are given for prednisolone equivalents. Reductions of GCs (marked in red) should be recommended only in the absence of any signs and symptoms of GCA (recommendation summarized from Table 7.4). *Mo* months, *wk* week

treatment-related adverse events, and comorbidities. The schedule for monitoring in relation to recommended dosages of GCs is depicted in Fig. 7.1. For monitoring after 18 months of disease duration, further clinical schedules depend on residual disease activity. Chest radiographs, echocardiography, PET, or MRI are recommended for early detection of an aortic aneurysm every 2–5 years, and additional bone mineral density may be needed.

Unfortunately, literature lays out that relapses of GCA under treatment with GCs occur in as many as 47.2% (95% confidence interval 40.0–54.3%) of patients, with more relapses reported in randomized-controlled trials (RCTs) than in observational studies and under shorter GC regimens (rate decrease of 1.7% for one additional month), but independent from initial GC doses (3). As a consequence, GCs alone appear to be insufficient for treatment of GCA in many patients, and GC-sparing agents may become necessary.

7.3   Glucocorticoid(GC)-Sparing Agents

Because of the wide spectrum of possible GC-related side effects, GC-sparing agents have always been considered as an important issue for treatment of GCA. Therefore, several synthetic and biological disease-modifying anti-rheumatic drugs (DMARDs) have been studied for the GC-sparing effects (Table 7.4). Overall, use of a GC-sparing agent beside GCs has been shown to be a protective factor both against new CV events (HR 0.44 (95% confidence interval (CI) 0.29–0.66)) as well as the development of aortic dilatation (HR 0.43 (CI 0.23–0.77)) [9]. Thus, GC-sparing agents should be considered especially for patients with insufficient response to GCs alone and patients with pre-existing comorbidities or high risk of GC-related side effects.

Recently, a meta-analysis comparing different GC-sparing agents showed that the two drugs tocilizumab (TCZ), a biological (b)DMARD, and methotrexate (MTX), a conventional (c)DMARD can be considered as GC-sparing agents. Both GC-sparing agents resulted in improved likelihoods of being relapse free with relative risks of 3.54 for TCZ and 1.54 for MTX [10]. At present, the bDMARD TCZ is the only FDA- and EMA-approved GC-sparing agent for the treatment of GCA—as an IL 6 R antagonist it showed efficacy in induction of sustained remission in both a phase II [11] and a phase III study (the GIACTA trial, [12]). The GIACTA trial showed that the risk of flares during TCZ treatment weekly and every other week decreases compared to the placebo group (HR 0.23 (CI 0.11–0.46) and 0.28 (CI, 0.12–0.66), respectively). TCZ co-treatment also resulted in lower cumulative prednisolone doses during trial duration ($p < 0.001$). To be remembered as a challenge of monitoring, is the suppressive effect of TCZ especially on the CRP biomarker. For monitoring of TCZ, it is important to early detect increased alanine aminotransferase (ALT) or aspartate aminotransferase (AST) >1.5-fold upper limit of normal, absolute neutrophil counts lower than $0.5–1.0 \times 10^9$/L, and platelet counts lower than $50–100 \times 10^3$/μL [13–16]. Blood count, liver function test, and lipid parameters should be evaluated 4–8 weeks after initiation and at 6-month interval thereafter. Live and live-attenuated vaccines should not be given concurrently with TCZ. Although the safety profile of TCZ in GCA appears similar to placebo with comparable numbers of adverse events per 100 patient years, longer follow-up periods in RCT trial are needed to underline its benefit-to-harm ratio [17].

Table 7.4 Summary of a meta-analysis (MA), a comparative MA (CMA), and additional randomized-controlled trials (RCTs, patient number >25) on treatment options for GCA, including conventional as well as biological disease-modifying anti-rheumatic drugs (cDMARDs and bDMARDs, respectively). *ABA* Abatacept, *ADA* Adalimumab, *CI* 95% confidence interval, *cDMARD* conventional DMARD, *bDMARD* biological DMARD, *ETA* etanercept, *GC* glucocorticoid, *HR* hazard ratio favoring MTX, *IFX* infliximab, *MTX* methotrexate, *mo* months, *n.s.* not significant, *Pl* placebo, *RR* relative risk to improve likelihood of being relapse free, *TCZ* tocilizumab, *vs* versus, *wks* weeks

Drug	MA/ RCT	Patients total [n]	Duration [months]	Results	Ref.
cDMARDs					
• MTX	MA	161	55 ± 39 wks	HR 1st relapse 0.65 (CI 0.44–0.98) HR 2nd relapse 0.49 (CI 0.27–0.89)	[18]
• MTX	CMA	161	55 ± 39 wks	RR 1.54 (CI 1.02–2.30)	[10]
bDMARDs					
IL6R blockade	CMA	281	52 wks	RR 3.54 (CI 2.25–5.51)	[10]
• TCZ	RCT	251	12 mo	*Sustained remission* $p \leq 0.001$: 56% (56/100) TCZ weekly 53% (26/49) TCZ every other week 14% (7/50) Pl; 26-week GC taper 18% (9/51) Pl; 52-week GC taper	[12]
• TCZ	RCT	30	12 mo	*Sustained remission* $p = 0.001$: 85% with TCZ ($n = 17/20$) 20% with GC ($n = 2/10$)	[11]
CTLA4-blockade	CMA	41	12 mo	RR 1.50 (CI 0.71–3.17)	[10]
• ABA	RCT	41	12 mo	*Sustained remission* $p = 0.049$: 48% with ABA vs. 31% with Pl	[20]
TNF-blockade	CMA	131	22–52 wks	RR 1.12 (0.79–1.58)	[10]
• IFX	RCT	44	22 wks.	*Relapse free* $p = 0.65$: 43% with IFX vs. 50% with Pl	[23]
• ADA	RCT	70	6 mo	*Sustained remission* $p = 0.46$: 20 (59%) with ADA vs. 18 (50%) with Pl	[24]
• ETA	RCT	17	1 year	*Controlled disease* $p = $ n.s.: 50% ETA and 22.2% placebo (n.s.)	[25]

As a consequence of this high level of evidence, the updated EULAR guidelines recommend that "adjunctive therapy should be used in selected patients with GCA (refractory or relapsing disease, the presence or an increased risk of GC-related adverse events or complications) using TCZ." MTX is only considered as an alternative (Table 7.5). MTX is not approved for the treatment of GCA and although lower dosages have not been shown to be effective, two independent meta-analyses of current literature revealed a beneficial effect of MTX in GCA [10, 18].

Only a few other agents have been tested as possible GC-sparing agents so far [19]. Although a randomized-controlled trial showed that the bDMARD abatacept

Table 7.5 Recommendations concerning GC-sparing agents (from EULAR and other national taskforces as indicated). Recommendations published before approval of TCZ for the indication of GCA are not included into this table. *TCZ* tocilizumab

Year	Recommendation	LoE	LoA (0–10)	Ref.
EULAR 2018/R5	Adjunctive therapy should be used in selected patients with GCA (refractory or relapsing disease, the presence or an increased risk of GC-related adverse effects or complications) using TCZ MTX may be used as an alternative	1b 1a	9.4 ± 0.8 9.4 ± 0.8	[1]
EULAR 2018/R7b	Initiation or modification of adjunctive therapy should be considered particularly after recurrent disease relapses	1b	9.6 ± 1.0	[1]
Sweden 2019/R6	In cases of newly diagnosed GCA, TCZ may be considered when there is a great risk of future side effects of GCs and pronounced clinical and laboratory signs of vascular inflammation			[4]
Sweden 2019/R5	The rationale for treating GCA with TCZ is primarily its GC-sparing effect over time. TCZ is recommended as supplement to prednisolone treatment in patients with recurrent or active illness during GC treatment, providing the criteria of relapse during GC treatment or relapse after completion of treatment with GC, large-vessel arteritis verified at some point with biopsy or with imaging of large vessels (MRI, PET-CT, or CTA), clinically active GCA, elevated CRP and ESR or obvious side effects of GC treatment or great risk of such side effects from future treatment with GCs are met			[4]
Sweden 2019/R7	Treatment with TCZ should be discontinued after 1 year. Longer periods of treatment cannot be recommended with our present state of knowledge. If inflammation persists after 1 year of treatment with TCZ, an individual assessment must be made by the treating physician			[4]

(ABA), an inhibitor of the T-cell receptor CTLA4, may be useful to maintain remission in GCA-patients [20], ABA was not so effective in this trial. Another open-label study suggested that the bDMARD ustekinumab, which targets the interleukins IL12 and IL23, could be useful for the treatment of patients with refractory GCA [21]. In cultured GCA arteries, inhibition of IL-12/IL-23p40 tended to reduce IFNγ and IL-17 mRNA production and to increase the Th17 inducers IL-1β and IL-6 [22]. Now, further studies are required to assess whether ABA and ustekinumab extend our repertoire of adjunctive therapies to reduce relapses or as a GC-sparing agents in GCA. The interleukin-1 binding bDMARD, anakinra has been successfully used only in a few patients with refractory GCA. Blockade of TNF-alpha turned out already earlier to be ineffective as a GC-sparing approach [23, 24].

7.4   Treatment of Comorbidities/Adjuvant Therapies

Comorbidities may occur as a consequence of higher age, as complications of GCA itself and GCA-treatment. For optimal treatment of GCA-patients, all of these issues have to be considered, and deterioration of only one of the comorbidities may result in severe complications with increased morbidity or even mortality.

Although treatment of comorbidities is essential for the optimal outcome of GCA, only a few recommendations refer to comorbidities (Tables 7.6):

1. Concerning the recommendations on antiplatelet and anticoagulant therapy, low-dose aspirin is advised or at least should be considered for GCA-patients without contraindication according to national guidelines, but the EULAR task force recommends low-dose aspirin or at least to consider it only for patients with other indications or in special situations (Table 7.6).
2. Bone protection is recommended by the UK guidelines for GCA.
3. Proton pump inhibitors for gastrointestinal protection should be considered according to the UK guidelines for GCA.
4. The systematic prescription of statins is not recommended by the French guidelines for GCA.
5. Recent evidence confirms the use of GC-sparing agents to reduce GCA-related comorbidities (see Sect. 7.3). Besides, monitoring is recommended especially for osteoporosis, CV-risk factors (including arterial hypertension and diabetes mellitus), and CV disease.

Further recommendations for other comorbidities are not included in the available EULAR and national GCA-specific recommendations, so that risk and comorbidity-specific recommendations have to be adapted for GCA-patients. For example, the risk of infections is estimated to be twofold increased in GCA-disease [26, 27], with the need of appropriate patients' information, monitoring and treatment, independent from the GCA-specific recommendations.

Table 7.6 Recommendations for additional treatments in GCA. *LoE* level of evidence, *LoA* level of agreement

Year	Recommendation	LoE	LoA (0–10)	Ref.
EULAR 2018/R8	Antiplatelet or anticoagulant therapy should not be routinely used unless it is indicated for other reasons (e.g., coronary heart disease or cerebrovascular disease). In special situations, such as vascular ischemic complications or high risk of cardiovascular disease, these might be considered on an individual basis	4	9.4 ± 0.8	[1]
France 2016/14a	Low-dose aspirin (75–300 mg/day) should be considered for every patient with newly diagnosed GCA upon benefit–risk assessment; for GCA with ophthalmic involvement, prescribing low-dose aspirin should be advised		100	[3]
UK 2010/R5	Low-dose aspirin should be considered in patients with GCA if no contraindications exist	C		[2]
France 2016/10c	Aspirin (75–300 mg/day) should be advised for GCA with ophthalmic involvement		96.8	[3]
France 2016/14b	The systematic prescription of an anticoagulant or a statin is not recommended		93.5	[3]
UK 2010/R4a	Patients should also receive bone protection. Proton pump inhibitors for gastrointestinal protection should be considered	C		[2]

References

1. Hellmich B, Agueda A, Monti S, et al. 2018 Update of the EULAR recommendations for the management of large vessel vasculitis. Ann Rheum Dis. 2020;79(1):19–30. https://doi.org/10.1136/annrheumdis-2019-215672.
2. Dasgupta B, Borg FA, Hassan N, et al. BSR and BHPR guidelines for the management of giant cell arteritis. Rheumatology (Oxford). 2010;49:1594–7.

3. Bienvenu B, Ly KHH, Lambert M, et al. Management of giant cell arteritis: recommendations of the French Study Group for Large Vessel Vasculitis (GEFA). Rev Med Interne. 2016;37:154–65.
4. Turesson C, Börjesson O, Larsson K, Mohammad AJ, Knight A. Swedish Society of Rheumatology 2018 guidelines for investigation, treatment, and follow-up of giant cell arteritis. Scand J Rheumatol. 2019;00:1–7.
5. Duru N, van der Goes MC, Jacobs JWG, et al. EULAR evidence-based and consensus-based recommendations on the management of medium to high-dose glucocorticoid therapy in rheumatic diseases. Ann Rheum Dis. 2013;72:1905–13.
6. Dejaco C, Ramiro S, Duftner C, et al. EULAR recommendations for the use of imaging in large vessel vasculitis in clinical practice. Ann Rheum Dis. 2018;77:636–43.
7. Slart RHJA, Glaudemans AWJM, Chareonthaitawee P, et al. FDG-PET/CT(A) imaging in large vessel vasculitis and polymyalgia rheumatica: joint procedural recommendation of the EANM, SNMMI, and the PET Interest Group (PIG), and endorsed by the ASNC. Eur J Nucl Med Mol Imaging. 2018;45:1250–69.
8. García-Martínez A, Arguis P, Prieto-González S, Espígol-Frigolé G, Alba MA, Butjosa M, Tavera-Bahillo I, Hernández-Rodríguez J, Cid MC. Prospective long term follow-up of a cohort of patients with giant cell arteritis screened for aortic structural damage (aneurysm or dilatation). Ann Rheum Dis. 2014;73:1826–32.
9. de Boysson H, Liozon E, Espitia O, et al. Different patterns and specific outcomes of large-vessel involvements in giant cell arteritis. J Autoimmun. 2019;103:102283. https://doi.org/10.1016/j.jaut.2019.05.011.
10. Berti A, Cornec D, Medina Inojosa JR, Matteson EL, Murad MH. Treatments for giant cell arteritis: meta-analysis and assessment of estimates reliability using the fragility index. Semin Arthritis Rheum. 2018;48:77–82.
11. Villiger PM, Adler S, Kuchen S, Wermelinger F, Dan D, Fiege V, Bütikofer L, Seitz M, Reichenbach S. Tocilizumab for induction and maintenance of remission in giant cell arteritis: a phase 2, randomised, double-blind, placebo-controlled trial. Lancet. 2016;387:1921–7.
12. Stone JH, Tuckwell K, Dimonaco S, et al. Trial of tocilizumab in giant-cell arteritis. N Engl J Med. 2017;377:317–28.
13. Shovman O, Shoenfeld Y, Langevitz P. Tocilizumab-induced neutropenia in rheumatoid arthritis patients with previous history of neutropenia: case series and review of literature. Immunol Res. 2015;61:164–8.
14. European Medicines Agency. Find medicine—RoActemra. http://www.ema.europa.eu/ema/index.jsp?curl=pages/medicines/human/medicines/000955/human_med_001042.jsp&mid=WC0b01ac058001d124. Accessed 18 Nov 2017.
15. Moots RJ, Sebba A, Rigby W, Ostor A, Porter-Brown B, Donaldson F, Dimonaco S, Rubbert-Roth A, van Vollenhoven R, Genovese MC. Effect of tocilizumab on neutrophils in adult patients with rheumatoid arthritis: pooled analysis of data from phase 3 and 4 clinical trials. Rheumatology. 2016;56:541–9.
16. Vitiello G, Orsi Battaglini C, Radice A, Carli G, Micheli S, Cammelli D. Sustained tocilizumab-induced hypofibrinogenemia and thrombocytopenia. Comment on: "Tocilizumab-induced hypofibrinogenemia: a report of 7 cases" by Martis et al., Joint Bone Spine 2016, doi: 10.1016/j.jbspin.2016.04.008. Joint Bone Spine. 2017;84:649–50.
17. Schirmer M, Muratore F, Salvarani C. Tocilizumab for the treatment of giant cell arteritis. Expert Rev Clin Immunol. 2018;14(5):339–49. https://doi.org/10.1080/1744666X.2018.1468251.
18. Mahr AD, Jover JA, Spiera RF, Hernández-García C, Fernández-Gutiérrez B, Lavalley MP, Merkel PA. Adjunctive methotrexate for treatment of giant cell arteritis: an individual patient data meta-analysis. Arthritis Rheum. 2007;56:2789–97.
19. Watelet B, Samson M, de Boysson H, Bienvenu B. Treatment of giant-cell arteritis, a literature review. Mod Rheumatol. 2017;27:747–54.
20. Langford CA, Cuthbertson D, Ytterberg SR, et al. A randomized, double-blind trial of abatacept (CTLA-4Ig) for the treatment of giant cell arteritis. Arthritis Rheumatol. 2017;69:837–45.

21. González-Gay MA, Pina T, Prieto-Peña D, Calderon-Goercke M, Blanco R, Castañeda S. The role of biologics in the treatment of giant cell arteritis. Expert Opin Biol Ther. 2019;19:65–72.
22. Espígol-Frigolé G, Planas-Rigol E, Lozano E, Corbera-Bellalta M, Terrades-García N, Prieto-González S, García-Martínez A, Hernández-Rodríguez J, Grau JM, Cid MC. Expression and function of IL12/23 related cytokine subunits (p35, p40, and p19) in giant-cell arteritis lesions: contribution of p40 to Th1- and Th17-mediated inflammatory pathways. Front Immunol. 2018;9:809.
23. Hoffman GS, Cid MC, Rendt-Zaga KE, et al. Infliximab for maintenance of glucocorticosteroid-induced remission of giant cell arteritis. Ann Intern Med. 2007;146:621–31.
24. Seror R, Baron G, Hachulla E, et al. Adalimumab for steroid sparing in patients with giant-cell arteritis: results of a multicentre randomised controlled trial. Ann Rheum Dis. 2014;73:2074–81.
25. Martínez-Taboada VM, Rodríguez-Valverde V, Carreño L, López-Longo J, Figueroa M, Belzunegui J, Mola EM, Bonilla G. A double-blind placebo controlled trial of etanercept in patients with giant cell arteritis and corticosteroid side effects. Ann Rheum Dis. 2008;67:625–30.
26. Mohammad AJ, Englund M, Turesson C, Tomasson G, Merkel PA. Rate of comorbidities in giant cell arteritis: a population-based study. J Rheumatol. 2017;44:84–90.
27. Petri H, Nevitt A, Sarsour K, Napalkov P, Collinson N. Incidence of giant cell arteritis and characteristics of patients: data-driven analysis of comorbidities. Arthritis Care Res. 2015;67:390. https://doi.org/10.1002/acr.22429.

Part II

Takayasu Arteritis

Classification Criteria, Epidemiology and Genetics; and Pathogenesis

8

Tanaz A. Kermani and Kenneth J. Warrington

Abstract

Takayasu arteritis (TAK) is a granulomatous large-vessel vasculitis, predominantly affecting the aorta and/or its major branches. Younger age is often used to distinguish it from patients with another form of large-vessel vasculitis, giant cell arteritis, but older age at onset has been well recognized. The incidence and prevalence of TAK varies by geographic region with the highest estimated prevalence in Japan at 40 per million. The strongest genetic susceptibility is with the major histocompatibility complex (MHC) Class I allele HLA-B52. The etiology of TAK is unknown and the pathogenesis is poorly understood. Histopathology of affected vessels show mixed inflammatory infiltrate comprising of macrophages with variable amounts of T- and B-lymphocytes and plasma cells. Cell-mediated autoimmunity appears to play a major role in TAK with recent studies demonstrating the importance of T-helper subsets Th1 and Th17.

Keywords

Epidemiology · Giant cell arteritis · Large-vessel vasculitis · Pathogenesis · Takayasu arteritis

T. A. Kermani (✉)
Division of Rheumatology, David Geffen School of Medicine, University of California, Los Angeles, CA, USA
e-mail: tkermani@mednet.ucla.edu

K. J. Warrington
Division of Rheumatology, Mayo Clinic, Rochester, MN, USA
e-mail: warrington.kenneth@mayo.edu

© Springer Nature Switzerland AG 2021
C. Salvarani et al. (eds.), *Large and Medium Size Vessel and Single Organ Vasculitis*, Rare Diseases of the Immune System, https://doi.org/10.1007/978-3-030-67175-4_8

8.1 Classification Criteria

The revised International Chapel Hill Consensus Conference (CHCC) on the Nomenclature of Systemic Vasculitides defines Takayasu arteritis (TAK) as "arteritis, often granulomatous, predominantly affecting the aorta and/or its major branches [1]." However, this form of large-vessel vasculitis (LVV) can be difficult to distinguish from giant cell arteritis (GCA) which is also a granulomatous LVV [1]. Age is often used to make the distinction although better classification criteria are being developed. The CHCC definition suggests age of onset typically before the age of 50 years for TAK compared to patients with GCA where onset is usually after age 50 years [1].

While CHCC provides a definition of TAK, the first diagnostic criteria for TAK were proposed in 1988 by Ishikawa [2]. This included the obligatory criterion of age ≤40 years with the presence of clinical laboratory and imaging parameters grouped as 2 major and 9 minor criteria, Table 8.1 [2]. Presence of 2 major criteria, 1 major and ≥2 minor criteria or ≥4 minor criteria was highly associated with probability of TAK [2]. The sensitivity of the criteria was 84% with the highest sensitivity (96%) in patients with active disease [2].

The 1990 American College of Rheumatology (ACR) classification criteria for TAK are listed in Table 8.2 [3]. In the data set used to develop these criteria, age at disease onset ≤40 years was the single most discriminatory variable in classifying patients with TAK from GCA [4]. The ACR classification criteria for giant cell

Table 8.1 Ishikawa Diagnostic Criteria for Takayasu arteritis[a] [2]

Obligatory criteria:
Age at disease onset ≤40 years
Major criteria:
Left mid-subclavian artery lesion
Right mid-subclavian artery lesion
Minor criteria:
Elevated sedimentation rate ≥20 mm/h
Common carotid artery tenderness
Hypertension
Aortic regurgitation or ectasia
Lesion[b] of:
Pulmonary artery
Left mid common carotid artery
Distal brachiocephalic trunk
Descending thoracic aorta
Abdominal aorta

[a]TAK highly likely when 2 major criteria, 1 major and ≥2 minor criteria or ≥4 minor criteria
[b]Based on angiography: abnormalities include stenosis, occlusion for the common carotid and brachiocephalic trunk, or, narrowing, dilatation, aneurysm, luminal irregularity for the pulmonary artery or aorta

Table 8.2 American College of Rheumatology Classification Criteria for Takayasu arteritis[a] [3]

1. Age at disease onset <40 years
2. Claudication of extremities
3. Decreased brachial artery pulse
4. Blood pressure difference >10 mmHg between arms
5. Bruit over subclavian arteries or aorta
6. Arteriogram abnormality

[a]Presence of three or more of the above criteria has a sensitivity of 90.5% and specificity of 97.8% for the diagnosis of Takayasu arteritis

arteritis (GCA), which is the other major form of LVV, uses age ≥50 years [5]. The classification of patients between 41 and 49 years with LVV remains problematic with recent studies suggesting they are more likely late-onset TAK than early onset GCA [6]. While the two main forms of LVV share similarities, there are genetic, epidemiologic, imaging and pathophysiologic differences between TAK and GCA [7].

Classification criteria have been validated for childhood TAK by the European League against Rheumatism, the Pediatric Rheumatology International Trials Organization, and the Pediatric Rheumatology European Society (EULAR/PRINTO/PRES) [8]. A diagnosis of TAK requires the presence of angiographic abnormalities of the aorta or its main branches and pulmonary arteries (mandatory criterion) and at least 1 of the following 5 criteria: (1) pulse deficit or claudication; (2) blood pressure discrepancy in any limb; (3) bruits; (4) hypertension; (5) elevated acute phase reactant.

The Diagnostic and Classification Criteria in Vasculitis (DCVAS) is a multinational collaborative effort to develop and validate diagnostic criteria, and, to improve and validate classification criteria for primary systemic vasculitis including TAK [9]. It is anticipated that updated classification criteria based on the DCVAS study will be published in the near future.

8.2 Epidemiology and Genetics

8.2.1 Incidence and Prevalence

TAK is an uncommon disease. An autopsy study from Japan found evidence of TAK was present in 0.033% cases [10].

Studies evaluating the incidence of TAK are sparse. The incidence varies by geographic region with annual estimates ranging from 0.8 to 3.4 per million. The reported annual incidences in Israel and the United States are 2.1–2.6 cases per million population per year [11, 12]. The lowest reported incidence was from a population-based study from the United Kingdom at 0.8 cases per million population [13]. A study from Norway found that the incidence of TAK between 1999 and 2003 was 1 per million/year and increased to 2 per million/year in the period

2008–2012. The exact reason for this increase was unclear although the greater availability of advanced imaging studies in recent years may have contributed to this observation [14]. In a population-based national database from Korea, the estimated incidence of TAK was 2.4 per million [15]. Hospital-based studies from Turkey have reported incidences ranging from 1.1 to 3.4 per million [16, 17].

Likewise, the prevalence of TAK varies by geographic location. A nationwide registry from Japan estimates the prevalence of TAK at >0.004% (40 per million) [18]. In Korea, the reported prevalence is 28.2 per million [15]. Studies from Turkey estimate the prevalence of TAK between 12.8 and 33 per million [16, 17]. In the study from the United Kingdom, the estimated prevalence was 4.7 per million while in a recent study from Norway the prevalence ranged from 22 to 25 per million (depending on criteria used to define TAK) [13, 14]. Furthermore, in the study from Norway, the highest prevalence was noted in residents of Asian and African descent [14].

8.2.2   Sex

TAK is a disease that predominantly affects females. In a large study of 1372 cases of TAK from the nationwide database in Japan, female:male ratio of 5:1 was reported though in a smaller study from Turkey, a female:male ratio as high as 12:1 was observed [17, 19].

8.2.3   Age at Diagnosis

TAK is a disease that predominantly affects younger individuals with peak onset in the second and third decades. Furthermore, criteria from Ishikawa and the ACR use a mandatory age $\leq$40 years for TAK [2, 3]. However, it is being increasingly recognized that TAK can also affect individuals >40 years of age. In clinical series of TAK, up to 13–43% of patients were >40 years old at diagnosis [14, 19–24]. In a large national registry of 1372 patients from Japan, age at onset >40 years was observed in 43% [19]. Furthermore, in this study, a bimodal peak for distribution of age at onset was observed with the major peak in the 15- to 29-year age group, and a minor broader peak in the 50- to 74-year age groups [19]. The median age at onset of male patients (43.5 years) was significantly higher than that of female patients (34 years), $p < 0.001$ [19].

In the nationwide registry from Japan, female patients with late-onset TAK also tended to have more coronary artery involvement [19]. In another multiethnic cohort of patients with TAK, a greater proportion of patients with TAK >40 years were White than non-White [20]. In one study, there was a longer delay in diagnosis of TAK in patients >40 years even though they had similar manifestations to those who presented at an earlier age [23]. One report found a higher prevalence of dyslipidemia in patients diagnosed with TAK >40 years while two other studies including a large national registry from Japan found a higher proportion of patients with TAK >40 years had hypertension [19, 23, 25].

8.2.4 Major Histocompatibility Complex

The strongest genetic susceptibility associated with TAK is with the Major Histocompatibility Complex (MHC) Class I allele HLA-B*52:01 [26–28]. This has been observed in patients with TAK from different ethnicities [29]. Furthermore, it is the only HLA-B allele associated with TAK at a genome-wide significance level [27, 28]. In patients with TAK, the presence of HLA-B*52:01 has been associated with higher risk of aortic regurgitation [30, 31].

Other HLA-B alleles associated with TAK include HLA-B*39 and HLA-B*67 in the Japanese population and HLA-B13 in the Turkish and European-American populations [27, 32–34]. HLA-Cw*07 also reached genome-wide significance for association in patients with TAK of Japanese, Turkish, and European-American descent, but this is possibly dependent on HLA-B*52 with which it is in high linkage disequilibrium [29].

HLA class II alleles HLA-DPB1*09 and HLA-DRB1*15 have been associated with TAK in the Japanese population, but this association may be related to HLA-B*52 susceptibility due to linkage disequilibrium [29]. Association with HLA-DRB1 and HLA-DQB1 was also reported at genome-wide significant levels in a study evaluating the Turkish and European-American populations [27]. HLA-DRB1*07 was associated with TAK susceptibility in a study from China [35].

Several studies have also found an association of HLA-B/MHC class I chain-related (MICA) polymorphisms with TAK [26, 27, 36, 37]. Increased MICA expression has been reported in aortic tissues from patients with TAK and may contribute to the disease pathogenesis [38].

8.2.5 Non-MHC

Interleukin (IL)-12B locus has been associated with TAK in Japanese and Chinese populations based on a recent meta-analysis using immunochip data [26, 28, 39]. Furthermore, in a study from Japan, IL12B had a synergistic effect on TAK susceptibility in combination with HLA-B*52:01 [28]. Presence of IL12B SNP has been associated with age of onset <20 years, relapses and resistance to glucocorticoid treatment [40]. IL12 encodes the IL12p40 which is a subunit of IL12 and IL23. IL12 plays a role in the proliferation of Th1 cells, and IL23 is important for survival and activation of Th17 [41]. Th1 and Th17 have been associated with many autoimmune diseases including TAK, and therefore this may play an important role in disease pathogenesis.

Fc fragment of IgG receptor IIa/IIa (FCGR2A/3A) has also been associated with TAK in a study evaluating Turkish and European-American populations, and, a study in the Chinese population [27, 42].

8.3   Pathogenesis

The etiology of TAK is unknown and the pathogenesis remains poorly understood. *Mycobacterium tuberculosis* infection has been proposed as a potential cause given the presence of granulomatous inflammation in TAK. In one series of 107 patients, 48% of patients with TAK had active tuberculosis [43]. Two recent series reported the prevalence of tuberculosis in patients with TAK at around 20% which is still higher than the general population [44, 45]. A higher frequency of IS6110 (a sequence which identifies the *Mycobacterium tuberculosis* complex), and, the HupB (differentiates *M. tuberculosis* from *M. bovis*) gene expression was noted in the aortic tissues from patients with TAK (70%) and tuberculosis (82%) and in only 32% of patients with atherosclerosis suggesting a link [46]. However, in other studies, mycobacterial DNA was not detectable in the peripheral blood and/or arteries from patients with TAK [47, 48].

Histopathology of the vessels affected by TAK show granulomatous inflammation with mixed inflammatory infiltrate comprising of macrophages with variable amounts of T- and B-lymphocytes, plasma cells, and eosinophils [49]. Medial necrosis may be present [49]. In the late phase of the disease, scarring can be seen in the media with disruption and disorganization of the remaining elastic fibers. The presence of dense adventitial fibrosis and significant intimal fibrous thickening with an overlap of fibroatheromatous plaques give a "tree bark" appearance to the intimal surface (Fig. 8.1). As opposed to GCA where the severe inflammation is predominantly in the inner media, severe adventitial scarring appears more common in TAK [49].

Cell-mediated autoimmunity appears to play a major role in TAK with immunohistochemical studies showing vascular infiltrates composed of macrophages, CD4+ T-cells, CD8+ T-cells, γδ T-cells, neutrophils, and natural killer (NK) cells [50–52]. The following sequence of events has been hypothesized in the pathogenesis of TAK [52]: An unknown stimulus triggers the expression of the 65 kDA heat-shock protein (HSP) in the aortic tissue which induces MICA on vascular cells [52]. The γδ T-cells and NK cells expressing NKG2D receptors recognize MICA on smooth muscle cells and release perforin causing acute vascular inflammation [52]. The release of proinflammatory cytokines causes recruitment of mononuclear cells, T-helper (Th)-1 and Th17 cells [52]. Th1 and Th17 pathways appear important in the pathogenesis and, have been associated with clinical disease activity in patients with TAK [53]. Two recent studies have also implicated the mammalian target of rapamycin (mTOR) pathway in the pathogenesis of TAK [54, 55].

The role of B cells in TAK remains controversial. B cells are not abundant in the inflammatory infiltrate in TAK lesions [49]. In a small study of seven patients, accumulation of memory/germinal center-like B cells was present in the adventitial layer

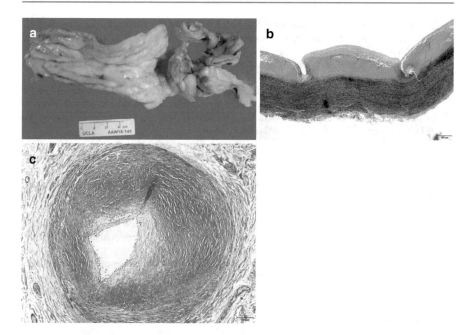

Fig. 8.1 "Tree barking" of the thoracic aorta in a patient with severe Takayasu arteritis (panel A); histopathology of the aorta in a patient with Takayasu arteritis showing intimal proliferation and scarring on elastin stain (panel B), and, histopathology of coronary artery involvement (trichrome stain) in a patient with Takayasu arteritis with medial attenuation and severe intimal fibrosis consistent with healed arteritis (panel C)

of aortic specimens from TAK [56]. Higher levels of circulating B-lymphocytes and anti-endothelial antibodies have been reported in patients with TAK [57]. Increased levels of B cell activating factor (BAFF) have also been reported in TAK in a study from Japan though in a study from India, the findings were not replicated [58, 59]. There are also reports of response of TAK to treatment with rituximab [60, 61].

References

1. Jennette JC. Overview of the 2012 revised International Chapel Hill Consensus Conference nomenclature of vasculitides. Clin Exp Nephrol. 2013;17(5):603–6.
2. Ishikawa K. Diagnostic approach and proposed criteria for the clinical diagnosis of Takayasu's arteriopathy. J Am Coll Cardiol. 1988;12(4):964–72.
3. Arend WP, Michel BA, Bloch DA, Hunder GG, Calabrese LH, Edworthy SM, et al. The American College of Rheumatology 1990 criteria for the classification of Takayasu arteritis. Arthritis Rheum. 1990;33(8):1129–34.
4. Michel BA, Arend WP, Hunder GG. Clinical differentiation between giant cell (temporal) arteritis and Takayasu's arteritis. J Rheumatol. 1996;23(1):106–11.
5. Hunder GG, Bloch DA, Michel BA, Stevens MB, Arend WP, Calabrese LH, et al. The American College of Rheumatology 1990 criteria for the classification of giant cell arteritis. Arthritis Rheum. 1990;33(8):1122–8.

6. Kermani TA, Crowson CS, Muratore F, Schmidt J, Matteson EL, Warrington KJ. Extra-cranial giant cell arteritis and Takayasu arteritis: how similar are they? Semin Arthritis Rheum. 2015;44(6):724–8.
7. Kermani TA. Takayasu arteritis and giant cell arteritis: are they a spectrum of the same disease? Int J Rheum Dis. 2019;22(Suppl 1):41–8.
8. Ozen S, Pistorio A, Iusan SM, Bakkaloglu A, Herlin T, Brik R, et al. EULAR/PRINTO/PRES criteria for Henoch-Schonlein purpura, childhood polyarteritis nodosa, childhood Wegener granulomatosis and childhood Takayasu arteritis: Ankara 2008. Part II: final classification criteria. Ann Rheum Dis. 2010;69(5):798–806.
9. Seeliger B, Sznajd J, Robson JC, Judge A, Craven A, Grayson PC, et al. Are the 1990 American College of Rheumatology vasculitis classification criteria still valid? Rheumatology (Oxford). 2017;56(7):1154–61.
10. Hotchi M. Pathological studies on Takayasu arteritis. Heart Vessels Suppl. 1992;7:11–7.
11. Hall S, Barr W, Lie JT, Stanson AW, Kazmier FJ, Hunder GG. Takayasu arteritis. A study of 32 North American patients. Medicine (Baltimore). 1985;64(2):89–99.
12. Nesher G, Ben-Chetrit E, Mazal B, Breuer GS. The incidence of primary systemic vasculitis in Jerusalem: a 20-year hospital-based retrospective study. J Rheumatol. 2016;43(6):1072–7.
13. Watts R, Al-Taiar A, Mooney J, Scott D, Macgregor A. The epidemiology of Takayasu arteritis in the UK. Rheumatology (Oxford). 2009;48(8):1008–11.
14. Gudbrandsson B, Molberg O, Garen T, Palm O. Prevalence, incidence, and disease characteristics of Takayasu arteritis by ethnic background: data from a large, population-based cohort resident in southern Norway. Arthritis Care Res (Hoboken). 2017;69(2):278–85.
15. Park SJ, Kim HJ, Park H, Hann HJ, Kim KH, Han S, et al. Incidence, prevalence, mortality and causes of death in Takayasu Arteritis in Korea—a nationwide, population-based study. Int J Cardiol. 2017;235:100–4.
16. Saritas F, Donmez S, Direskeneli H, Pamuk ON. The epidemiology of Takayasu arteritis: a hospital-based study from northwestern part of Turkey. Rheumatol Int. 2016;36(7):911–6.
17. Birlik M, Kucukyavas Y, Aksu K, Solmaz D, Can G, Taylan A, et al. Epidemiology of Takayasu's arteritis in Turkey. Clin Exp Rheumatol. 2016;34(3 Suppl 97):S33–9.
18. JCS Joint Working Group. Guideline for management of vasculitis syndrome (JCS 2008). Japanese Circulation Society. Circ J. 2011;75(2):474–503.
19. Watanabe Y, Miyata T, Tanemoto K. Current clinical features of new patients with Takayasu arteritis observed from cross-country research in Japan: age and sex specificity. Circulation. 2015;132(18):1701–9.
20. Arnaud L, Haroche J, Limal N, Toledano D, Gambotti L, Costedoat Chalumeau N, et al. Takayasu arteritis in France: a single-center retrospective study of 82 cases comparing white, North African, and black patients. Medicine (Baltimore). 2010;89(1):1–17.
21. Kerr GS, Hallahan CW, Giordano J, Leavitt RY, Fauci AS, Rottem M, et al. Takayasu arteritis. Ann Intern Med. 1994;120(11):919–29.
22. Ohigashi H, Haraguchi G, Konishi M, Tezuka D, Kamiishi T, Ishihara T, et al. Improved prognosis of Takayasu arteritis over the past decade—comprehensive analysis of 106 patients. Circ J. 2012;76(4):1004–11.
23. Schmidt J, Kermani TA, Bacani AK, Crowson CS, Cooper LT, Matteson EL, et al. Diagnostic features, treatment, and outcomes of Takayasu arteritis in a US cohort of 126 patients. Mayo Clin Proc. 2013;88(8):822–30.
24. Vanoli M, Daina E, Salvarani C, Sabbadini MG, Rossi C, Bacchiani G, et al. Takayasu's arteritis: a study of 104 Italian patients. Arthritis Rheum. 2005;53(1):100–7.
25. Yoshida N, Watanabe R, Ishii T, Machiyama T, Akita K, Fujita Y, et al. Retrospective analysis of 95 patients with large vessel vasculitis: a single center experience. Int J Rheum Dis. 2016;19(1):87–94.
26. Carmona FD, Coit P, Saruhan-Direskeneli G, Hernandez-Rodriguez J, Cid MC, Solans R, et al. Analysis of the common genetic component of large-vessel vasculitides through a meta-Immunochip strategy. Sci Rep. 2017;7:43953.

27. Saruhan-Direskeneli G, Hughes T, Aksu K, Keser G, Coit P, Aydin SZ, et al. Identification of multiple genetic susceptibility loci in Takayasu arteritis. Am J Hum Genet. 2013;93(2):298–305.
28. Terao C, Yoshifuji H, Kimura A, Matsumura T, Ohmura K, Takahashi M, et al. Two susceptibility loci to Takayasu arteritis reveal a synergistic role of the IL12B and HLA-B regions in a Japanese population. Am J Hum Genet. 2013;93(2):289–97.
29. Renauer P, Sawalha AH. The genetics of Takayasu arteritis. Presse Med. 2017;46(7–8 Pt 2):e179–e87.
30. Kitamura H, Kobayashi Y, Kimura A, Numano F. Association of clinical manifestations with HLA-B alleles in Takayasu arteritis. Int J Cardiol. 1998;66(Suppl 1):S121–6.
31. Yajima M, Numano F, Park YB, Sagar S. Comparative studies of patients with Takayasu arteritis in Japan, Korea and India—comparison of clinical manifestations, angiography and HLA-B antigen. Jpn Circ J. 1994;58(1):9–14.
32. Kimura A, Kitamura H, Date Y, Numano F. Comprehensive analysis of HLA genes in Takayasu arteritis in Japan. Int J Cardiol. 1996;54(Suppl):S61–9.
33. Takamura C, Ohhigashi H, Ebana Y, Isobe M. New human leukocyte antigen risk allele in Japanese patients with Takayasu arteritis. Circ J. 2012;76(7):1697–702.
34. Yoshida M, Kimura A, Katsuragi K, Numano F, Sasazuki T. DNA typing of HLA-B gene in Takayasu's arteritis. Tissue Antigens. 1993;42(2):87–90.
35. Lv N, Wang Z, Dang A, Zhu X, Liu Y, Zheng D, et al. HLA-DQA1, DQB1 and DRB1 alleles associated with Takayasu arteritis in the Chinese Han population. Hum Immunol. 2015;76(4):241–4.
36. Kimura A, Ota M, Katsuyama Y, Ohbuchi N, Takahashi M, Kobayashi Y, et al. Mapping of the HLA-linked genes controlling the susceptibility to Takayasu's arteritis. Int J Cardiol. 2000;75 Suppl 1:S105–10; discussion S11–2.
37. Wen X, Chen S, Li J, Li Y, Li L, Wu Z, et al. Association between genetic variants in the human leukocyte antigen-B/MICA and Takayasu arteritis in Chinese Han population. Int J Rheum Dis. 2018;21(1):271–7.
38. Seko Y, Sugishita K, Sato O, Takagi A, Tada Y, Matsuo H, et al. Expression of costimulatory molecules (4-1BBL and Fas) and major histocompatibility class I chain-related A (MICA) in aortic tissue with Takayasu's arteritis. J Vasc Res. 2004;41(1):84–90.
39. Wen X, Chen S, Li P, Li J, Wu Z, Li Y, et al. Single nucleotide polymorphisms of IL12B are associated with Takayasu arteritis in Chinese Han population. Rheumatol Int. 2017;37(4):547–55.
40. Matsumura T, Amiya E, Tamura N, Maejima Y, Komuro I, Isobe M. A novel susceptibility locus for Takayasu arteritis in the IL12B region can be a genetic marker of disease severity. Heart Vessel. 2016;31(6):1016–9.
41. Teng MW, Bowman EP, McElwee JJ, Smyth MJ, Casanova JL, Cooper AM, et al. IL-12 and IL-23 cytokines: from discovery to targeted therapies for immune-mediated inflammatory diseases. Nat Med. 2015;21(7):719–29.
42. Chen S, Wen X, Li J, Li Y, Li L, Tian X, et al. Association of FCGR2A/FCGR3A variant rs2099684 with Takayasu arteritis in the Han Chinese population. Oncotarget. 2017;8(10):17239–45.
43. Lupi-Herrera E, Sanchez-Torres G, Marcushamer J, Mispireta J, Horwitz S, Vela JE. Takayasu's arteritis. Clinical study of 107 cases. Am Heart J. 1977;93(1):94–103.
44. Lim AY, Lee GY, Jang SY, Gwag HB, Choi SH, Jeon ES, et al. Comparison of clinical characteristics in patients with Takayasu arteritis with and without concomitant tuberculosis. Heart Vessel. 2016;31(8):1277–84.
45. Mwipatayi BP, Jeffery PC, Beningfield SJ, Matley PJ, Naidoo NG, Kalla AA, et al. Takayasu arteritis: clinical features and management: report of 272 cases. ANZ J Surg. 2005;75(3):110–7.
46. Soto ME, Del Carmen Avila-Casado M, Huesca-Gomez C, Alarcon GV, Castrejon V, Soto V, et al. Detection of IS6110 and HupB gene sequences of Mycobacterium tuberculosis and bovis in the aortic tissue of patients with Takayasu's arteritis. BMC Infect Dis. 2012;12:194.
47. Arnaud L, Cambau E, Brocheriou I, Koskas F, Kieffer E, Piette JC, et al. Absence of Mycobacterium tuberculosis in arterial lesions from patients with Takayasu's arteritis. J Rheumatol. 2009;36(8):1682–5.

48. Carvalho ES, de Souza AW, Leao SC, Levy-Neto M, de Oliveira RS, Drake W, et al. Absence of mycobacterial DNA in peripheral blood and artery specimens in patients with Takayasu arteritis. Clin Rheumatol. 2017;36(1):205–8.
49. Stone JR, Bruneval P, Angelini A, Bartoloni G, Basso C, Batoroeva L, et al. Consensus statement on surgical pathology of the aorta from the Society for Cardiovascular Pathology and the Association for European Cardiovascular Pathology: I. Inflammatory diseases. Cardiovasc Pathol. 2015;24(5):267–78.
50. Seko Y, Minota S, Kawasaki A, Shinkai Y, Maeda K, Yagita H, et al. Perforin-secreting killer cell infiltration and expression of a 65-kD heat-shock protein in aortic tissue of patients with Takayasu's arteritis. J Clin Invest. 1994;93(2):750–8.
51. Chauhan SK, Singh M, Nityanand S. Reactivity of gamma/delta T cells to human 60-kd heat-shock protein and their cytotoxicity to aortic endothelial cells in Takayasu arteritis. Arthritis Rheum. 2007;56(8):2798–802.
52. Arnaud L, Haroche J, Mathian A, Gorochov G, Amoura Z. Pathogenesis of Takayasu's arteritis: a 2011 update. Autoimmun Rev. 2011;11(1):61–7.
53. Saadoun D, Garrido M, Comarmond C, Desbois AC, Domont F, Savey L, et al. Th1 and Th17 cytokines drive inflammation in Takayasu arteritis. Arthritis Rheumatol. 2015;67(5):1353–60.
54. Hadjadj J, Canaud G, Mirault T, Samson M, Bruneval P, Regent A, et al. mTOR pathway is activated in endothelial cells from patients with Takayasu arteritis and is modulated by serum immunoglobulin G. Rheumatology (Oxford). 2018;57(6):1011–20.
55. Maciejewski-Duval A, Comarmond C, Leroyer A, Zaidan M, Le Joncour A, Desbois AC, et al. mTOR pathway activation in large vessel vasculitis. J Autoimmun. 2018;94:99–109.
56. Clement M, Galy A, Bruneval P, Morvan M, Hyafil F, Benali K, et al. Tertiary lymphoid organs in Takayasu arteritis. Front Immunol. 2016;7:158.
57. Wang H, Ma J, Wu Q, Luo X, Chen Z, Kou L. Circulating B lymphocytes producing autoantibodies to endothelial cells play a role in the pathogenesis of Takayasu arteritis. J Vasc Surg. 2011;53(1):174–80.
58. Nishino Y, Tamai M, Kawakami A, Koga T, Makiyama J, Maeda Y, et al. Serum levels of BAFF for assessing the disease activity of Takayasu arteritis. Clin Exp Rheumatol. 2010;28(1 Suppl 57):14–7.
59. Zanwar A, Jain A, Gupta L, Chaurasia S, Kumar S, Misra DP, et al. Serum BAFF and APRIL levels in Indian patients with Takayasu arteritis. Clin Rheumatol. 2018;37(12):3439–42.
60. Hoyer BF, Mumtaz IM, Loddenkemper K, Bruns A, Sengler C, Hermann KG, et al. Takayasu arteritis is characterised by disturbances of B cell homeostasis and responds to B cell depletion therapy with rituximab. Ann Rheum Dis. 2012;71(1):75–9.
61. Pazzola G, Muratore F, Pipitone N, Crescentini F, Cacoub P, Boiardi L, et al. Rituximab therapy for Takayasu arteritis: a seven patients experience and a review of the literature. Rheumatology (Oxford). 2018;57(7):1151–5.

Clinical Manifestations, Differential Diagnosis, and Laboratory Markers

9

Fatma Alibaz-Oner and Haner Direskeneli

Abstract

As a large-vessel arteritis, Takayasu's arteritis (TAK) predominantly affects aorta and its major branches. Arterial stenosis, occlusion, and aneurysms lead to various signs and symptoms such as consitutional features, extremity pain, claudication, light-headedness, bruits, absent or diminished pulses, and loss of blood pressure. As acute-phase reactants, ESR and C-reactive protein are frequently advocated for disease assessment of TAK. Recently, a member of pentraxin family, PTX-3 was suggested to be a discriminative marker for active disease in TAK, with controversial results. Giant-cell arteritis, accelerated atherosclerosis, and various non-inflammatory vascular disorders have clinical similarities with TAK and should be investigated in the differential diagnosis.

Keywords

Clinical manifestations · Acute-phase response · Differential diagnosis

Takayasu's arteritis (TAK) is a rare, chronic granulomatous large-vessel arteritis that predominantly affects aorta and its major branches which may lead to segmental stenosis, occlusion, dilatation and/or aneurysm formation. TAK, also known as *"pulseless disease," "aortic arch syndrome,"* or *"occlusive thromboarthropathy,"* was first described by Mikito Takayasu who is a Japanese ophthalmologist, as a case of retinal vasculitis with pulselessness in 1908 [1]. Although all large arteries

F. Alibaz-Oner · H. Direskeneli (✉)
Division of Rheumatology, Department of Internal Medicine, Marmara University, School of Medicine, Istanbul, Turkey

© Springer Nature Switzerland AG 2021
C. Salvarani et al. (eds.), *Large and Medium Size Vessel and Single Organ Vasculitis*, Rare Diseases of the Immune System,
https://doi.org/10.1007/978-3-030-67175-4_9

including pulmonary arteries as well as medium-sized coronary arteries can be affected, aorta, subclavian, and carotid arteries are the most commonly involved (60–90%) [2, 3].

9.1 Clinical Manifestations

The clinical manifestatations of TAK changes according to the involved arteries (Table 9.1). Arterial stenosis, occlusion, and aneurysms lead to various signs and symptoms such as extremity pain, claudication, light-headedness, constitutional features (such as fever, malaise, anorexia, and weight loss), bruits, absent or diminished pulses, and loss of blood pressure. TAK generally follows an insidious course at onset but presentation with atypical and/or catastrophic disease such as acute visual loss or stroke may also occur. Unfortunately, many patients experience considerable delay in diagnosis since there are no specific diagnostic laboratory tests, biomarkers, or autoantibodies [4].

The clinical course of TAK generally have three phases. The first phase is characterized with nonspecific constitutional inflammatory symptoms such as fever, weight loss, and fatigue. In the second phase, inflammation of arterial walls is prominent, causing carotidynia, neck pain, and sometimes back pain in thoracic and dorsal area. The third phase, thought as the late phase of the disease, is characterized with bruits, decreased or absence of pulses and blood pressure difference between arms and extremity claudication [5]. In an inception cohort from Turkey, signs and symptoms of "systemic inflammation" such as carotidynia and claudication were found to be more prominent in newly diagnosed TAK patients whereas vascular

Table 9.1 Symptoms and signs in Takayasu's arteritis according to involved arteries

Arterial territory	Symptoms	Signs
Subclavian artery	Upper extremity claudication, Raynaud phenomenon, numbness	Bruit, pulseless, decreased pulse and/or blood pressure, muscle atrophy compared to contralateral extremity
Aorta	Chest pain, back pain, dyspnea	Bruit, aortic valve insufficiency
Common carotid artery	Carotidynia, vertigo, dizziness, visual changes, syncope, transient schemic attacks, stroke	Bruit, pulseless
Renal artery	Hypertension	Bruit, rarely renal failure
Vertebral artery	Visual changes, dizziness	
Celiac/mesenteric artery	Abdominal angina, nausea, vomiting	Bruit
Common iliac artery	Lower extremity claudication, numbness	Bruit, pulseless, decreased pulse, and/or blood pressure
Pulmonary artery	Atypical chest pain, dyspnea, rarely hemoptysis	Pulmonary hypertension
Coronary artery	Angina, dyspnea	Myocardial infarction, congestive heart failure

Table 9.2 Clinical characteristics of Inception and Retrospective Cohorts from Turkey

	Inception cohort (*n* = 170)	Retrospective cohort (Bıçakçıgil et al.) (*n* = 248)
Constitutional symptoms	115/165 (69.6%)	163/248 (66%)
Limb claudication	87/131 (66.4%)	119/248 (48%)
Carotidynia	31/130 (18.2%)	–
Pulseless	45/130 (34.6%)	218/248 (88%)
Musculoskeletal manifestations	90/163 (52.9%)	104/248 (42%)
Mucocutaneous manifestations	30/162 (17.6%)	22/248 (8.8%)
Respiratory manifestations	47/163 (28.8%)	22/184 (12%)
Neurologic manifestations	69/163 (40.6%)	156/248 (63%)
Cardiac involvement	64/146 (43.8%)	141/248 (57%)
Ophthalmologic involvement	27/166 (16.2%)	57/248 (36%)

extent and damage accumulates in retrospectively followed cases during the disease course [6] (Table 9.2). During the diagnostic phase, 10–20% of patients with TAK are asymptomatic. Those patients were diagnosed as TAK when their abnormal vascular findings such as pulseless and blood pressure difference between arms were detected incidentally on examination [2].

Active inflammation in the vessel wall can cause tenderness over the vessel. Carotidynia occurs in 2–32% of patients. Stenosis or aneurysm formation as a result of vessel inflammation may cause decreased circulation. This manifests as typical intermittent claudication in extremities. Vertebral and carotid involvement may be asymptomatic or present with transient ischemic attacks, stroke, dizziness, syncope, headache, or visual changes. Mesenteric involvement is common, but gastrointestinal symptoms such as nausea, diarrhea, vomiting, and ischemic abdominal pain are not seen frequently [7]. Hypertension may be seen due to atypical coarctation of the aorta, aortic valve regurgitation related to aortitis or renal artery stenosis [8, 9].

Cardiac involvement is present in about one-third of patients [5, 10]. In a large cohort including 411 patients cardiac involvement was present in 39%. Among this group, valvular abnormalities were found in 82%, myocardial abnormalities in 16%, and coronary artery abnormalities in 12% [11]. In a retrospective study of 1069 patients over 25 years, 70% of patients had aortic regurgitation and nearly half had moderate to severe aortic regurgitation [12]. Pulmonary arterial involvement may not be clinically apparent, but it ranges among 20–56% in autopsy series [13, 14]. Pulmonary hypertension due to vasculits is present in 0–42% in different series [15] and increases the mortality [11].

Takayasu retinopathy and scleritis are uncommon manifestations of the disease [3, 16]. Retinopathy is low in recent series (<10%); however, hypertensive retinopathy associated with poorly regulated hypertension is common as blood pressure monitorization is especially difficulty in cases with bilateral subclavian occlusion. Cutaneous manifestations range between 3 and 28% of patients, the most common one is erythema nodosum. Other skin manifestations such as pyoderma gangrenosum, Raynoud's phenomenon, livedo reticularis, and purpura can be rarely seen in

TAK [17, 18]. Joint involvement may present as arthritis and arthralgia in almost half of the patients, but it does not have a progressive and destructive pattern [3, 19].

There are an increasing number of studies reporting inflammatory bowel disease and other spondyloarthropathy features in TAK [20–22]. In a Turkish study including 69 TAK patients, 14 (20.3%) fulfilled the Assessment of Spondyloarthritis international Society (ASAS) criteria for spondyloarthropathy. Patients having both diseases were required more biologic treatments compared to patients having TAK alone (64.3% vs 29.1%, $p = 0.014$) [23]. It seems that the association between TAK and spondyloarthropathies is more than a simple coincidence. Further investigations are needed focusing on possible shared immuno-pathogenic or genetic processes.

9.2   Physical Examination

Physical examination for new vascular signs is the first step for disease assessment in TAK. Palpation of arterial pulses, blood pressure measurements of all extremities and cardiac, neck and abdominal auscultation for detecting bruits are crucial parts of the physical examination. However, the limitations of physical examination for assessing disease extent was shown by Grayson et al. Although abnormal findings on vascular physical examination are highly associated with the presence of arterial lesions in imaging, at least 30% of arteriographic lesions can be missed with only physical examination [24]. In a recent study, a high specificity was detected for *newly developed* clinical symptoms and concurrent vascular imaging findings. Vascular imaging abnormalities are often present in a patient presenting with a specific head, neck, and arm symptom. However, the presence of ischemic symptoms or even signs may not always indicate active inflammation of the vessel wall. In this context, carotidynia may be considered as a strong indicator of active inflammation whereas limb claudication is usually a sign of vasculitis-associated damage in TAK [25].

9.3   Laboratory: Role of Acute-Phase Response

Erythrocyte sedimentation rate (ESR) and C-reactive protein are frequently advocated for disease assessment of TAK [26], despite being shown to be neither sensitive nor specific enough to monitor disease activity [27, 28]. In one study, active disease was present in the setting of normal laboratory parameters in 23% of patients [29]. Similarly, ESR was elevated in only 72% of patients considered to have active disease and was still high in 44% of patients considered to be in remission [1]. Serum autoantibodies such as anti-aorta or anti-endothelial antibodies [30–32] and serum biomarkers such as IL-6, IL-8, IL-18, and BAFF are shown to be elevated in TAK, but are not disease specific [33–37].

Pentraxin (PTX) superfamily is a group of proteins recognizing a wide range of exogenous pathogenic substances and behaving as acute-phase response mediators [38]. PTX-3 was suggested to be a discriminative marker for active disease in TAK

[39, 40]. In a Turkish TAK cohort, patients had higher serum PTX-3 levels compared to healthy controls, but PTX-3 levels did not differ between patients in active and inactive phases [41]. In an Italian TAK cohort, Tombetti et al. reported that only CRP was higher in active disease and PTX-3 levels were similar between active and inactive patients, similar to the Turkish study. However, significantly higher PTX-3 levels were observed in a subset of patients with "detectable signs of vascular inflammation" shown with vascular imaging [42]. The results with the PTX-3 for activity assessment are controversial and need to be further investigated especially longitudinally.

9.4   Differential Diagnosis

Currently, there are no universally accepted diagnostic criteria for systemic vasculitides, including TAK. 1990 American College of Rheumatology (ACR) criteria, the most widely used in clinical studies, requires the presence of three of six criteria to differentiate TAK from other systemic vasculitis [43] (Table 9.3). However, this criteria set mainly covers late stage of disease and includes conventional angiography as the only imaging modality. In the presence of typical symptoms and physical findings such as loss of pulses and/or decreased arterial blood pressure and elevated acute-phase responses, the diagnosis can be confirmed easily by angiographic imaging modalities. In a young patient with unexplained systemic inflammation, nine red flags should remind TAK to the clinician (Table 9.4) [44]. When the possibility of TAK comes to the mind of the clinician, the diagnosis should be confirmed by the imaging methods—discussed and compared with each other in the following section. Overall, narrowing or occlusion of the aortic arch and proximal parts of its branches is highly suggestive of TAK. Involvement of subclavian arteries, especially the left side, and of common/internal carotid arteries are typical for TAK. Cluster analysis also revealed that TAK lesions mostly develop in a symmetric manner in paired vascular territories and disease extension is contiguous in the aorta [45].

One of the most important disease in differential diagnosis of TAK as a large-vessel vasculitis is GCA. There is an ongoing debate whether they are in a spectrum of the same large-vessel disease or are different entities. Disease onset in young age

Table 9.3   1990 criteria for the classification of Takayasu's arteritis

Age of 40 years or younger at disease onset
Claudication of the extremities
Decreased pulsation of one or both brachial arteries
Difference of at least 10 mmHg in systolic blood pressure between arms
Bruit over one or both subclavian arteries or the abdominal aorta
Arteriographic narrowing or occlusion of the entire aorta, its primary branches, or large arteries in the upper or lower extremities that is not due to arteriosclerosis, fibromuscular dysplasia, or other causes
At least 3 of 6 criteria are necessary for classification

Table 9.4 Red flags to investigate Takayasu's arteritis in a
young patient with otherwise
unexplained   systemic
inflammation

Carotidynia
Hypertension
Angina pectoris
Vertigo and syncope
Extremity claudication
Absent/weak peripheral pulses
Discrepant blood pressure in the upper limbs (>10 mmHg)

(<40), striking female predominence and ethnic discrimination are important dif-
fereneces of TAK. Also, aorta and its main branch involvement is more typical for
TAK. While internal carotid artery branches are involved mostly by TAK, external
carotid artery involvement is more typical for GCA [46, 47]. Grayson et al. also
reported that carotid and mesenteric arterial involvement were more common in
TAK, whereas axillary disease was more common in GCA. Subclavian artery
involvement tended to be asymmetric in TAK with a high frequency of left subclavian artery disease, symmetric subclavian with concomitant axillary involvement
was observed more frequently in GCA [48].

Differentiation of atherosclerotic vascular lesions from vasculitis is another very
important problem for the diagnosis of a patient suspected with TAK. Even if imaging modalities may help in discrimination, it is not always possible in especially
elderly patients having risk factors for atherosclerotic vascular disease. Involvement
of upper extremity vessels is thought to be more typical for TAK, but it may also be
observed in atherosclerosis. While the vasculitic involvement is generally located in
the proximal part of vessels, atherosclerotic lesions are generally located in bifurca-
tion sites and ostia of the vessels. In the vessel wall, vasculitic involvement leads to
diffuse and homogeneous thickening, whereas atherosclerosis leads more localized,
irregular and non-homogeneous thickening. Punctate, linear calcification, and
patchy involvement also suggest atherosclerosis, in contrast to mural and circumferential calcification suggesting diffuse involvement in vasculitis [49].

In the differential diagnosis of TAK, there are many rare entities leading to aortitis. Aortitis can be infectious or non-infectious. The most frequent infectious
agents are salmonella, staphylococcus aureus, streptococcus pneumonia, mycobacterium tuberculosis, human immunodeficiency virus, and rarely Treponema palli-
dum [50]. Non-infectious aortitis may be seen in many inflammatory rheumatologic
diseases such as Behçet's disease [51, 52], IgG4-related disease [53], rheumatoid
arthritis [54], systemic lupus erythematosus [55, 56], Sjögren's syndrome [57],
ANCA-associated vasculitides [58], HLA-B27-associated spondyloarthropathies
[59], psoriatic arthritis [60], sarcoidosis [61], Cogan's syndrome [62], relapsing
polychondritis [63], and inflammatory bowel diseases [64, 65]. Isolated inflammatory aortitis should also be thought in the differential diagnosis of TAK if there is
only aortic involvement. Most of the data for isolated aortitis comes from surgical
case studies, with a prevalence ranging between 4 and 8%. The isolated aortitis is
generally seen in males and older patients in contrast to TAK. Aortic arch, thoracic,
and abdominal aorta are involved in both, but aortic branches are generally spared
in isolated aortitis [66].

9.5   Large-Vessel Vasculitis Mimickers in the Differential Diagnosis of TAK

In a patient presenting with large-vessel vasculitis (LVV) with the history of previous malignity, it should be kept in mind that radiotherapy can cause damage in vascular endothelial cells leading intimal thickening and irregularity with focal fibrosis and necrosis [67].

Congenital aortic coarctation may also be in differential diagnosis in a young TAK patient. It is commonly located in the junction of distal aortic arch and descending aorta, after the origin of the left subclavian artery. However, it is more common in males in contrast to TAK and there is no systemic inflammation. It is often associated with several other cardiac and vascular abnomalies, such as bicuspid aortic valve, ventricular septal defect, patent ductus arteriosus, and aortic arch hypoplasia [68].

Middle aortic syndrome is a clinical condition characterized with segmental narrowing of the abdominal or distal descending thoracic aorta. Segmental aortic stenosis may be located at the suprarenal, inter-renal or infrarenal aorta, with also concomitant stenoses in both the renal (63%) and visceral (33%) arteries. TAK can cause middle aortic syndrome but also various pathologies such as neurofibromatosis, fibromuscular dysplasia, Marfan syndrome, Ehler–Danlos syndrome retroperitoneal fibrosis, mucopolysaccharidosis, Williams syndrome, or congenital, developmental dorsal aorta abnormality [69].

Fibromuscular dysplasia (FMD) is another important clinical entity in the differential diagnosis of TAK in especially a young woman. It is a non-atherosclerotic non-inflammatory vasculapathy primarily affecting women aged between 20 and 60. It most commonly affects the renal and carotid arteries, but almost every artery in the body may be affected. Stenosis, aneurysm, dissection, and occlusion may ocur. Most common presentation is hypertension due to renal artery involvement. The patient also can frequently present with transient ischemic attack, stroke, or dissection due to carotid and/or vertebral involvement. Erythrocyte sedimentation rate and C-reactive protein are usually within normal reference ranges in FMD unless there is infarction of the kidney or bowel. Middle and distal portions of renal, internal carotid, and vertebral arteries are most commonly affected in FMD. Also aortic involvement is rare. Classical imaging findings such as "string-of-beads" appearance, focal concentric narrowing, and diffuse tubular stenosis are discriminative features for FMD. There are also no arterial wall thickening, edema, or contrast uptake on magnetic resonance angiography [70–72].

Segmental arterial mediolysis (SAM) is a rare non-atherosclerotic, non-inflammatory vasculopathy with unknown etiology. It is characterized by lysis of the medial layer of the arterial wall, often resulting in dissection, aneurysm, occlusion, or stenosis [73]. It is controversial whether SAM is a distinct vasculopathy or a subtype of FMD [74]. SAM should also be kept in mind when aneurysms, stenoses, and occlusions are identified in medium and large vessels, especially when these lesions are limited to one anatomic location. Histopathology is gold standard for diagnosis [75]. There is also no significant concurrent arterial wall thickening (<3 mm) or elevation of ESR and C-reactive protein levels in SAM [76].

Table 9.5 Differential features of genetic disorders mimicking Takayasu's arteritis

	Characteristic features	Differential features from TAK
Marfan syndrome	Autosomal dominant disorder of connective tissue matrix with the mutations in the fibrillin-1 gene Aneurysm formation, dissection, and aortic regurgitation can occur due to effects on thoracic aorta wall	No systemic inflammation No arterial wall thickening or stenosis with imaging Histopathology: Cystic medial necrosis without inflammation Typical Marfanoid body status and clinical features including lens Dislocation
Ehlers–Danlos Syndrome Type IV	Autosomal dominant disorder of the connective tissue matrix with the mutations in the type III procollagen gene Dissection, rupture, or aneurysm can occur due to effects on descending and abdominal aorta wall	No systemic inflammation No arterial wall thickening or stenosis with imaging Histopathology: Cystic medial necrosis without inflammation
Loeys–Dietz syndrome	Genetic disorder of the connective tissue matrix with the mutations in the TGF-β receptor gene Tortuosity, aneurysms, and dissections can occur in thoracic and abdominal aorta	No systemic inflammation Clinical features including hypertelorism, bifid uvula, cleft palate, and bicuspid aortic valve
Neurofibromatosis type 1 (NF1) (von Recklinghausen's disease)	Vascular aneurysms/arteriovenous malformations, renal artery stenosis, coarctation of aorta, or segmental narrowing of abdominal or distal descending thoracic aorta	No systemic inflammation Neurocutaneous tumors, plexiform tumors, optic gliomas, hamartomatous Lisch nodules in the iris, café au lait macules, and learning disabilities
Erdheim–Chester disease (ECD)	Non-Langerhans histiocytosis Periarterial thickening, stenosis/occlusion in whole aorta	Histopathology: Xanthogranulomatous infiltration of foamy histiocytes surrounded by fibrosis Cortical osteosclerosis and typical pain of long bones

Rare genetic disorders such as Marfan Syndrome [77, 78], Ehlers–Danlos Syndrome Type IV [75, 79], Loeys–Dietz syndrome (LDS) [75, 80], Neurofibromatosis type 1 (NF1) [81, 82], and Erdheim–Chester disease [83] may mimic Takayasu's arteritis. The differential features of these genetic disorders are summarized in Table 9.5.

References

1. Numano F. The story of Takayasu arteritis. Rheumatology (Oxford). 2002;41:103–6.
2. Kerr GS, Hallahan CW, Giordano J, Leavitt RY, Fauci AS, et al. Takayasu arteritis. Ann Intern Med. 1994;120(11):919–29.

3. Bıcakcıgil M, Aksu K, Kamalı S, Ozbalkan Z, Ates A, et al. Takayasu's arteritis in Turkey—clinical and angiographic features of 248 patients. Clin Exp Rheumatol. 2009;27:S59–64.
4. Alibaz-Oner F, Aydin SZ, Direskeneli H. Advances in the diagnosis, assessment and outcome of Takayasu's arteritis. Clin Rheumatol. 2013;32(5):541–6.
5. Li J, Li H, Sun F, Chen Z, Yang Y, et al. Clinical characteristics of heart involvement in Chinese patients with Takayasu arteritis. J Rheumatol. 2017;44(12):1867–74.
6. Alibaz-Oner F, On behalf of Turkish Vasculitis Study Group. Vascular damage is less present in an early inception cohort in Takayasu's arteritis [abstract]. Arthritis Rheumatol. 2019;71(Suppl 10).
7. Langford C. Takayasu arteritis. In: Hochberg MC, editor. Rheumatology. 7th ed. Philadelphia: Elsevier; 2019. p. 1378–83.
8. Park MC, Lee SW, Park YB, Chung N, Lee SK. Clinical characteristics and outcomes of Takayasu's arteritis: analysis of 108 patients using standardized criteria for diagnosis, activity assessment, and angiographic classification. Scand J Rheumatol. 2005;34:284–92.
9. Vanoli M, Daina E, Salvarani C, Sabbadini M, Rossi C, et al. Takayasu's arteritis: a study of 104 Italian patients. Arthritis Rheum. 2005;53:100–7.
10. Park YB, Hong SK, Choi KJ, Sohn DW, Oh BH, et al. Takayasu arteritis in Korea. Clinical and angiographic features. Heart Vessels Suppl. 1992;7:55–9.
11. He Y, Lv N, Dang A, Cheng N. Pulmonary artery involvement in patients with Takayasu arteritis. J Rheumatol. 2019. pii: jrheum.190045.
12. Zhang Y, Yang K, Meng X, Tian T, Fan P, et al. Cardiac valve involvement in Takayasu arteritis is common: a retrospective study of 1,069 patients over 25 years. Am J Med Sci. 2018;356(4):357–64.
13. Hotchi M. Pathological studies on Takayasu arteritis. Heart Vessels Suppl. 1992;7:11–7.
14. Sharma BK, Jain S, Radotra BD. An autopsy study of Takayasu arteritis in India. Int J Cardiol. 1998;66(Suppl 1):S85–91.
15. Kalfa M, Emmungil H, Musayev O, Gündüz ÖS, Yılmaz Z, et al. Frequency of pulmonary hypertension in transthoracic echocardiography screening is not increased in Takayasu arteritis: experience from a single center in Turkey. Eur J Rheumatol. 2018;5(4):249–53.
16. Esen F, Ergelen R, Alibaz-Öner F, Çelik G, Direskeneli H, Kazokoğlu H. Ocular findings and blood flow in patients with Takayasu arteritis: a cross-sectional study. Br J Ophthalmol. 2019;103(7):928–32.
17. Francès C, Boisnic S, Blétry O, Dallot A, Thomas D, et al. Cutaneous manifestations of Takayasu arteritis. A retrospective study of 80 cases. Dermatologica. 1990;181(4):266–72.
18. Pascual-López M, Hernández-Núñez A, Aragüés-Montañés M, Daudén E, Fraga J, García-Díez A. Takayasu's disease with cutaneous involvement. Dermatology. 2004;208(1):10–5.
19. Lupi-Herrera E, Sanchez-Torres G, Marchushamer J, et al. Takayasu's arteritis: clinical study of 107 cases. Am Heart J. 1977;93:94–103.
20. Riviere E, Arnaud L, Ebbo M, Allanore Y, Claudepierre P, Dernis E, et al. Takayasu arteritis and spondyloarthritis: coincidence or association? A study of 14 cases. J Rheumatol. 2017;44:1011–7.
21. Kilic L, Kalyoncu U, Karadag O, Akdogan A, Dogan I, et al. Inflammatory bowel diseases and Takayasu's arteritis: coincidence or association? Int J Rheum Dis. 2016;19(8):814–8.
22. Kanıtez NA, Toz B, Güllüoğlu M, Erer B, Esen BA, et al. Microscopic colitis in patients with Takayasu's arteritis: a potential association between the two disease entities. Clin Rheumatol. 2016;35(10):2495.
23. Güzel Esen S, Armagan B, Atas N, Ucar M, Varan Ö, et al. Increased incidence of spondyloarthropathies in patients with Takayasu arteritis: a systematic clinical survey. Joint Bone Spine. 2019;86(4):497–501.
24. Grayson PC, Tomasson G, Cuthbertson D, Carette S, Hoffman GS, Khalidi NA, et al. Vasculitis Clinical Research Consortium. Association of vascular physical examination findings and arteriographic lesions in large vessel vasculitis. J Rheumatol. 2012;39(2):303–9.
25. Michailidou D, Rosenblum JS, Rimland CA, Marko J, Ahlman MA, Grayson PC. Clinical symptoms and associated vascular imaging findings in Takayasu's arteritis compared to giant cell arteritis. Ann Rheum Dis. 2020;79(2):262–7. https://doi.org/10.1136/annrheumdis-2019-216145.

26. Salvarani C, Cantini F, Boiardi L, Hunder GG. Laboratory investigations useful in giant cell arteritis and Takayasu's arteritis. Clin Exp Rheumatol. 2003;21(Suppl 32):S23–8.
27. Mason JC. Takayasu arteritis-advances in diagnosis and management. Nat Rev Rheumatol. 2010;6(7):406–15.
28. Hoffman GS, Ahmed AE. Surrogate markers of disease activity in patients with Takayasu arteritis. A preliminary report from The International Network for the Study of the Systemic Vasculitides (INSSYS). Int J Cardiol. 1998;66(Suppl 1):S191–5.
29. Maksimowicz-Mckinnon K, Clark TM, Hoffman GS. Limitations of therapy and a guarded prognosis in an American cohort of Takayasu arteritis patients. Arthritis Rheum. 2007;56:1000–9.
30. Dhingra R, Talwar KK, Chopra P, Kumar R. An enzyme linked immunosorbent assay for detection of anti-aorta antibodies in Takayasu arteritis patients. Int J Cardiol. 1993;40:237–42.
31. Lee SK. Anti-endothelial cell antibodies and antiphospholipid antibodies in Takayasu's arteritis: correlations of their titers and isotype distributions with disease activity. Clin Exp Rheumatol. 2006;24(Suppl 41):S10–6.
32. Chauhan SK, Tripathy NK, Nityanand S. Antigenic targets and pathogenicity of antiaortic endothelial cell antibodies in Takayasu arteritis. Arthritis Rheum. 2006;54:2326–33.
33. Noris M, Daina E, Gamba S, Bonazzola S, Remuzzi G. Interleukin-6 and RANTES in Takayasu arteritis: a guide for therapeutic decisions? Circulation. 1999;100:55–60.
34. Park MC, Lee SW, Park YB, Lee SK. Serum cytokine profiles and their correlations with disease activity in Takayasu's arteritis. Rheumatology. 2006;45:545–8.
35. Tripathy N, Sinha N, Nityanand S. Interleukin-8 in Takayasu's arteritis: plasma levels and relationship with disease activity. Clin Exp Rheumatol. 2004;22:S27–30.
36. Nishino Y, Tamai M, Kawakami A, et al. Serum levels of BAFF for assessing the disease activity of Takayasu arteritis. Clin Exp Rheumatol. 2010;28:14–7.
37. Alibaz-Oner F, Yentur SP, Saruhan-Direskeneli G, Direskeneli H. Serum cytokine profiles in Takayasu's arteritis: a search for a biomarker. Clin Exp Rheumatol. 2015;33(Suppl 89):32–5.
38. Garlanda C, Bottazzi B, Bastone A, Mantovani A. Pentraxins at the crossroads between innate immunity, inflammation, matrix deposition, and female fertility. Annu Rev Immunol. 2005;23:337–66.
39. Ishihara T, Haraguchi G, Kamiishi T, Tezuka D, Inagaki H, Isobe M. Sensitive assessment of activity of Takayasu's arteritis by pentraxin3, a new biomarker. J Am Coll Cardiol. 2011;57(16):1712–3. No abstract available.
40. Dagna L, Salvo F, Tiraboschi M, Bozzolo EP, Franchini S, et al. Pentraxin-3 as a marker of disease activity in Takayasu arteritis. Ann Intern Med. 2011;155(7):425–33.
41. Alibaz-Oner F, Aksu K, Yentur SP, Keser G, Saruhan-Direskeneli G, Direskeneli H. Plasma pentraxin-3 levels in patients with Takayasu's arteritis during routine follow-up. Clin Exp Rheumatol. 2016;34(Suppl 97):S73–6.
42. Tombetti E, Di Chio MC, Sartorelli S, Papa M, Salerno A, et al. Systemic pentraxin-3 levels reflect vascular enhancement and progression in Takayasu arteritis. Arthritis Res Ther. 2014;16:479.
43. Arent WP, Michel BA, Bloch DA, Hunder GG, Calabrese LH, et al. The American College of Rheumatology 1990 criteria for the classification of Takayasu arteritis. Arthritis Rheum. 1990;33:1129–34.
44. Nazareth R, Mason J. Takayasu arteritis: severe consequences of delayed diagnosis. QJM. 2010;104:797–800.
45. Arnaud L, Haroche J, Mathian A, Gorochov G, Amoura Z. Pathogenesis of Takayasu's arteritis: a 2011 update. Autoimmun Rev. 2011;11:61–7.
46. Maksimowicz-McKinnon K, Clark TM, Hoffman GS. Takayasu arteritis and giant cell arteritis: a spectrum within the same disease? Medicine. 2009;88:221–6.
47. Furuta S, Cousins C, Chaudhry A, Jayne D. Clinical features and radiological findings in large vessel vasculitis: are Takayasu arteritis and giant cell arteritis 2 different diseases or a single entity? J Rheumatol. 2015;42:300–8.

48. Grayson PC, Maksimowicz-McKinnon K, Clark TM, Tomasson G, Cuthbertson D, et al. Distribution of arterial lesions in Takayasu's arteritis and giant cell arteritis. Ann Rheum Dis. 2012;71:1329–34.
49. Keser G, Aksu K, Direskeneli H. Takayasu arteritis: an update. Turk J Med Sci. 2018;48(4):681–97.
50. Tavora F, Burke A. Review of isolated ascending aortitis: differential diagnosis, including syphilitic, Takayasu's and giant cell aortitis. Pathology (Phila). 2006;38(4):302–8.
51. Tsui KL, Lee KW, Chan WK, Chan HK, Hon SF, et al. Behçet's aortitis and aortic regurgitation: a report of two cases. J Am Soc Echocardiogr. 2004;17(1):83–6.
52. Sahutoglu T, Artim Esen B, Aksoy M, Kurtoglu M, Poyanli A, Gul A. Clinical course of abdominal aortic aneurysms in Behçet disease: a retrospective analysis. Rheumatol Int. 2019;39(6):1061–7.
53. Stone JH, Khosroshahi A, Deshpande V, Stone JR. IgG4-related systemic diseaseaccounts for a significant proportion of thoracic lymphoplasmacytic aortitis cases. Arthritis Care Res. 2010;62(3):316–22.
54. Kaneko S, Yamashita H, Sugimori Y, Takahashi Y, Kaneko H, et al. Rheumatoid arthritis-associated aortitis: a case report and literature review. Springerplus. 2014;3:509.
55. Brinster DR, Grizzard JD, Dash A. Lupus aortitis leading to aneurysmal dilatation in the aortic root and ascending aorta. Heart Surg Forum. 2009;12(2):E105–8.
56. Sokalski D, Spring TC, Roberts W. Large artery inflammation in systemic lupus erythematosus. Lupus. 2013;22(9):953–6.
57. Loricera J, Blanco R, Hernández JL, Carril JM, Martínez-Rodríguez I, et al. Non-infectious aortitis: a report of 32 cases from a single tertiary centre in a 4-year period and literature review. Clin Exp Rheumatol. 2015;33(2 Suppl 89):S-19–31. Epub 2014 Dec 1.
58. Chirinos JA, Tamariz LJ, Lopes G, Del Carpio F, Zhang X, et al. Large vessel involvement in ANCA-associated vasculitides: report of a case and review of the literature. Clin Rheumatol. 2004;23(2):152–9.
59. Grewal GS, Leipsic J, Klinkhoff AV. Abdominal aortitis in HLA-B27+ spondyloarthritis: case report with 5-year follow-up and literature review. Semin Arthritis Rheum. 2014;44(3):305–8.
60. Tufan A, Tezcan ME, Kaya A, Mercan R, Oner Y, Ozturk MA. Aortitis in a patient with psoriatic arthritis. Mod Rheumatol. 2012;22(5):774–7.
61. Chapelon-Abric C, Saadoun D, Marie I, Comarmond C, DesboisAC, et al. Sarcoidosis with Takayasu arteritis: a model of overlapping granulomatosis. A report of seven cases and literature review. Int J Rheum Dis. 2018;21(3):740–5.
62. Gasparovic H, Djuric Z, Bosnic D, Petricevic M, Brida M, et al. Aortic root vasculitis associated with Cogan's syndrome. Ann Thorac Surg. 2011;92(1):340–1.
63. Erdogan M, Esatoglu SN, Hatemi G, Hamuryudan V. Aortic involvement in relapsing polychondritis: case-based review. Rheumatol Int. 2019. https://doi.org/10.1007/s00296-019-04468-5.
64. Delay C, Schwein A, Lejay A, Gaertner S, Aleil B, et al. Aortitis and aortic occlusion in Crohn disease. Ann Vasc Surg. 2015;29(2):365.e5–9.
65. Kudo T, Aoyagi Y, Fujii T, Ohtsuka Y, Nagata S, Shimizu T. Ulcerative colitis and aortitis syndrome. Pediatr Int. 2010;52(1):e43–5.
66. Talarico R, Boiardi L, Pipitone N, d'Ascanio A, Stagnaro C, et al. Isolated aortitis versus giant cell arteritis: are they really two sides of the same coin? Clin Exp Rheumatol. 2014;32(3 Suppl 82):S55–8.
67. Mertz LE, Conn DL. Vasculitis associated with malignancy. Curr Opin Rheumatol. 1992;4(1):39–46.
68. Dijkema EJ, Leiner T, Grotenhuis HB. Diagnosis, imaging and clinical management of aortic coarctation. Heart. 2017;103(15):1148–55.
69. Delis KT, Gloviczki P. Middle aortic syndrome: from presentation to contemporary open surgical and endovascular treatment. Perspect Vasc Surg Endovasc Ther. 2005;17(3):187–203.
70. Olin JW, Sealove BA. Diagnosis management, and future developments offibromuscular dysplasia. J Vasc Surg. 2011;53(3):826–36.e1.

71. Slovut DP, Olin JW. Fibromuscular dysplasia. N Engl J Med. 2004;350:1862–71.
72. Keser G, Aksu K. Diagnosis and differential diagnosis of large-vessel vasculitides. Rheumatol Int. 2019;39(2):169–85.
73. Shenouda M, Riga C, Naji Y, et al. Segmental arterial mediolysis: a systematic review of 85 cases. Ann Vasc Surg. 2014;28:269–77.
74. Slavin RE, Saeki K, Bhagavan B, Maas AE. Segmental arterial mediolysis: a precursor to fibromuscular dysplasia? Mod Pathol. 1995;8:287–94.
75. Baker-LePain JC, Stone DH, Mattis AN, Nakamura MC, Fye KH. Clinical diagnosis of segmental arterial mediolysis: differentiation from vasculitis and other mimics. Arthritis Care Res (Hoboken). 2010;62(11):1655–60.
76. Skeik N, Olson SL, Hari G, Pavia ML. Segmental arterial mediolysis (SAM): systematic review and analysis of 143 cases. Vasc Med. 2019;24(6):549–63.
77. Khasnis A. Mimics of primary systemic vasculitides. Int J Clin Rheumatol. 2009;4(5):597–609.
78. Milewicz DM, Dietz HC, Miller DC. Treatment of aortic disease in patients with Marfan syndrome. Circulation. 2005;111(11):e150–7.
79. Pepin M, Schwarze U, Superti-Furga A, Byers PH. Clinical and genetic features of Ehlers–Danlos syndrome type IV, the vascular type. N Engl J Med. 2000;342(10):673–80.
80. Loeys BL, Schwarze U, Holm T, Callewaert BL, Thomas GH, et al. Aneurysm syndromes caused by mutations in the TGF-βreceptor. N Engl J Med. 2006;355(8):788–98.
81. Williams VC, Lucas J, Babcock MA, Gutmann DH, Korf B, Maria BL. Neurofibromatosis type 1 revisited. Pediatrics. 2009;123(1):124–33.
82. Borofsky S, Levy LM. Neurofibromatosis: types 1 and 2. Am J Neuroradiol. 2013;34(12):2250–1.
83. Estrada-Veras JI, O'Brien KJ, Boyd LC, Dave RH, Durham BH, et al. The clinical spectrum of Erdheim–Chester disease: an observational cohort study. Blood Adv. 2017;1(6):357–66.

Imaging

10

Fatma Alibaz-Oner and Haner Direskeneli

Abstract

Conventional digital subtraction angiography (DSA) used to be the "gold standard" for the diagnosis of TAK. However, MR angiography has become the most preferred imaging tool for the diagnosis of TAK and is suggested to be the first-choice of modality in recent EULAR guidelines for imaging in LVV. CT angiography is also helpful as a cheap and fast tool to determine the damage associated with vascular stenosis and occlusion. FDG-PET-CT, detecting the vascular distribution of 18-F-FDG, assesses the metabolic, usually inflammatory activity in aorta and its major branches and demonstrate early vascular changes before occlusions or aneursym development during the clinical course of TAK patients. Finally, Doppler US with contrast enhancement is helpful for carotid lesions. The role of imaging to evaluate disease activity is currently an area of promising research, especially for therapeutic clinical trials.

Keywords

Digital subtraction angiography · MR angiography · CT angiography
FDG-PET-CT · CDUS

Angiographic imaging modalities are essential for both the diagnosis and the follow-up of Takayasu Arteritis (TAK) [1]. Ideally, imaging modality in TAK should assess both the arterial lumen and the arterial wall. Luminal changes can be detected only after stenosis, occlusion, or dilatation has occurred. On the other hand, arterial

F. Alibaz-Oner · H. Direskeneli (✉)
Division of Rheumatology, Department of Internal Medicine, Marmara University, School of Medicine, Istanbul, Turkey

© Springer Nature Switzerland AG 2021
C. Salvarani et al. (eds.), *Large and Medium Size Vessel and Single Organ Vasculitis*, Rare Diseases of the Immune System,
https://doi.org/10.1007/978-3-030-67175-4_10

wall changes detected with positron emission tomography (PET), magnetic resonance (MR) imaging, ultrasound (US), or computerized tomography (CT) may reveal pre-stenotic disease which is thought to be the earlier phase of disease [2]. The first detectable vascular abnormality in TAK is usually the thickening of the vessel wall caused by inflammation. The vessel wall thickness can be detected with MR angiography (MRA), US, and to a lesser degree, CT angiography (CTA). Contrast-enhanced MRA or CTA allow non-invasive imaging of the aorta and its major branches. Conventional digital subtraction angiography (DSA) which was thought to be the "gold standard" until recently for the diagnosis of TAK, detects well stenosis, occlusions and aneurysms which usually represents the latter stages of TAK. However, it is the least sensitive method for visualizing wall thickness [3] and is not routinely recommended in recent EULAR guidelines for imaging in LVV [4].

10.1   CTA

CTA shows vascular lumen and the arterial wall well and allows early diagnosis before the development of significant luminal remodeling [5]. In a study including patients with suspected TAK, CTA had a sensitivity of 95% and specificity of 100% for diagnosing TAK compared to clinical criteria [6]. While performing CTA, both early "arterial" and "delayed" phase are acquired following infusion of iodinated contrast. The acquisition of "delayed" phase images is needed to assess late contrast enhancement to evaluate the presence of a double-ring appearance. In delayed images, vessel wall thickening with enhancement and low attenuation ring is indicative for active disease [7, 8]. The presence of low attenuation ring have 100% specificity for active disease assessed by clinical evaluation and acute phase reactants; however the sensitivity is quite low (34–57%). On the other hand, wall thickening together with enhancement has a sensitivity of 88% and a specificity of 75% [9, 10]. In a study using electron beam CTA, there was no association between vessel abnormalities and disease activity by the NIH criteria [11]. The same group also published the follow-up data of five TAK patients having new active CTA lesions but considered inactive by clinical criteria. These patients had complications attributable to these lesions during the follow-up with changes in medical therapy leading to improvement in the CTA findings [12].

An important advantage of CTA is its value in differentiating TAK from atherosclerosis. Vascular calcification can be seen with CTA due to several reasons such as chronic renal failure, atherosclerosis, and rarely vasculitis. However, the radiological appearance of aortic calcification caused by vasculitis seems to differ from atherosclerosis. A circumferential calcification pattern is observed only in TAK [13]. Thoracic aorta involvement was also more common in TAK compared to SLE in the same study. Assessing coronary artery calcification is also possible with CTA [14].

The clinical utility of CTA is similar to MRA both in the diagnosis and the assessment during the follow-up of patients with TAK. An important advantage of

CTA over MRA is its shorter acquisition time in daily practice. However, exposure to large amounts of radiation and iodinated contrast limits the usefulness of CTA in routine follow-up [15].

10.2 MRA

Currently, MRA has become the most preferred imaging tool for the diagnosis of TAK and is suggested to be the first-choice of modality in EULAR guidelines [4]. Lack of radiation exposure allows multiple longitudinal evaluations in young patients. Contrast-enhanced MRA also allow non-invasive imaging of the aorta and its major branches, defining better the features of thickened arterial wall. But this type of assessment needs longer duration compared to standard analysis. In MRA assessment, T1-weighted imaging is used to localize arterial wall lesions. For detecting changes suggestive of active inflammation in arterial vessel wall, T2-weighted and contrast-enhanced T1-weighted imagings are used to assess wall edema and late contrast enhancement, respectively [2]. In a meta-analysis of three studies ($n = 182$) investigating the utility of MRA (1.5 T) for the diagnosis of TAK compared to DSA to detect vessel stenosis, occlusion, or dilatation, the pooled sensitivity and specificities were 79% and 97%, respectively. Vessel wall abnormalities not visualized by DSA were detected by MRA with a specificity of 92% (five studies, total $n = 152$) [15]. Although not yet formally studied, the circumferential or crescentic wall thickening observed in long irregular lesions can be considered pathognomonic for large-vessel vasculitis [5, 16].

MRA can also localize fibro-inflammatory lesions and give detailed information on whether these are limited to the vessel wall or extend to peri-adventitial tissues, determining the disease extent. However, overlap between active and inactive disease remains also challenging with MRA [17]. The wall thickness and enhancement in MRA were proposed to represent active disease. Some studies also defined new vascular dilatation, stenosis, occlusion, or wall irregularity as active disease. Tso et al. [18] performed MRA scans on 24 patients with TAK. The scans of 94% of the patients revealed vessel wall edema during periods of unequivocally active disease and 56% showed them during apparent clinical remission. Andrews et al. [19] and Choe et al. [20] detected that edema and enhancement of vascular wall, as well as a reduction of the mural diameter on MR images are associated with disease activity. Furthermore, these studies suggest that there is a close correlation between wall thickness and/or edema of the vessel, enhancement of wall detected by MR imaging and acute phase reactants. Another study analyzed the imaging manifestations of contrast-enhanced MRA to quantitatively measure and assess disease activity of TAK with an MRA scoring system. MRA scores moderately correlated to CRP, platelet count, and fibrinogen levels ($p < 0.05$) and pointed that the MRA scoring system of lumen stenosis, wall thickness, and wall enhancement could be a non-invasive approach to facilitate assessment in TAK activity [21].

Two other scoring systems aiming to assess vascular damage with MRA for large-vessel vasculitis is also proposed recently. Combined Arteritis Damage Score (CARDS) is a numerical damage index assessing the cumulative number of regions with stenosis, occlusions, and aneurysms [22]. Another composite score also evaluates arterial dilatation and stenosis in 17 arterial territories. Longitudinal changes in these scores correlated with disease activity and mirrored arterial disease evolution [23].

In a recent study, MRA was also found to be active in most patients with clinical remission [24]. In three studies assessing intima media thickness (IMT) by MRA in TAK, IMT was observed to be higher in active patients than inactives (pooled mean difference in IMT of 1.78 mm) [15]. On the other hand, there are a few studies reporting lower association between vessel wall thickening/enhancement and the active disease. Eshet et al. reported a lower sensitivity of 44% and specificity of 65% [25]. Heterogeneity between studies due to lack of validated activity assessment tools and medications lead differences in study results. But it is clear that MRA became the routine imaging method in the longitudinal follow-up of patients with TAK as a safe, non-invasive tool. But it is still a matter of debate whether MRA can reflect disease activity with cross-sectional, single time point assessments of arterial wall edema or post-contrast enhancement. Finally, "pseudostenosis" as an MRA artifact mimicking real arterial stenosis, should also be kept in mind during MRA assessments in LVV [26].

10.3 FDG-PET

FDG-PET-CT is a non-invasive and widely used imaging modality in oncological diseases to detect the regional distribution of 18-F-FDG visualizing the metabolic status of the body. It has promising results in LVV based on the interpretation of FDG uptake by metabolically active inflammatory cells in vessel walls [27]. Some studies used semiquantitative analysis comparing the 18F-FDG uptake of a vascular region of interest (ROI) with that of the liver. The level of large-vessel 18F-FDG uptake was visually graded using a four-point scale: 0 = no uptake present, I = low-grade uptake (uptake present but lower than liver uptake), II = intermediate-grade uptake (similar to liver uptake) and III = high-grade uptake (uptake higher than liver uptake)] [12, 28] while others quantified. 18F-FDG uptake using methods such as standard uptake value (SUV) [29, 30]. Webb et al. [31] were the first to report the diagnostic accuracy of FDG-PET in 18 TAK cases. Their sensitivity was 92%, and specificity was 100%. Kobayashi et al. [29] were the first to establish a cut-off for max SUV (strong accumulation: SUV >2, weak accumulation: SUV: 1.2–2.3) in their study of 14 TAK patients. Their sensitivity was 90.9%, and specificity 88.8%, however with defining active disease as the clinical requirement to use prednisolone. Walter et al. [32] described the qualitative utility of FDG-PET in 26 cases with giant cell arteritis ($n = 20$) or TAK ($n = 6$), and the visual grade of FDG uptake (grades I to III) correlated significantly with both CRP and ESR. Arnaud et al. [33] showed a lack of correlation between 18F-FDG uptake, clinical disease activity and levels of markers of inflammation. This study depended exclusively on clinical symptoms without markers of inflammation when assessing clinical disease activity and reported that FDG-PET scan had a sensitivity of 69.2% and a specificity of 33.3% for clinically active TAK [34]. Tezuka et al. [35] measured the mean SUV in the center of the inferior vena cava in all cases and target/background ratio was calculated as max SUV in arterial wall/mean SUV in inferior vena cava. They suggested that max SUV may provide a valid means of comparing patients with active vs. inactive TAK. Max SUV obtained with FDG-PET/CT had a high sensitivity and specificity for detecting subtle TAK activity in this study and ROC curve indicated that this approach may be superior to both ESR and CRP. The diagnostic accuracy of max SUV was also shown in relapsing TAK cases with a max SUV cut-off of 2.1 proposed to discriminate active inflammation of TAK. In another study, Zhang et al. [36] showed that SUV max, SUV mean, and SUV ratios were significantly higher in clinically active group compared to the inactives and with a 2.1 SUV max cut-off they reported 86.2% sensitivity and 90% specificity. Finally, a meta-analysis including eight studies assessing the performance of FDG-PET for detecting vasculitis in LVV showed a pooled sensitivity of 76% (95% CI 69, 82) and specificity of 93% (95% CI 89, 96) [37].

Recently, Grayson et al. Developed a scoring system labeled PETVAS, which is a total quantitative score of most commonly involved nine arteries in LVV. Active FDG-PET/CT differentiated clinically active LVV patients from comparators with a sensitivity and specificity of over 80% in this study. However, more than half of the patients (58%) who were in clinical remission according to NIH criteria were also interpreted to have active FDG-PET-CT. The specificity of FDG-PET-CT in distinguishing clinically active patients was therefore only 42%. In the comparator group who did not have an LVV diagnosis, 17% of patients were also found to have active vasculitic lesions. When a cut-off value of >20 was used, the sensitivity increased to 68% and specificity raised to 71%. Among patients who underwent PET during clinical remission, future clinical relapse was more common in patients with a high PETVAS (>20) compared to low PETVAS group (55% versus 11%; $p = 0.03$) over a median follow-up of 15 months [38]. Previous reports suggested that corticosteroid (CS) treatment reduces the FDG uptake [39]. In the study by Grayson et al., PETVAS scores decreased after CS and/or ISs treatments [38]. However, in a recent study from our center, we did not find any difference in PETVAS scores between patients with and without CS or IS use (*Kaymaz-Tahra S, unpublished*).

In a recent study, Banerjee et al. used a combined assessment of imaging, clinical and biomarker use to observe the effects of treatments in LVV patients. Increases in treatment led to a significant reduction in disease activity, whereas all three assessments of disease activity remained similarly unchanged when treatments were unaltered. When treatment was reduced, PET activity significantly worsened but clinical and serologic activity did not significantly change. Treatment of GCA with tocilizumab and of TAK with tumor necrosis factor inhibitors resulted in significant improvement in imaging and clinical assessments of disease activity, but only rarely did the assessments both become normal [40].

Without an histopathological confirmation, it is difficult to clarify whether increased FDG uptake in the vascular wall in patients with LVV in clinical remission is due to subclinical vasculitis [41] or to secondary processes such as vascular remodeling, hypoxia [42], atherosclerosis [43], or a combination of these factors. The interpretation of FDG-PET-CT has also some technical challenges. One of the main limitations is the lack of standardization for the time interval between the FDG administration and acquisition in LVV. According to the "EULAR recommendations for the use of imaging in LVV in clinical practice," a minimum of 60 min between intravenous FDG administration and acquisition is recommended. However, a delayed acquisition may increase the sensitivity of detecting FDG uptake [4]. Most of PET studies in the literature was performed at 1-h, but the data comparing the first hour and delayed acquisition is conflicting [44, 45] (*Kaymaz-Tahra S, unpublished*). In two recent studies, it was reported that PET assessment at 2 h time point would capture more active patients with LVV compared to 1 h time point assessments [46, 47].

PET scan is also an expensive imaging tool. In many countries, even in developed ones, access to PET scanning is very limited in any disease other than malignancies. Radiation exposure during PET-CT scan imaging may be another disadvantage which may be decreased with PET-MRA technique [48]. FDG uptake in all active cells other than inflammatory vessel wall is also an important restriction and there is ongoing research for new ligand options in PET scanning [2]. Therefore, despite the promising results both in the diagnosis and activity assessment, PET scan is still not a standardized imaging tool in TAK and its value in especially long-term follow-up of TAK patients needs to be further investigated.

10.4 Ultrasonography

The role of ultrasonography (US) is less established in TAK compared to other modalities. Doppler US performs well for carotid lesions with a high sensitivity (90%) and specificity (91%) in detecting stenotic lesions [49]. However, aortic and subclavian arteries are more difficult to visualize by US, with poorer detection of lesions. US may also help in determining inflammatory activity, demonstrating hypoechogenicity and mural thickening in active lesions [50]. Contrast-enhanced ultrasound (CEUS) may allow the identification of inflammation-driven hyperemia and neovascularization, a potential marker of disease activity [51]. In a recent study including 159 carotid artery CEUS from 86 patients with TAK, the enhanced intensity of carotid artery wall was higher in active patients and had a high predictive value for disease activity with area under the curve (AUC) of 86.3%, sensitivity of 88.0%, and specificity of 79.1%. This high predictive value did not increase by addition of ESR, CRP, and arterial wall thickness. Qualitative grading of wall vascularization based on the visual appearance of contrast enhancement within the lesion was also found higher in active patients [52]. In a prospective study including 31 patients with LVV, a graded vascularization score with CEUS of the carotid arteries was used as an index of disease activity which correlated closely with

18FDG-PET [53]. There are few case reports showing decreased artery wall thickness after corticosteroid treatment [54].

Being an operator-dependent imaging modality is an important restriction for US and its usage is mainly limited to carotid, vertebral, subclavian, and axillary arteries. However, it may also be used for abdominal aorta [55]. However, as US is a noninvasive, cheap and widely accessible imaging modality, further studies are warranted to confirm the potential of this technique for monitoring disease activity and response to treatment in TAK.

10.5 Conclusion

In summary, conventional angiography is no longer considered as the gold standard for the diagnosis of TAK. Currently, many physicians prefer to use MRA or CTA with FDG-PET-CT in selected cases for establishing the diagnosis of TAK. MRA is the gold standard modality for the longitudinal follow-up patients with TAK. Compared with DSA, three-dimensional MRA can effectively show vessel wall thickening, whereas contrast-enhanced MRA allows better soft-tissue differentiation. Exposure to large amounts of radiation and iodinated contrast limit the usefulness of CTA in routine follow-up. Recently, exciting preliminary reports have come up with PET-MRA with comparable visual and quantitative results to PET-CT. Improved soft-tissue resolution and definition of anatomy was reported with PET-MRA assessment using lower total radiation doses [56, 57]. Further prospective research is needed with PET-MR focusing on clinical activity assessment and changes with immunosuppressive treatments (Figs. 10.1, 10.2, 10.3, 10.4, 10.5, and 10.6).

Fig. 10.1 3D reconstruction of CT angiographic data demonstrating a high grade stenosis in left subclavian artery

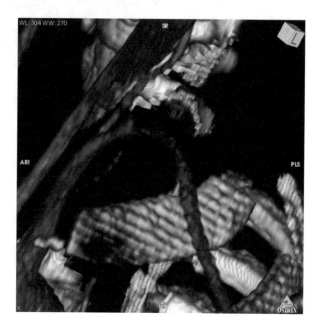

Fig. 10.2 CT angiographic image demonstrating occlusion in left subclavian artery

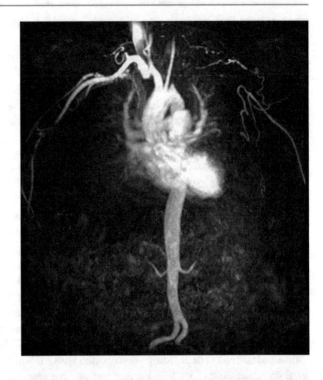

Fig. 10.3 MR angiographic image demonstrating a high grade stenosis in right subclavian artery and brachial artery

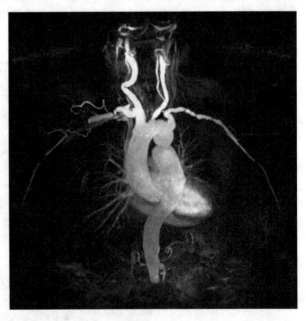

Fig. 10.4 MR
angiographic image
demonstrating bilateral
common carotid artery
stenosis and right
subclavian arteriel stenosis

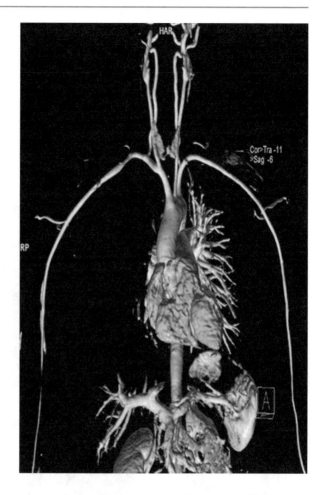

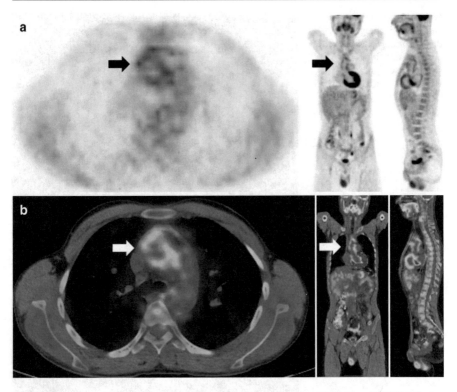

Fig. 10.5 Axial, coronal and sagittal positron emission tomography (PET) (**a**) and PET/CT fusion (**b**) images of the same patient shows fluorine-18 fluorodeoxyglucose (FDG) uptake at the level of the ascending aorta and the aortic arch (arrows) consistent with activated disease

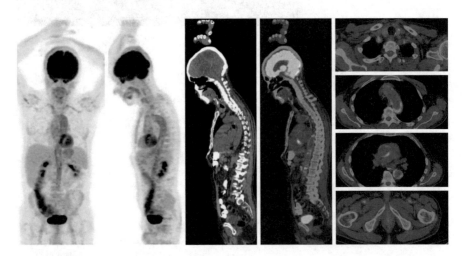

Fig. 10.6 PET/CT Images of a patient showing increased 3 fluorine-18 fluorodeoxyglucose (FDG) uptake (higher than liver uptake) in biateral carotid, subclavian, axillary, iliac, femoral arteries and assending-arcus-abdominal aorta

References

1. Quinn KA, Grayson PC. The role of vascular imaging to advance clinical care and research in large-vessel vasculitis. Curr Treat Opt Rheumatol. 2019;5(1):20–35.
2. Tombetti E, Mason JC. Application of imaging techniques for Takayasu arteritis. Presse Med. 2017;46(7–8 Pt 2):e215–23. Epub 2017 Jul 28.
3. Alibaz-Öner F, Aydın SZ, Direskeneli H. Recent advances in Takayasu's arteritis. Eur J Rheumatol. 2015;2(1):24–30. Epub 2015 Mar 1.
4. Dejaco C, Ramiro S, Duftner C, Besson FL, Bley TA, Blockmans D, et al. Eular recommendations for the use of imaging in large vessel vasculitis in clinical practice. Ann Rheum Dis. 2018;77:636–43.
5. Gotway MB, Araoz PA, Macedo TA, Stanson AW, Higgins CB, Ring EJ, et al. Imaging findings in Takayasu's arteritis. Am J Roentgenol. 2005;184:1945–50.
6. Yamada I, Nakagawa T, Himeno Y, Numano F, Shibuya H. Takayasu arteritis: evaluation of the thoracic aorta with CT angiography. Radiology. 1998;209:103–9.
7. Yoshida S, Akiba H, Tamakawa M, Yama N, Takeda M, Hareyama M, et al. The spectrum of findings in supra-aortic Takayasu's arteritis as seen on spiral CT angiography and digital subtraction angiography. Cardiovasc Intervent Radiol. 2001;24:117–21.
8. Yamazaki M, Takano H, Miyauchi H, Daimon M, Funabashi N, Nagai T, et al. Detection of Takayasu arteritis in early stage by computed tomography. Int J Cardiol. 2002;85:305–7.
9. Kim SY, Park JH, Chung JW, Kim HC, Lee W, So YH, et al. Follow-up CT evaluation of the mural changes in active Takayasu arteritis. Korean J Radiol. 2007;8:286–94.
10. Park JH, Chung JW, Im JG, Kim SK, Park YB, Han MC. Takayasu arteritis: evaluation of mural changes in the aorta and pulmonary artery with CT angiography. Radiology. 1995;196:89–93.
11. Paul JF, Hernigou A, Lefebvre C, Blétry O, Piette JC, Gaux JC, et al. Electron beam CT features of the pulmonary artery in Takayasu's arteritis. AJR Am J Roentgenol. 1999;173:89–93.
12. Paul JF, Fiessinger JN, Sapoval M, Hernigou A, Mousseaux E, Emmerich J, et al. Follow-up electron beam CT for the management of early phase Takayasu arteritis. J Comput Assist Tomogr. 2001;25:924–31.
13. Seyahi E, Ucgul A, Cebi Olgun D, Ugurlu S, Akman C, Tutar O, et al. Aortic and coronary calcifications in Takayasu arteritis. Semin Arthritis Rheum. 2013;43:96–104.
14. Banerjee S, Bagheri M, Sandfort V, Ahlman MA, Malayeri AA, et al. Vascular calcification in patients with large-vessel vasculitis compared to patients with hyperlipidemia. Semin Arthritis Rheum. 2019;48(6):1068–73.
15. Barra L, Kanji T, Malette J, Pagnoux C, CanVasc. Imaging modalities for the diagnosis and disease activity assessment of Takayasu's arteritis: a systematic review and meta-analysis. Autoimmun Rev. 2018;17(2):175–87. Epub 2017 Dec 5.
16. Matsunaga N, Hayashi K, Sakamoto I, Matsuoka Y, Ogawa Y, Honjo K, et al. Takayasu arteritis: MR manifestations and diagnosis of acute and chronic phase. J Magn Reson Imaging. 1998;8:406–14.
17. Li D, Lin J, Yan F. Detecting disease extent and activity of Takayasu arteritis using whole body magnetic resonance angiography and vessel wall imaging as a 1-stop solution. J Comput Assist Tomogr. 2011;35:468–74.
18. Tso E, Flamm SD, White RD, Schvartzman PR, Mascha E, Hoffman GS. Takayasu arteritis: utility and limitations of magnetic resonance imaging in diagnosis and treatment. Arthritis Rheum. 2002;46:1634–42.
19. Andrews J, Al-Nahhas A, Pennell DJ, Hossain MS, Davies KA, Haskard DO, et al. Non-invasive imaging in the diagnosis and management of Takayasu's arteritis. Ann Rheum Dis. 2004;63:995–1000.
20. Choe YH, Han BK, Koh EM, Do YS, Lee WR. Takayasu's arteritis: assessment of disease activity with contrast enhanced MRA imaging. Am J Roentgenol. 2000;175:505–11.
21. Jiang L, Li D, Yan F, Dai X, Li Y, Ma L. Evaluation of Takayasu arteritis activity by delayed contrast-enhanced magnetic resonance imaging. Int J Cardiol. 2012;155(2):262–7. Epub 2010 Nov 6.

22. Nakagomi D, Cousins C, Sznajd J, Furuta S, Mohammad AJ, et al. Development of a score for assessment of radiologic damage in large-vessel vasculitis (Combined Arteritis Damage Score, CARDS). Clin Exp Rheumatol. 2017;35 Suppl 103(1):139–45.
23. Tombetti E, Godi C, Ambrosi A, Doyle F, Jacobs A, et al. Novel angiographic scores for evaluation of large vessel vasculitis. Sci Rep. 2018;8(1):15979.
24. Quinn KA, Ahlman MA, Malayeri AA, Marko J, Civelek AC, et al. Comparison of magnetic resonance angiography and ^{18}F-fluorodeoxyglucose positron emission tomography in large-vessel vasculitis. Ann Rheum Dis. 2018;77(8):1165–71. Epub 2018 Apr 17.
25. Eshet Y, Pauzner R, Goitein O, Langevitz P, Eshed I, Hoffmann C, et al. The limited role of MRI in long-term follow-up of patients with Takayasu's arteritis. Autoimmun Rev. 2011;11:132–6.
26. Marinelli KC, Ahlman MA, Quinn KA, Malayeri AA, Evers R, Grayson PC. Stenosis and pseudostenosis of the upper extremity arteries in large-vessel vasculitis. ACR Open Rheumatol. 2019;1(3):156–63.
27. Danve A, O'Dell J. The role of 18f fluorodeoxyglucose positron emission tomography scanning in the diagnosis and management of systemic vasculitis. Int J Rheum Dis. 2015;18:714–24.
28. De Leeuw K, Bijl M, Jager PL. Additional value of positron emission tomography in diagnosis and follow-up of patients with large vessel vasculitides. Clin Exp Rheumatol. 2004;22:S21–6.
29. Kobayashi Y, Ishii K, Oda K, Nariai T, Tanaka Y, Ishiwata K, et al. Aortic wall inflammation due to Takayasu arteritis imaged with 18F-FDG PET coregistered with enhanced CT. J Nucl Med. 2005;46:917–22.
30. Meller J, Strutz F, Siefker U, Scheel A, Sahlmann CO, Lehmann K, et al. Early diagnosis and follow-up of aortitis with [18F]FDG PET and MRI. Eur J Nucl Med Mol Imaging. 2003;30:730–6.
31. Webb M, Chambers A, Al-Nahhas A, et al. The role of 18F-FDG PET in characterizing disease activity in Takayasu arteritis. Eur J Nucl Med Mol Imaging. 2004;31:627–34.
32. Walter MA, Melzer RA, Schindler C, Muller-Brand J, Tyndall A, Nitzsche AU. The value of [18F] FDG-PET in the diagnosis of large-vessel vasculitis and the assessment of activity and extent of disease. Eur J Nucl Med Mol Imaging. 2005;32:674–81.
33. Arnaud L, Haroche J, Malek Z, Archambaud F, Gambotti L, et al. Is (18)F-fluorodeoxyglucose positron emission tomography scanning a reliable way to assess disease activity in Takayasu arteritis? Arthritis Rheum. 2009;60(4):1193–200.
34. Lee KH, Cho A, Choi YJ, Lee SW, Ha YJ, et al. The role of (18) F-fluorodeoxyglucose-positron emission tomography in the assessment of disease activity in patients with Takayasu arteritis. Arthritis Rheum. 2012;64(3):866–75.
35. Tezuka D, Haraguchi G, Ishihara T, Ohigashi H, Inagaki H, Suzuki J, Hirao K, Isobe M. Role of FDG PET-CT in Takayasu arteritis: sensitive detection of recurrences. JACC Cardiovasc Imaging. 2012;5(4):422–9.
36. Zhang X, Zhou J, Sun Y, Shi H, Ji Z, Jiang L. 18F-FDG-PET/CT: an accurate method to assess the activity of Takayasu's arteritis. Clin Rheumatol. 2018;37:1927–35.
37. Lee YH, Choi SJ, Ji JD, Song GG. Diagnostic accuracy of 18F-FDG PET or PET/CT for large vessel vasculitis: a meta-analysis. Z Rheumatol. 2016;75:924–31.
38. Grayson PC, Alehashemi S, Bagheri AA, Civelek AC, Cupps TR, et al. (18) f-fluorodeoxyglucose-positron emission tomography as an imaging biomarker in a prospective, longitudinal cohort of patients with large vessel vasculitis. Arthritis Rheumatol. 2018;70:439–49.
39. Blockmans D, de Ceuninck L, Vanderschueren S, Knockaert D, Mortelmans L, Bobbaers H. Repetitive 18f-fluorodeoxyglucose positron emission tomography in giant cell arteritis: a prospective study of 35 patients. Arthritis Rheum. 2006;55:131–7.
40. Banerjee S, Quinn KA, Gribbons KB, Rosenblum JS, Civelek AC, et al. Effect of treatment on imaging, clinical, and serologic assessments of disease activity in large-vessel vasculitis. J Rheumatol. 2020;47(1):99–107. https://doi.org/10.3899/jrheum.181222.
41. Newman KA, Ahlman MA, Hughes M, Malayeri AA, Pratt D, Grayson PC. Diagnosis of giant cell arteritis in an asymptomatic patient. Arthritis Rheumatol. 2016;68:1135.

42. Folco EJ, Sheikine Y, Rocha VZ, Christen T, Shvartz E, et al. Hypoxia but not inflammation augments glucose uptake in human macrophages: implications for imaging atherosclerosis with 18fluorine-labeled 2-deoxy-D-glucose positron emission tomography. J Am Coll Cardiol. 2011;58:603–14.
43. Rosenbaum D, Millon A, Fayad ZA. Molecular imaging in atherosclerosis: FDG PET. Curr Atheroscler Rep. 2012;14:429–37.
44. Slart R, Writing Group, Reviewer Group, Members of EANM Cardiovascular, Members of EANM Infection & Inflammation, et al. Fdg-pet/ct(a) imaging in large vessel vasculitis and polymyalgia rheumatica: joint procedural recommendation of the eanm, snmmi, and the pet interest group (pig), and endorsed by the asnc. Eur J Nucl Med Mol Imaging. 2018;45:1250–69.
45. Bucerius J, Mani V, Moncrieff C, Machac J, Fuster V, et al. Optimizing 18f-fdg pet/ct imaging of vessel wall inflammation: the impact of 18f-fdg circulation time, injected dose, uptake parameters, and fasting blood glucose levels. Eur J Nucl Med Mol Imaging. 2014;41:369–83.
46. Rosenblum JS, Quinn KA, Rimland CA, Mehta NN, Ahlman MA, Grayson PC. Clinical factors associated with time-specific distribution of 18F-fluorodeoxyglucose in large-vessel vasculitis. Sci Rep. 2019;9(1):15180.
47. Quinn KA, Rosenblum JS, Rimland CA, Gribbons KB, Ahlman MA, et al. Imaging acquisition technique influences interpretation of positron emission tomography vascular activity in large-vessel vasculitis. Semin Arthritis Rheum. 2020;50(1):71–6. pii: S0049-0172(19)30411-1.
48. Padoan R, Crimì F, Felicetti M, Padovano F, Lacognata C, et al. Fully integrated 18F-FDG PET/MR in large vessel vasculitis. Q J Nucl Med Mol Imaging. 2019. https://doi.org/10.23736/S1824-4785.19.03184-4.
49. Raninen RO, Kupari MM, Pamilo MS, et al. Ultrasonography in the quantification of arterial involvement in Takayasu's arteritis. Scand J Rheumatol. 2000;29:56–61.
50. Park S, Chung JW, Lee JW, Han MH, Park JH. Carotid artery involvement in Takayasu's arteritis: evaluation of the activity by ultrasonography. J Ultrasound Med. 2001;20:371–8.
51. Magnoni M, Dagna L, Coli S, Cianflone D, Sabbadini MG, Maseri A. Assessment of Takayasu arteritis activity by carotid contrast-enhanced ultrasound. Circ Cardiovasc Imaging. 2011;4(2):e1–2.
52. Huang Y, Ma X, Li M, Dong H, Wan Y, Zhu J. Carotid contrast assessment of disease activity in Takayasu arteritis. Eur Heart J Cardiovasc Imaging. 2019;20(7):789–95.
53. Germano G, Macchioni P, Possemato N, Boiardi L, Nicolini A, Massimiliano C, et al. Contrast-enhanced ultrasound of the carotid artery in patients with large vessel vasculitis: correlation with positron emission tomography findings. Arthritis Care Res (Hoboken). 2016;69:143–9.
54. Fukudome Y, Abe I, Onaka U, Fujii K, Ohya Y, Fukuhara M, et al. Regression of carotid wall thickening after corticosteroid therapy in Takayasu's arteritis evaluated by B-mode ultrasonography: report of 2 cases. J Rheumatol. 1998;25:2029–32.
55. Schmidt WA. Imaging in vasculitis. Best Pract Res Clin Rheumatol. 2013;27:107–18.
56. Zeimpekis KG, Barbosa F, Hullner M, ter Voert E, Davison H, Veit-Haibach P, et al. Clinical evaluation of PET image quality as a function of acquisition time in a new TOF-PET/MRI compared to TOF-PET/CT—initial results. Mol Imaging Biol. 2015;17:735–44.
57. Einspieler I, Thurmel K, Pyka T, Eiber M, Wolfram S, Moog P, et al. Imaging large vessel vasculitis with fully integrated PET/MRI: a pilot study. Eur J Nucl Med Mol Imaging. 2015;42:1012–24.

Prognosis and Disease Activity

11

Fatma Alibaz-Oner and Haner Direskeneli

Keywords

Prognosis · Disease assessment · Damage

Correct assessment of the extent of arterial involvement, clinical activity and damage in Takayasu's Arteritis (TAK) is essential for treatment or surgical intervention decisions during the disease course [1]. However, there are no widely accepted and validated definitions of "disease activity" or "response to treatment". One of the major difficulties is the differentiation between ongoing activity and vascular damage in TAK. Vascular stenosis may occur as a result of active inflammation or be a sign of disease-related damage due to scarring in the vessel wall [2]. Atherosclerosis is another important clinical problem in the assessment of TAK, especially in patients having long-standing disease or normal acute-phase response. There is a clear need and ongoing efforts to develop a validated set of outcome measures for use in clinical trials of TAK.

11.1 Disease Activity Assessment

11.1.1 Physical Examination in Clinical Activity Assessment

Physical examination for new or worsened vascular signs such as bruits, pulse or blood pressure difference between extremities is the first step for disease assessment in TAK. However, the limitations of physical examination for assessing disease

F. Alibaz-Oner · H. Direskeneli (✉)
Division of Rheumatology, Department of Internal Medicine, Marmara University,
School of Medicine, Istanbul, Turkey

© Springer Nature Switzerland AG 2021
C. Salvarani et al. (eds.), *Large and Medium Size Vessel and Single Organ Vasculitis*, Rare Diseases of the Immune System,
https://doi.org/10.1007/978-3-030-67175-4_11

extent was shown by Grayson et al. Although abnormal findings on vascular physical examination are highly associated with the presence of arterial lesions in imaging, at least 30% of arteriographic lesions can be missed with only physical examination [3]. In a recent study, a high specificity was detected between *newly developed* clinical symptoms and concurrent vascular imaging findings. Vascular imaging abnormalities are often present in a patient presenting with a specific head, neck and arm symptoms. However, presence of ischemic symptoms or even signs may not always indicate active inflammation of the vessel wall. In this context, carotidynia may be considered as a strong indicator of active inflammation, whereas limb claudication is usually a sign of vasculitis-associated damage in TAK [4].

11.1.2 Laboratory in Disease Activity Assessment

Erythrocyte sedimentation rate (ESR) and C-reactive protein are frequently advocated for disease assessment of TAK [5], despite being shown to be neither sensitive nor specific enough to monitor disease activity [6, 7]. In one study, active disease was present in the setting of normal laboratory parameters in 23% of the patients [8]. Similarly, ESR was elevated in only 72% of patients considered to have active disease and was still high in 44% of patients considered to be in remission [9]. Serum autoantibodies such as anti-aorta or anti-endothelial antibodies [10–12] and serum biomarkers such as TNF-α, IL-6, IL-8, IL-18, IFN-γ, MMP-2, MMP-9, YKL-40, APRIL and BAFF are shown to be elevated in TAK, but are not disease-specific [13–20]. Soluble IL-6R was recently suggested as a potential biomarker for disease activity in TAK patients [21]. In a recent study, it was suggested that increased serum FGF-2 level may distinguish TAK from giant cell arteritis, but needs to be confirmed [22].

Pentraxin (PTX) superfamily is a group of proteins recognizing a wide range of exogenous pathogens and behave as acute-phase response mediators [23]. PTX-3 was suggested to be a discriminative marker for active disease in TAK [24–26]. In a Turkish TAK cohort, patients had higher serum PTX-3 levels compared to healthy controls, but PTX-3 levels did not differ between active and inactive phases [27]. In an Italian TAK cohort, Tombetti et al. reported that only CRP was higher in active disease and PTX-3 levels were similar between active and inactive patients, similar to the Turkish study. However, significantly higher PTX-3 levels were observed in a subset of patients with 'detectable signs of vascular inflammation' shown with vascular imaging [28]. In a recent Chinese study, Serum PTX-3 level was found significantly higher in active TAK patients, but it was not superior to ESR or hsCRP for activity assessment in TAK [29]. Pulsatelli L. et al. recently assessed angiogenic markers in 33 TAK patients and reported that VEGF and PTX-3 significantly associated with disease activity determined by PET scan and activity indices (NIH, ITAS2010) [30]. The role of PTX-3 for activity assessment in TAK and its association with, especially, active lesions at imaging needs to be further investigated longitudinally.

11.1.3 Imaging in Disease Activity Assessment

Currently, conventional angiography is no longer considered as the 'gold standard' imaging tool for the diagnosis of TAK. Many physicians prefer to use MRA or CTA with FDG-PET-CT in selected cases for establishing the diagnosis of TAK. MRA is currently the 'gold standard' modality for the longitudinal follow-up of patients with TAK. Compared with DSA, three-dimensional MRA can effectively show vessel wall thickening, whereas contrast-enhanced MRA allows better soft-tissue differentiation.

Exposure to large amounts of radiation and iodinated contrast limit the usefulness of CTA in routine follow-up. Recently, exciting preliminary reports have come up with PET-MRA with visual and quantitative results comparable to PET-CT. Improved soft-tissue resolution and definition of anatomy was reported with PET-MRA assessment using lower total radiation doses [31, 32]. However, further prospective research is needed with PET-MRA before it can replace other modalities for activity assessment. Imaging tools for the assessment of clinical activity in TAK were discussed in detail in the previous chapter.

11.1.4 Outcome Measures in Disease Activity Assessment

The simple definition of "active disease" that was used in a study from the National Institute of Health (NIH): "presence of constitutional symptoms, new-bruits, APR or new angiographic features" is commonly applied in clinical studies [33]. Birmingham Vasculitis Activity Score (BVAS), documenting evidence of active vasculitis on a simple one-page form [34], is designed to apply to all vasculitides. However, BVAS is mostly used in therapeutic trials of ANCA-associated vasculitis and is validated for use only in small- and medium-vessel vasculitis. Most of the 11 organ systems in BVAS are not involved in TAK [35] and only two studies have used BVAS [36, 37]. The "disease extent index for Takayasu's arteritis (DEI.TAK)" was developed as an assessment/disease extent tool in which items corresponding to large arterial disease carry greater weights than general items of the disease and changes in the prior 3 months in the physical examination are the basis of evaluation [38]. In a study from Turkey, most patients with slow progression of disease demonstrated no change in the DEI.TAK score. As DEI.TAK was substantially derived from BVAS, most items are related to small-vessel vasculitis and were not involved or did not change in patients with TAK. Furthermore, discriminant ability of the instrument was not high. Among the DEI.TAK (−) group, 31% were felt to have "active/persistent" disease according to the physician's global assessment (PGA) while 18% of patients with a DEI.TAK score ≥1 were considered inactive by PGA. PGA and DEI.TAK had only modest agreement (68%) [35].

In 2010, a new version of DEI.TAK, the Indian Takayasu's Arteritis Score (ITAS) was introduced [39]. ITAS2010 has only six systems and scoring is weighted for vascular items (0–2). ITAS2010 seems to have a sufficient comprehensiveness and the inter-rater agreement is better than (PGA) (0.97 vs 0.82). However, convergent validity, when assessed by comparison to PGA, is quite low at the initial evaluation but improved at subsequent study visits ($r = 0.51$, 0.64, and 0.72). Although CRP and ESR had weak correlations with ITAS2010, the authors also incorporated acute-phase response to the score (ITAS2010-A) by adding an extra 1–3 points for elevated ESR or CRP. This change resulted in higher ITAS2010-A scores both in active and inactive patients, and a cut-off of 4 points is suggested for a definition of active disease [40]. In a study of Turkish patients during routine follow-up, ITAS2010 was significantly higher in patients with active disease. However, total agreement between ITAS2010 and PGA was again moderate (66.4%), but was better between ITAS2010 and NIH score (82.8%). During follow-up, 14 of 15 patients showing vascular progression with imaging were categorized as having inactive disease according to ITAS2010. Low correlation of ITAS2010 with PGA suggests that physicians seem to accept some patients only with increased APR or new abnormalities on vascular imaging studies (such as new vessel wall enhancement or thickening observed by MRI or PET) as "active," which were below the cut-off values of ITAS2010 for active disease [41]. In a recent study, ITAS2010 was combined with imaging. A total of 410 visits in 52 patients were evaluated with 3–6 monthly B-mode/Doppler ultrasonography (US) and 6–12 monthly MRI/MRA. An additional point was added to ITAS2010-A if there is radiologically active disease which was defined as the presence of new major involvement and mural contrast enhancement/edema on MRI/MRA, or arterial wall thickness on US compared to the previous assessment. This new scoring was labeled as ITAS-A-Rad. The agreement was found to be 76% between Rad-Active and PGA, 83% between Rad-Active and Kerr et al.'s criteria. Both the agreements of ITAS2010 and acute-phase reactants with PGA (69% and 60, respectively) and also Kerr et al.'s criteria (78% and 42%, respectively) were lower compared to those of Rad-Active. Mean ITAS-A-Rad scores were higher in visits with active disease according to PGA and Kerr et al.'s criteria [42]. This study showed that imaging should be a part of activity assessment in TAK. Further prospective validation studies are needed to confirm these results.

The OMERACT Vasculitis Working Group completed a Delphi exercise to determine a consensus for candidate outcomes for disease activity assessment in large-vessel vasculitis (LVV) in clinical trials and a set of important items to measure were identified. However, as all items are not required to be included in an activity index, a data-driven approach for item reduction is needed [43].

Recently, EULAR suggested new definitions for active disease, relapse, and remission (Tables 11.1 and 11.2). But these new definitions are consensus-based and do not derive from a systematic literature review. EULAR suggest using the term "relapse" and avoiding the term "flare." These definitions seem acceptable, but needs to be tested in prospective studies [44].

Table 11.1 EULAR consensus definitions for disease activity states in large-vessel vasculitis

Activity state	EULAR consensus definition

	1. The presence of typical signs or symptoms of active LVV (Table 11.2)
	2. At least one of the following:
	   (a) Current activity on imaging or biopsy
	   (b) Ischemic complications attributed to LVV
	   (c) Persistently elevated inflammatory markers (after other causes have been excluded)

Flare	We do not recommend use of this term
Relapse	We recommend use of the terms major relapse or minor relapse as defined below
Major relapse	Recurrence of active disease with either of the following: (a) Clinical features of ischemia (including jaw claudication, visual symptoms, visual loss attributable to GCA, scalp necrosis, stroke, limb claudication) (b) Evidence of active aortic inflammation resulting in progressive aortic or large-vessel dilatation, stenosis, or dissection
Minor relapse	Recurrence of active disease, not fulfilling the criteria for a major relapse
Refractory	Inability to induce remission (with evidence of reactivation of disease, as defined above in "Active disease") despite the use of standard care therapy
Remission	Absence of all clinical signs and symptoms attributable to active LVV and normalization of ESR and CRP; in addition, for patients with extracranial disease there should be no evidence of progressive vessel narrowing or dilatation (frequency of repeat imaging to be decided on an individual basis)
Sustained remission	1. Remission for at least 6 months 2. Achievement of the individual target GC dose
Glucocorticoid-free remission	Sustained remission Discontinued GC therapy (but could still be receiving other immunosuppressive therapy)

Table 11.2 Key symptoms and clinical findings suggestive of active large-vessel vasculitis

Takayasu arteritis
Key symptoms
• New onset or worsening of limb claudication
• Constitutional symptoms (e.g., weight loss >2 kg, low-grade fever, fatigue, night sweats)
• Myalgia, arthralgia, arthritis • Severe abdominal pain
• Stroke, seizures (non-hypertensive), syncope, dizziness
• Paresis of extremities
• Myocardial infarct, angina
• Acute visual symptoms such as amaurosis fugax or diplopia
Key findings on clinical examination
• Hypertension (>140/90 mmHg)
• New loss of pulses, pulse inequality
• Bruits
• Carotidynia

11.2 Prognosis

11.2.1 Disease Course

TAK generally has a relapsing-remitting course leading to prolonged periods of seemingly clinically "inactive" disease during which arterial damage can still progress. Due to lack of standardized assessment tools, physicians generally manage the cases with TAK according to PGA as the "gold standard" in daily practice, combining subjective clinical symptoms, laboratory markers and imaging. Relapses are frequent in TAK during the disease course [45]. A significant subset of TAK patients (44%) developed new severe manifestations during their follow-up in the VCRC cohort from the USA [46]. In a series of Korean patients in remission, 22% had a relapse during a follow-up of 37 months, which is mainly associated with Type V disease, suggesting that low-level inflammation is associated with the extent of the disease [47]. Interestingly, disease starting >40 years is observed to have fewer relapses with lower initial doses of corticosteroids for remission induction in Japan [48]. In a retrospective French cohort including 318 patients, during a median follow-up of 6.1 years, relapses were observed in 43%, vascular complications in 38%, retinopathy in 4%, and death in 5%. The 5- and 10-year relapse-free survivals were 36.4% (30.3; 43.9) and 69.9% (64.3; 76.0), respectively. Multivariate analysis showed that relapses were more common in patients with elevated CRP levels, carotidynia, and male gender. This study also showed that almost half of patients with TAK will relapse and experience a vascular complication ≤10 years from diagnosis [49]. In a recent, retrospective Korean study, it was reported that statins may be beneficial in reducing relapse rate after achieving remission [50].

As in other inflammatory disorders, accelerated atherosclerosis is a possible risk factor for increased morbidity and mortality in TAK. There are very few data about the risk of cardiovascular (CV) disease and atherosclerotic burden in TAK. Seyahi et al. first showed that the frequency of atherosclerotic plaques is increased in TAK, similar to SLE a disease associated with systemic premature atherosclerosis [51]. Da Silva et al. also found a high prevalence of metabolic syndrome in patients with TAK [52]. There are also a few studies favoring the use of antiplatelet agents in TAK [53–55]. Recently, in a comparative study of patients from the USA and Turkey, CV risk factors were more common in patients with TAK, particularly hypertension. The Framingham 10-year general CV risk score at the time of diagnosis and the cumulative incidence of CV events were higher during follow-up in patients with TAK. However, aspirin usage had no significant effect on the risk of CV event development [56]. In another study from Brasil, aspirin usage with doses of 100–200 mg/day reduced the risk of ischemic events in TAK [57]. According to 2018 Update of the EULAR recommendations for the management of large-vessel vasculitis, aspirin should not be routinely used for the treatment of LVV unless it is indicated for other reasons (e.g., coronary heart disease, cerebrovascular disease) [37]. Overall, current data suggest that patients with TAK should undergo careful assessment of CV risk factors, and an aggressive risk modification approach is warranted.

11.2.2 Damage Assessment in TAK

Treatment of TAK is usually focused on the prevention of disease-related damage [58]. But, it is critical to differentiate irreversible damage from disease activity and thus avoid potential over-treatment with toxic agents such as corticosteroids. Angiographic findings may not demonstrate whether changes in the vessel wall are associated with active vascular inflammation or irreversible damage [59]. Vasculitis Damage Index (VDI) has been the standard tool for assessing damage in small-vessel vasculitis. In the development and validation study of VDI which had only six TAK patients out of 100, 95% had at least one damage item at baseline [60]. In a large series from Turkey, VDI was assessed in 165 TAK patients with a mean follow-up of 60 months. VDI scores in TAK were moderately high (mean: 4 (1–12)) and were mainly due to the disease itself with major vessel occlusion. Still, 39% also had treatment-related damage with osteoporosis/vertebral fractures the main causes. Age, resistant disease course, disease duration, and cumulative corticosteroid doses were independently associated with damage, suggesting that, even in experienced centers, accumulation of damage is a major challenge in the management of TAK patients [61].

Another damage score, Takayasu Arteritis Damage Score (TADS), derived from DEI.TAK, was developed to evaluate the cumulative damage in only TAK patients. The scoring system consists of seven categories, which are mainly focused on the cardiovascular system [35, 62]. In a recent study comparing VDI and TADS, median VDI score was 4 (1–8) and median TADS score was 7 (1–15) at baseline assessment. At the end of the follow-up (app. 77 months), the median VDI score was 5.0 (1–17) and median TADS score was 8.0 (1–19). The median number of disease-related items were higher in TADS scoring (8 items vs 4 items). At least 1 new corticosteroid-related damage item occurred in 35 patients (31%). Older age at symptom-onset and cumulative CS doses were predictor factors for higher VDI score (≥5). Also, age at symptom-onset and disease duration were associated with an increase in TADS (≥8). Gender and number of relapses were not found to be associated with damage scores. The results confirmed that damage assessment with VDI seems to be predominantly evaluating the treatment-related damage, whereas TADS provides more detailed information on disease-related damage in TAK (*Kaymaz-Tahra S, unpublished*). Therefore, both disease-related and treatment-related damage must be considered while monitoring the disease. Another assessment tool for damage, large-vessel vasculitis index of damage (LVVID) score, are in the development phases by VCRC. LVVID includes additional items in the ocular, cardiac, and peripheral arterial categories which are mainly involved in large-vessel vasculitis and are missing on the VDI [63].

11.2.3 Mortality

Although data is showing better prognosis in recent studies, there is still a significant delay in the diagnosis of TAK. Both morbidity and mortality rate is still high due to new and severe manifestations after diagnosis [64]. In an old study, Ishikawa et al. developed a prognostic scoring system with three stages based on three different parameters, namely the presence or absence of major complications (defined as at least one of the following: microaneurysm formation, severe hypertension, grade 3 or 4 aortic regurgitation), presence or absence of progressive disease course, and age at diagnosis. Survival rate at 15 years was 43% in stage 3 (major complication, progressive course with/without high ESR). But, in stage 1 (patients without major complications nor progressive course with high ESR or patients with only low ESR, or patients with progressive disease, high ESR but without major complications), 15 years survival rate was 100%. Major causes of death were congestive heart failure, acute myocardial infarction, cerebrovascular accidents, and postoperative complications [65]. Soto et al. reported a decrease in overall survival rates over time, 92%, 81%, and 73%, respectively, at 2, 5, and 10 years after diagnosis in Mexican TAK patients. Systemic arterial hypertension, coronary heart disease, and aortic valve regurgitation were found as predictors for mortality [66]. In a large series with a long follow-up from the Mayo Clinic, USA, overall survival was much better compared to earlier series (97% at 10 and 86% at 15 years), but mortality was still increased compared to the general population [67]. In a recent French TAK cohort including 299 patients, 47 (16%) TAK patients presented at least one ischemic or aneurysmal complication or died during follow-up. The 5- and 10-years event-free survival was 81% (95% CI: 76–87) and 75% (95% CI: 68–82) in TAK [68]. Secondary hypertension, congestive heart failure, and longer disease duration were main factors for mortality in another series of Chinese patients [69]. In recent French Vasculitis Network series assessing 318 patients, mortality was 5% in a median follow-up of 6.1 years. In multivariate analysis, progressive disease course at diagnosis, thoracic aorta involvement, and retinopathy were independently associated with death and complication-free survival. The authors suggested a prognostic score based on this model as low and high risk for the probability of death and complication-free survival according to the presence of progressive disease course, thoracic aorta involvement, and retinopathy. If there is none of the three selected factors or presence of one factor at diagnosis, score is categorized as low risk. If there is 2 or 3 factors, the score is categorized as high risk. The probability of death and complication-free survival at 1 year in the low risk vs. high risk groups was 90.7% vs. 78.6% and at 5 years 78.4% vs. 51.5% [70]. Differences of mortality rates reported in different series may be explained by diverse disease phenotypes and severities due to ethnicity. Differences in medical therapy (e.g., less or more frequent use of CSs and cytotoxic agents) and variations in access to endovascular or surgical therapy may also affect the mortality rates [71].

11.3 Conclusion

Biomarkers (ESR, CRP) have limited value for activity assessment in TAK. PTX-3 was recently suggested as a discriminative test for clinical activity, but the results are controversial and needs to be further investigated—especially longitudinally.

Currently, conventional angiography is no longer considered as the "gold standard" imaging tool for the diagnosis of TAK. Many physicians prefer to use MRA or CTA with FDG-PET-CT in selected cases for establishing the diagnosis of TAK. MRA is the gold standard modality for the longitudinal follow-up patients with TAK. Compared to DSA, three-dimensional MRA can effectively show vessel wall thickening, whereas contrast-enhanced MRA allows better soft-tissue differentiation for the assessment of disease activity. Exposure to large amounts of radiation and iodinated contrast limit the usefulness of CTA in routine follow-up. Recently, exciting preliminary reports have come up with PET-MRA with comparable visual and quantitative results to PET-CT. Improved soft-tissue resolution and definition of anatomy was reported with PET-MRA assessment using lower total radiation doses. New tools for disease assessment such as ITAS2010 aim to better characterize and quantify disease activity.

Prognosis is recently possibly getting better with lower mortality, but a substantial damage is present even in early cases. There is a clear need to develop a validated set of outcome measures to be used in clinical trials of TAK. The OMERACT Vasculitis Working Group has taken on this task, finished a Delphi exercise with experts and aims to develop a core set of outcomes for LVV.

References

1. Keser G, Direskeneli H, Aksu K. Management of Takayasu arteritis: a systematic review. Rheumatology (Oxford). 2014;53:793–801.
2. Direskeneli H. Clinical assessment in Takayasu's arteritis: major challenges and controversies. Clin Exp Rheumatol. 2017;35 Suppl 103(1):189–93. Epub 2017 Mar 27. Review.
3. Grayson PC, Tomasson G, Cuthbertson D, Carette S, Hoffman GS, Khalidi NA, et al. Vasculitis Clinical Research Consortium. Association of vascular physical examination findings and arteriographic lesions in large vessel vasculitis. J Rheumatol. 2012;39(2):303–9.
4. Michailidou D, Rosenblum JS, Rimland CA, Marko J, Ahlman MA, Grayson PC. Clinical symptoms and associated vascular imaging findings in Takayasu's arteritis compared to giant cell arteritis. Ann Rheum Dis. 2020;79(2):262–7. https://doi.org/10.1136/annrheumdis-2019-216145.
5. Salvarani C, Cantini F, Boiardi L, Hunder GG. Laboratory investigations useful in giant cell arteritis and Takayasu's arteritis. Clin Exp Rheumatol. 2003;21(Suppl 32):S23–8.
6. Mason JC. Takayasu arteritis-advances in diagnosis and management. Nat Rev Rheumatol. 2010;6(7):406–15.
7. Hoffman GS, Ahmed AE. Surrogate markers of disease activity in patients with Takayasu arteritis. A preliminary report from The International Network for the Study of the Systemic Vasculitides (INSSYS). Int J Cardiol. 1998;66(Suppl 1):S191–5.
8. Maksimowicz-Mckinnon K, Clark TM, Hoffman GS. Limitations of therapy and a guarded prognosis in an American cohort of Takayasu arteritis patients. Arthritis Rheum. 2007;56:1000–9.
9. Numano F. The story of Takayasu arteritis. Rheumatology (Oxford). 2002;41:103–6.
10. Dhingra R, Talwar KK, Chopra P, Kumar R. An enzyme linked immunosorbent assay for detection of anti-aorta antibodies in Takayasu arteritis patients. Int J Cardiol. 1993;40:237–42.
11. Lee SK. Anti-endothelial cell antibodies and antiphospholipid antibodies in Takayasu's arteritis: correlations of their titers and isotype distributions with disease activity. Clin Exp Rheumatol. 2006;24(Suppl 41):S10–6.

12. Chauhan SK, Tripathy NK, Nityanand S. Antigenic targets and pathogenicity of antiaortic endothelial cell antibodies in Takayasu arteritis. Arthritis Rheum. 2006;54:2326–33.
13. Tamura N, Maejima Y, Tezuka D, Takamura C, Yoshikawa S, Ashikaga T, et al. Profiles of serum cytokine levels in Takayasu arteritis patients: potential utility as biomarkers for monitoring disease activity. J Cardiol. 2017;70(3):278–85.
14. Rodriguez-Pla A, Warner RL, Cuthbertson D, Carette S, Khalidi NA, Koening CL, et al. Vasculitis Clinical Research Consortium. Evaluation of potential serum biomarkers of disease activity in diverse forms of vasculitis. J Rheumatol. 2020;47(7):1001–10. https://doi.org/10.3899/jrheum.190093.
15. Park MC, Lee SW, Park YB, Lee SK. Serum cytokine profiles and their correlations with disease activity in Takayasu's arteritis. Rheumatology. 2006;45:545–8.
16. Sun Y, Kong X, Wu S, Ma L, Yan Y, Lv P, Jiang L. YKL-40 as a new biomarker of disease activity in Takayasu arteritis. Int J Cardiol. 2019;293:231–7.
17. Zanwar A, Jain A, Gupta L, Chaurasia S, Kumar S, Misra DP, et al. Serum BAFF and APRIL levels in Indian patients with Takayasu arteritis. Clin Rheumatol. 2018;37(12):3439–42.
18. Alibaz-Oner F, Yentur SP, Saruhan-Direskeneli G, Direskeneli H. Serum cytokine profiles in Takayasu's arteritis: a search for a biomarker. Clin Exp Rheumatol. 2015;33(Suppl 89):32–5.
19. Savioli B, Abdulahad WH, Brouwer E, Kallenberg CGM, de Souza AWS. Are cytokines and chemokines suitable biomarkers for Takayasu arteritis? Autoimmun Rev. 2017;16(10):1071–8.
20. Goel R, Kabeerdoss J, Ram B, Prakash JA, Babji S, Nair A, et al. Serum cytokine profile in Asian Indian patients with Takayasu arteritis and its association with disease activity. Open Rheumatol J. 2017;11:23–9.
21. Pulsatelli L, Boiardi L, Assirelli E, Pazzola G, Muratore F, Addimanda O, et al. Interleukin-6 and soluble interleukin-6 receptor are elevated in large-vessel vasculitis: a cross-sectional and longitudinal study. Clin Exp Rheumatol. 2017;35 Suppl 103(1):102–10. Epub 2017 Apr 20.
22. Fukui S, Kuwahara-Takaki A, Ono N, Sato S, Koga T, Kawashiri SY, et al. Serum levels of fibroblast growth factor-2 distinguish Takayasu arteritis from giant cell arteritis independent of age at diagnosis. Sci Rep. 2019;9(1):688.
23. Garlanda C, Bottazzi B, Bastone A, Mantovani A. Pentraxins at the crossroads between innate immunity, inflammation, matrix deposition, and female fertility. Annu Rev Immunol. 2005;23:337–66.
24. Ishihara T, Haraguchi G, Kamiishi T, Tezuka D, Inagaki H, Isobe M. Sensitive assessment of activity of Takayasu's arteritis by pentraxin3, a new biomarker. J Am Coll Cardiol. 2011;57(16):1712–3. No abstract available.
25. Dagna L, Salvo F, Tiraboschi M, Bozzolo EP, Franchini S, et al. Pentraxin-3 as a marker of disease activity in Takayasu arteritis. Ann Intern Med. 2011;155(7):425–33.
26. Ishihara T, Haraguchi G, Tezuka D, Kamiishi T, Inagaki H, Isobe M. Diagnosis and assessment of Takayasu arteritis by multiple biomarkers. Circ J. 2013;77(2):477–83. Epub 2012 Oct 26.
27. Alibaz-Oner F, Aksu K, Yentur SP, Keser G, Saruhan-Direskeneli G, Direskeneli H. Plasma pentraxin-3 levels in patients with Takayasu's arteritis during routine follow-up. Clin Exp Rheumatol. 2016;34(Suppl 97):S73–6.
28. Tombetti E, Di Chio MC, Sartorelli S, Papa M, Salerno A, et al. Systemic pentraxin-3 levels reflect vascular enhancement and progression in Takayasu arteritis. Arthritis Res Ther. 2014;16:479.
29. Chen Z, Hu C, Sun F, Li J, Yang Y, Tian X, Zeng X. Study on the association of serum pentraxin-3 and lysosomal-associated membrane protein-2 levels with disease activity in Chinese Takayasu's arteritis patients. Clin Exp Rheumatol. 2019;37 Suppl 117(2):109–15. Epub 2019 Mar 19.
30. Pulsatelli L, Boiardi L, Assirelli E, Pazzola G, Muratore F, Addimanda O. Imbalance between angiogenic and anti-angiogenic factors in sera from patients with large-vessel vasculitis.Clin Exp Rheumatol. 2020;38 Suppl 124(2):23–30.
31. Zeimpekis KG, Barbosa F, Hullner M, ter Voert E, Davison H, Veit-Haibach P, et al. Clinical evaluation of PET image quality as a function of acquisition time in a new TOF-PET/MRI compared to TOF-PET/CT—initial results. Mol Imaging Biol. 2015;17:735–44.

32. Einspieler I, Thurmel K, Pyka T, Eiber M, Wolfram S, Moog P, et al. Imaging large vessel vasculitis with fully integrated PET/MRI: a pilot study. Eur J Nucl Med Mol Imaging. 2015;42:1012–24.
33. Kerr GS, Hallahan CW, Giordano J, Leavitt RY, Fauci AS, Rottem M, Hoffman GS. Takayasu arteritis. Ann Intern Med. 1994;120(11):919–29.
34. Mukhtyar C, Lee R, Brown D, Carruthers D, Dasgupta B, Dubey S, et al. Modification and validation of the Birmingham Vasculitis Activity Score (version 3). Ann Rheum Dis. 2009;68:1827–32.
35. Aydin SZ, Yilmaz N, Akar S, Aksu K, Kamali S, Yucel E, et al. Assessment of disease activity and progression in Takayasu's arteritis with Disease Extent Index-Takayasu. Rheumatology (Oxford). 2010;49(10):1889–93.
36. Ureten K, Oztürk MA, Onat AM, Oztürk MH, Ozbalkan Z, Güvener M, et al. Takayasu's arteritis: results of a university hospital of 45 patients in Turkey. Int J Cardiol. 2004;96:259–64.
37. Henes JC, Müller M, Krieger J, Balletshofer B, Pfannenberg AC, Kanz L, et al. (18F) FDG-PET/CT as a new and sensitive imaging method for the diagnosis of large vessel vasculitis. Clin Exp Rheumatol. 2008;26(Suppl 49):S47–52.
38. Sivakumar MR, Misra RN, P. A. Bacon for the IRAVAS Group. The Indian perspective of Takayasu arteritis and developmentof a disease extent index (DEI.Tak) to assess Takayasu arteritis. Rheumatology. 2005;44(Suppl 3):iii6–7.
39. Mishra R, Danda D, Jayaseelan L, Sivakumar R, Lawrence A, Bacon PA. ITAS & DEI. TAK—scores for clinical diseaseactivity and damage extent in Takayasu's aortoarteritis (TA). Rheumatology. 2008;47:ii:101.
40. Misra R, Danda D, Rajappa SM, Ghosh A, Gupta R, Mahendranath KM, et al. Indian Rheumatology Vasculitis (IRAVAS) group. Development and initial validation of the Indian Takayasu Clinical Activity Score (ITAS2010). Rheumatology. 2013;52:1795–801.
41. Alibaz-Oner F, Aydin SZ, Akar S, Aksu K, Kamali S, Yucel E, et al. Assessment of patients with Takayasu arteritis in routine practice with Indian Takayasu clinical activity score. J Rheumatol. 2015;42(8):1443–7.
42. Kenar G, Karaman S, Çetin P, Yarkan H, Akar S, Can G, et al. Imaging is the major determinant in the assessment of disease activity in Takayasu's arteritis. Clin Exp Rheumatol. 2020;38 Suppl 124(2):55–60.
43. Aydin SZ, Direskeneli H, Merkel PA. International Delphi on disease activity assessment in large-vessel vasculitis. Assessment of disease activity in large-vessel vasculitis: results of an international Delphi exercise. J Rheumatol. 2017;44(12):1928–32.
44. Hellmich B, Agueda A, Monti S, Buttgereit F, de Boysson H, Brouwer E, et al. 2018 Update of the EULAR recommendations for the management of large vessel vasculitis. Ann Rheum Dis. 2020;79(1):19–30.
45. Bicakcigil M, Aksu K, Kamali S, Ozbalkan Z, Ates A, Karadag O, et al. Takayasu's arteritis in Turkey—clinical and angiographic features of 248 patients. Clin Exp Rheumatol. 2009;27(1 Suppl 52):S59–64.
46. Grayson PC, Cuthbertson D, Carette S, Hoffman GS, Khalidi NA, Koening CL, et al. Vasculitis Clinical Research Consortium. New features of disease after diagnosis in 6 forms of systemic vasculitis. J Rheumatol. 2013;40:1905–12.
47. Hong S, Bae SH, Ahn SM, Lim DH, Kim YG, Lee CK, et al. Outcome of takayasu arteritis with inactive disease at diagnosis: the extent of vascular involvement as a predictor of activation. J Rheumatol. 2015;42:489–94.
48. Fukui S, Iwamoto N, Shimizu T, Umeda M, Nishino A, Koga T, et al. Fewer subsequent relapses and lower levels of IL-17 in Takayasu arteritis developed after the age of 40 years. Arthritis Res Ther. 2016;18:293.
49. Comarmond C, Biard L, Lambert M, Mekinian A, Ferfar Y, Kahn JE, et al. Long-term outcomes and prognostic factors of complications in Takayasu arteritis: a multicenter study of 318 patients. Circulation. 2017;136:1114–22.
50. Kwon OC, Oh JS, Park MC, Hong S, Lee CK, Yoo B, et al. Statins reduce relapse rate in Takayasu arteritis. Int J Cardiol. 2019;287:111–5.

51. Seyahi E, Ugurlu S, Cumali R, Balci H, Seyahi N, Yurdakul S, et al. Atherosclerosis in Takayasu arteritis. Ann Rheum Dis. 2006;65:1202–7.
52. da Silva TF, Levy-Neto M, Bonfá E, Pereira RM. High prevalence of metabolic syndrome in Takayasu arteritis: increased cardiovascular risk and lower adiponectin serum levels. J Rheumatol. 2013;40:1897–904.
53. Numano F, Shimokado K, Kishi Y, Nishiyama K, Turkoglu C, Yajima M, et al. Changes in the plasma levels of thromboxane B2 and cyclic nucleotides in patients with Takayasu disease. Jpn Circ J. 1982;46:16–20.
54. Kasuya N, Kishi Y, Isobe M, Yoshida M, Numano F. P-selectin expression, but not GPIIb/IIIa activation, is enhanced in the inflammatory stage of Takayasu's arteritis. Circ J. 2006;70:600–4.
55. Akazawa H, Ikeda U, Yamamoto K, Kuroda T, Shimada K. Hypercoagulable state in patients with Takayasu's arteritis. Thromb Haemost. 1996;75:712–6.
56. Alibaz-Oner F, Koster MJ, Unal AU, Yildirim HG, Çikikçi C, Schmidt J, et al. Assessment of the frequency of cardiovascular risk factors in patients with Takayasu's arteritis. Rheumatology (Oxford). 2017;56(11):1939–44.
57. de Souza AW, Machado NP, Pereira VM, Arraes AE, Reis Neto ET, Mariz HA, et al. Antiplatelet therapy for the prevention of arterial ischemic events in Takayasu arteritis. Circ J. 2010;74:1236–41.
58. Seo P, Jayne D, Luqmani R, Merkel PA. Assessment of damage in vasculitis: expert ratings of damage. Rheumatology (Oxford). 2009;48:823–7.
59. Kermani TA, Dasgupta B. Current and emerging therapies in large-vessel vasculitis. Rheumatology (Oxford). 2018;57:1513–24.
60. Exley AR, Bacon PA, Luqmani RA, Kitas GD, Gordon C, Savage CO, et al. Development and initial validation of the Vasculitis Damage Index for the standardized clinical assessment of damage in the systemic vasculitides. Arthritis Rheum. 1997;40(2):371–80.
61. Omma A, Erer B, Karadag O, Yilmaz N, Alibaz-Oner F, Yildiz F, et al. Remarkable damage along with poor quality of life in Takayasu arteritis: cross-sectional results of a long-term followed-up multicentre cohort. Clin Exp Rheumatol. 2017;35 Suppl 103(1):77–82. Epub 2016 Nov.
62. Misra DP, Aggarwal A, Lawrence A, Agarwal V, Misra R. Pediatric-onset Takayasu's arteritis: clinical features and short-term outcome. Rheumatol Int. 2015;35:1701–6.
63. Kermani TA, Sreih AG, Cuthbertson D, Carette S, Hoffman GS, Khalidi NA, et al. Vasculitis Clinical Research Consortium. Evaluation of damage in giant cell arteritis. Rheumatology (Oxford). 2018;57(2):322–8.
64. Ohigashi H, Haraguchi G, Konishi M, Tezuka D, Kamiishi T, Ishihara T, et al. Improved prognosis of Takayasu arteritis over the past decade—comprehensive analysis of 106 patients. Circ J. 2012;76:1004–11.
65. Ishikawa K, Maetani S. Long-term outcome for 120 Japanese patients with Takayasu's disease. Clinical and statistical analyses of related prognostic factors. Circulation. 1994;90:1855–60.
66. Soto ME, Espinola N, Flores-Suarez LF, Reyes PA. Takayasu arteritis: clinical features in 110 Mexican Mestizo patients and cardiovascular impact on survival and prognosis. Clin Exp Rheumatol. 2008;26(3 Suppl 49):S9–15.
67. Schmidt J, Kermani TA, Bacani AK, Crowson CS, Cooper LT, Matteson EL, et al. Diagnostic features, treatment, and outcomes of Takayasu arteritis in a US cohort of 126 patients. Mayo Clin Proc. 2013;88:822–30.
68. Vautier M, Dupont A, de Boysson H, Comarmond C, Mirault T, Mekinian A, et al. Prognosis of large vessel involvement in large vessel vasculitis. J Autoimmun. 2020;108:102419.
69. Li J, Zhu M, Li M, Zheng W, Zhao J, Tian X, et al. Cause of death in Chinese Takayasu arteritis patients. Medicine (Baltimore). 2016;95(27):e4069.
70. Mirouse A, Biard L, Comarmond C, Lambert M, Mekinian A, Ferfar Y, et al. French Takayasu network. Overall survival and mortality risk factors in Takayasu's arteritis: a multicenter study of 318 patients. J Autoimmun. 2019;96:35–9.
71. Alibaz-Oner F, Direskeneli H. Update on Takayasu's arteritis. La Presse Médicale. 2015;44:e259–65.

Treatment

12

Fatma Alibaz-Oner and Haner Direskeneli

Abstract

Glucocorticoids (GC) are required for remission-induction in patients with Takayasu's arteritis. Remission is usually achieved with high-dose (1 mg/kg/day or pulse) regimens. A non-biologic disease modifying agent such as methotrexate, azathioprine or leflunomide is suggested as a first-line approach. In relapsing or refractory patients biologic agents tumor necrosis factor inhibitors or tocilizumab are chosen as second-line treatments. Except in acute ischemic episodes, vascular interventions should be performed in remission phases and under immunosuppressive regimens.

Keywords

Glucocorticoids · Biologic agents · Tumor necrosis factor inhibitors · Tocilizumab

Glucocorticoids are the mainstay of treatment for remission induction in Takayasu's arteritis (TAK). Early intensive therapy with high-dose glucocorticoids (GC) induces remission in most patients with large vessel vasculitis (LVV) [1–3]. The initial dose of prednisolone is 1 mg/kg/day (maximum 60 mg/day). The initial high dose should be maintained for a month and tapered gradually [4]. Generally, two-thirds of the total daily dose is given early in the morning and the rest of one-third in the evening after meals [5].

Despite the high response with GCs in TAK, there is a high relapse rate while gradually tapering the glucocorticoids. There are no studies comparing different GC

F. Alibaz-Oner · H. Direskeneli (✉)
Division of Rheumatology, Department of Internal Medicine, Marmara University, School of Medicine, Istanbul, Turkey

© Springer Nature Switzerland AG 2021
C. Salvarani et al. (eds.), *Large and Medium Size Vessel and Single Organ Vasculitis*, Rare Diseases of the Immune System, https://doi.org/10.1007/978-3-030-67175-4_12

tapering protocols in TAK. In a randomized controlled study (RCT) of tociluzumab, GC tapering in the placebo group by 10% per week after 4 weeks led to around 80% relapse during weeks 8–16 [6]. A similar relapse rate was observed with GC mono-therapy in a recent RCT of abatacept in TAK [7]. According to the 2018 update of the "*EULAR recommendations for the management of LVV*," it was recommended that in patients who have reached 15–20 mg daily GC dose after 2–3 months, GCs should be decreased slowly targeting ≤10 mg/day at the end of 1 year [8]. However, ≤10 mg/day doses of GCs in long-term remission are possibly too high compared to the recommendations in other disorders such as rheumatoid arthritis (usually ≤5 mg/day) and should be individually assessed in each patient according to the risk of GC-associated complications.

Long-term treatment with GCs causes many side effects. Therefore, many physicians prefer to start a conventional immunosuppressive (IS) agents while tapering GCs in daily practice despite the lack of randomized controlled study of any agent showing additional benefit in TAK. EULAR also recommends usage of non-biologic disease-modifying agents in addition to GC in all patients with TAK.

12.1 Non-biologic Disease-Modifying Agents

12.1.1 Methotrexate

Methotrexate (MTX) is a cheap, widely used and relatively safe agent in rheumatology. Therefore, it is generally the first choice of many physicians in daily practice. However, data about MTX usage in TAK comes from only open small studies [9–11]. In an open prospective series of 18 patients with TAK, the use of weekly oral MTX plus standard GC (started at 0.3 mg/kg/week with the initial dose not to exceed 15 mg/week) had favorable clinical response and regression of angiographic progression in 13 patients during a follow-up of mean 2.8 years. GC dosage could also be tapered in about half of the patients [12].

12.1.2 Azathioprine

Azathioprine (AZA) is another widely used IS agent in rheumatology; however, there is only one open study with AZA for the treatment of TAK. In this study, 65 IS-naive patients were given 2 mg/kg/day AZA in addition to GC treatment for 1 year. At the end of first year, acute phase responses were significantly reduced and no adverse events occurred. There was no progression in follow-up angiography. However, long-term follow-up of these patients was not reported [13]. In a large series of 251 TAK patients from India, almost all patients were given IS agents in addition to GC treatment. Fifty-four (21.5%) of these patients used AZA and all patients except 1 had complete remission with AZA treatment [14].

12.1.3 Leflunomide

Leflunomide (LEF) is an important disease-modifying agent for the treatment of rheumatoid arthritis. There are case reports and open studies showing benefical effects of LEF for the treatment of TAK [15, 16]. In the first open-label study, 15 TAK patients with active disease despite GC and IS treatments were given leflunomide 20 mg daily. One patient had intolerance to LEF. In a follow-up of mean 9.1 months later, significant improvement in disease activity (93% vs. 20%, $p = 0.002$) and CRP (10.3 vs. 5.3 mg/L, $p = 0.012$) was observed, and the mean daily dose of prednisone (34.2 vs. 13.9 mg, $p < 0.001$) decreased. In two (13.3%) patients, new angiographic lesions developed in the follow-up imaging [17]. In the extended phase of this study, follow-up data could be retrieved from 12 out of 15 patients. The mean follow-up time was 43.0 ± 7.6 months. Five (41.6%) of 12 patients remained on leflunomide therapy during the follow-up, while 7 (58.3%) patients had to change to treatment due to relapses in 6 patients and toxicity in one patient. Baseline clinical characteristics and cumulative GC dosage at the last visit were similar between patients remaining on LEF and changing the treatment [18]. In a very recent case series from China, 56 patients with TAK treated with LEF for at least 3 months were reported. Fourty-one of these patients were newly diagnosed, while 15 were cyclophosphamide (CYC)-resistant. Complete remission was achieved in 67.8% at 6 months. At the end of first year, complete remision rate was 55.3%. At the end of the follow-up period (14.4 ± 6 months), 48 patients (85.7%) were still under LEF treatment with good tolerance. Leflunomide was switched to another IS agent in 5 patients (2 patients due to relapse, 3 patients due to side effects) [19].

12.1.4 Mycophenolate Mofetil

Mycophenolate mofetil (MMF), a widely used agent effective in the treatment of lupus nephritis, is also reported as a promising agent in TAK [20]. In the first open study, ten patients with treatment-resistant TAK were given MMF for a mean period of 23 months. MMF resulted in a significant reduction in acute phase response. Five patients had received MMF as the first IS agent in addition to GC, while the others were refractory to other IS agents. Remission was achieved in all patients with MMF therapy, except one patient [21]. Goel et al. reported the data of 21 Indian TAK patients using MMF for 9.6 ± 6.4 months. Among those patients, ten had been resistant to GC plus AZA treatment. Disease activity was controlled together with decreasing GC requirement. The only adverse event reported was skin rash in a single patient [22]. In another long-term follow-up results of 251 TAK patients from India, 235 (93.6%) patients were given IS agents in addition to GC treatment. MMF was the most frequently preferred IS agent (161/235) in this group and 72% of these patients achieved complete remission with MMF treatment [14]. In a recent Chinese study of 30 TAK patients, MMF was combined with GCs. If clinical remission could not be achieved, another traditional ISs were added on current treatment. Overall, 16 patients were given MMF + GCs, while 14 patients were given MTX or AZA in addition to MMF + GC treatment. MMF + GCs was effective in 12 patients. When MMF was combined with methotrexate less than 15 mg/week, it was effective in nine patients (partial response in 3) and with AZA 100–150 mg/day in three patients (partial response in one). The authors suggested that MMF may be effective in controlling disease activity in up to 80%, either combined with low-dosage GCs or with MTX or AZA. Four patients stopped MMF due to side effects [23]. However, combination of different IS agents in TAK should still be considered with caution due to lack of convincing data and safety issues.

12.1.5 Cyclophosphamide

Cyclophosphamide (CYC) has been used in adults with TAK resistant to GCs in a small open-label study. In this study, 6 out of 20 patients who were refractory to GC treatment were given 2 mg/kg oral CYC daily. Four of these six patients had no vascular progression under CYC, while two had vascular progression [24]. CYC is generally preferred in the presence of severe life and/or vital organ-threatening conditions, including retinal vasculitis, pulmonary artery involvement with/without aneurysm, severe aortic regurgitation, or myocarditis [25–27]. In another open study, eight patients with TAK having myocardial involvement were reported to experience clinical hemodynamic and morphological improvement using GCs + CYC treatment [28]. Recently, Sun Y. et al. reported an open prospective observational cohort study assessing efectiveness and safety of CYC and MTX as induction therapy for TAK. There were 46 patients in CYC and 12 in MTX group. CYC group had more severe disease at baseline with higher Kerr activity score (≥ 3) and higher acute phase response compared to MTX group. At the 6-month evaluation, patients in CYC group had higher decrease in activity indices together with a decrease in acute phase response and radiologic improvement (wall enhancement scores: 4.2 ± 2.3 vs. 10.3 ± 3.8, $p = 0.03$). However, remission rate was similar between CYC and MTX groups (71.7% vs 75%, respectively). The authors concluded that CYC may be a better option than MTX for remission induction in more severe Takayasu's arteritis [29]. But differences of baseline characteristics and patient numbers in groups are very important limitations of this study.

12.1.6 Other Non-biologic Disease-Modifying Agents

Tacrolimus [30, 31] and cyclosporine [32–34] which are calcineurin inhibitors widely used in tranplant patients were reported as effective in selected cases with TAK. Shimizu M. et al. reported a TAK patient refractory to a combination of GCs, MTX, and infliximab and effectively treated with tacrolimus and mizoribin combination [35]. Tofacitinib is also reported as an effective treatment option for TAK in two case reports [36, 37].

12.2 Biologic Disease-Modifying Agents

12.2.1 Tumor Necrosis Factor Inhibitors

Tumor Necrosis Factor (TNF) inhibitors are the first biologic agents used for the treatment of TAK. In contrast to the experience in GCA, they seem quite effective in TAK; however, all evidence for TNF inhibitors come from open-label studies. In an early study, Hoffman et al. [38] reported the use of etanercept (ETN) and inflximab (IFX) in 15 refractory TAK patients, with 10 patients achieving complete remission without GCs. Still, 9 of the 14 responders required an increase in the TNF inhibitor dosage in order to attain remission and progression developed in 4 out of 15 patients despite apparent complete or partial remission. There are further many retrospective case series reporting TNF inhibitor usage in mainly refractory TAK patients not responding to conventional treatments and demonstrating clinical efficacy [39–44].

IFX was the mostly preferred TNF inhibitor (80%) in an analysis including 120 refractory TAK patients receiving TNF inhibitors. The remaining patients in this analysis had used either ETN or adalimumab (ADA). Overall response rate was 80% and GC dose could be reduced or discontinued in over 40% of the patients. However, relapses occurred in 37% and nearly 50% of relapsing patients required either an increase in dose or frequency, or were switched to a different TNF inhibitor [45]. Certolizumab [46, 47] and golimumab [48] were also reported as effective TNF inhibitors in selected cases.

A recent retrospective, longitudinal follow-up cohort from Norway reported less angiographic progression at 2 years in TAK patients receiving TNF inhibitors (10%) compared to conventional ISs (40%). In this study, angiographic progression rate was 90% in patients receiving GC treatment only [49]. Overall, TNF inhibitor usage in refractory TAK patients seem a highly effective option. However, different definitions of activity and refractory disease, concomitant usage of high-dose GCs should be kept in mind while interpreting these open studies. There is still a need for randomized, controlled, long studies to clarify the efficacy and safety of TNF inhibitors in TAK.

12.2.2 Tociluzumab

The critical role of Interlukin-6 (IL-6) in the pathogenesis of LVV is well known [50]. The clinical efficacy of Tociluzumab (TCZ) which is an IL-6 blocking agent was first reported in TAK by Nishimoto et al. in 2008 [51]. Then, many open case series reported the efficacy of TCZ in refractory TAK. In a very recent systematic review of 105 patients, TCZ was used in 72% for patients refractory to conventional treatments. Clinical improvement was present within 3 months in 90 (85.7%) and GC dose could be decreased in 75 patients. Imaging results were available in 66 patients, 43 (65.2%) had radiological improvement. Relapse under TCZ treatment was observed in 7 (9%) patients, in 6 after TCZ discontinuation with a median time of 5 months. Side effects were noted in 18%, with TCZ interruption in seven cases [52]. This review confirms that TCZ is a safe and effective agent in refractory TAK, but relapses seem an important issue after TCZ discontinuation in almost half of the patients.

TCZ was recently studied in a double-blind RCT for the treatment of TAK in Japan. In this study, 36 patients which relapsed within the last 12 weeks and gone into remission with oral GC treatment, were enrolled. Patients were randomized 1:1 to TCZ 162 mg/week or placebo subcutaneously. Oral GCs were tapered 10% weekly started from week 4 to a minimum of 0.1 mg/kg daily until 19 patients relapsed. The primary endpoint was "time to relapse" which was defined as ≥ 2 of the following: objective systemic symptoms, subjective systemic symptoms, elevated inflammation markers, vascular signs and symptoms, or ischemic symptoms. This study did not reach to the primary endpoint (intention-to-treat analysis: HR for time to relapse 0.41, 95% CI 0.15–1.10; $p = 0.0596$). However, a trend favoring TCZ over placebo was suggested (per protocol set: HR 0.34, 95% CI 0.11–1.00; $p = 0.0345$). There were no safety alerts with TCZ in the study group [6]. All 36 patients involved in this RCT were followed in open-label extension phase. Twenty-eight patients received weekly 162 mg tocilizumab for 96 weeks. The median GC dose was 0.22 mg/kg/day before the study entry and was 0.105 mg/kg/day after 96 weeks. Overall, 46.4% of patients reduced their GC dose to <0.1 mg/kg/day. The authors concluded that TCZ might have steroid-sparing effects with no safety concerns [53].

Overall, data with TCZ usage in refractory TAK patients show that TCZ may be another effective option. However, quick relapses after TCZ discontinuation seem as an important clinical problem. There is, again, a need for randomized, controlled long-term follow-up studies for the assessment efficacy and safety of TCZ usage and especially optimal treatment duration for sustained remission in TAK.

12.2.3 Rituximab

Hoyer et al. [54] first suggested a prominent role for B cells in the pathogenesis of TAK and recently, novel autoantibodies regulating endothelial activation are described [55]. Three active, refractory TAK patients responding to rituximab (RTX) therapy are first described, with later also isolated case reports [56–60]. The biggest series was reported by Pazzola et al. and included seven patients, six of them having refractory disease unresponsive to high-dose GCs and conventional immunosuppressive and/or biologic agents. Only three patients achieved complete remission after RTX treatment. Persistent disease activity and/or radiographic disease progression were observed in the remaining four patients [61]. Therefore, this limited experience of RTX do not support a role for RTX as the first- or second-line biologic therapy in TAK patients. But RTX may be an option in patients with TAK refractory to TNF inhibitors and TCZ, or intolerance and side effects of these agents.

12.2.4 Other Biologic Disease-Modifying Agents

Genome-wide association studies (GWAS) determined IL12B as a susceptibility gene for TAK. A single nucleotide polymorphism (SNP) in IL12B is also strongly associated with disease activity and a synergistic effect in combination with human leucocyte antigen (HLA)-B*52:01 was suggested in Japanese population [62, 63]. Therefore, IL-12/23p40, encoded by IL12B, may have a crucial role in TAK pathophysiology. The usage of ustekinumab, which is a monoclonal antibody against IL-12/23p40, was reported first in three TAK patients refractory to GCs and conventional ISs. Ustekinumab was given 45 mg subcutaneously at day 0 and day 28. When clinical, laboratory, and MRI findings at day 0 and day 84 were assessed, a significant decrease in inflammatory markers with no suppression of vascular lesions in MRI was observed [64]. Recently, another case with TAK and psoriasis treated with ustekinumab was published. Three month later after 90 mg ustekinumab treatment, a significant decrease in GC dose and normalization of acute phase response with no constitutional symptoms were reported [65].

In a double-blind RCT, 34 patients with TAK were treated with abatacept at a dose of 10 mg/kg on days 1, 15, 29 and at 8 weeks. At week 12, patients in remission were randomized to either receive placebo ($n = 15$) or monthly abatacept ($n = 11$) and followed up until 12 months. The primary endpoint was the "duration of remission" (relapse-free survival). The relapse-free survival rate at 12 months was 22% for those receiving abatacept and 40% for those receiving placebo ($p = 0.853$). There was also no difference regarding duration of remission between the two groups [66].

There is only one study reporting anakinra (IL-1Ra) usage in refractory TAK. In this case study, four patients were given anakinra due to unresponsiveness to conventional treatments and biologics. It was discontinued in two patients due to ineffectivity, in one patient due to side effects and in one patient due to other reasons. In this study, 86 biologic DMARD courses of 50 patients were also assessed retrospectively. In 86 biologic DMARD courses, 61 of them were TNF inhibitors, while 17 were TCZ. In head-to-head comparison, drug survival rate of TNF inhibitors was significantly higher than TCZ (67.2% vs 41.1%, $p = 0.028$). Concomitant conventional DMARD usage at baseline had a positive effect on drug survival rate (HR = 3.79, 95% CI = 1.49–9.60, $p = 0.005$) [67].

12.3 Vascular Interventions and Surgical Therapy

Except in emergency conditions, open or endovascular vascular interventions should be thought as the last option in case of medical treatment failure for preventing ischemic arterial symptoms or injury in TAK. As a general rule, such interventions should be avoided during the active phase of the disease and should be tried only after suppression of vascular inflammation by appropriate IS treatment [68]. If there is active arteritis and need for emergency surgery, some experts suggest to use intravenous biologic treatments with TCZ or TNF inhibitors in the preoperative period to decrease inflammatory burden [69, 70]. Major complications of surgical intervention in TAK are relatively rare, but active disease at the time of surgery represents a major risk factor [71]. In long-term follow-up results of 60 interventions (in 42 patients), revision rates at 5 and 10 years were zero in inactive patients with no GCs, 5% at 5 years, and 19% at 10 years in those patients with inactive disease under maintenance GCs compared to 43% at both 5 and 10 years in patients having active disease with GCs and 67% at both 5 and 10 years in those having active disease not prescribed GCs [72].

According to data coming from case series, main indications for surgery are as follows: refractory hypertension related to renal artery stenosis, aortic disease including coarctation and ascending aortic dilatation ± aortic valve regurgitation, ischemic heart disease, supra-aortic disease with cerebral ischemia, mesenteric ischemia, severe limb-threatening claudication, and aneurysm repair [1, 73–77].

Outcomes of endovascular interventions generally depend on involved area and the length of involved segment. In short segment involvement, balloon angioplasty or stent graft replacement may be better options. Percutaneous transluminal angioplasty is a less invasive and safe method compared to open surgery [78, 79]. However, angioplasty and stenting have a higher rate of restenosis than surgical reconstruction [80, 81]. In a recent meta-analysis comparing balloon angioplasty and stenting outcomes, balloon angioplasty was performed in 186 and stenting in 130 lesions. There were no significant differences in the incidence of restenosis and other complications overall ($p = 0.38$), but restenosis risk in stenting was significantly higher than balloon angioplasty (OR = 4.40, 95% CI = 2.14–9.02, $p < 0.001$) in renal stenosis. Acute vascular complications were significantly fewer in stenting than in balloon angioplasty (OR = 0.07, 95% CI = 0.02–0.29, $p < 0.001$) [82]. In long-segment involvement with extensive periarterial fibrosis or occlusion, surgical bypass of involved segment in especially lower limb and renal arteries is the best option. Also it is clearly associated with better outcomes compared to endovascular interventions [76, 83]. Although drug-eluting balloons and/or stents were offered to avoid or increase the stent restenosis, the results are controversial [78, 84, 85]. Antiplatelet treatment may decrease restenosis development after vascular interventions [86].

12.4 Conclusion

There are only two RCTs not reaching primary endpoints for the management of TAK. Majority of current data comes from case series and open studies. Therefore, level of evidence for TAK management is low and expert opinion is still the main determinant while managing TAK patients during daily practice. Glucocorticoids are the mainstay of treatment, but a conventional IS agent should be added on GCs. MTX, AZA, MMF, or LEF could be chosen as the first-line IS agent. If there is a treatment failure with first-line agents, switch to biologic treatments can be thought. According to EULAR recommendations, TCZ or TNF inhibitors can be considered equally at this point [8]. In an indirect comparison of small retrospectve series, all comparisons such as disease activity and acute phase response were found similar between TNF inhibitors and TCZ [87]. However, TCZ did not reach to the primary endpoint in an RCT [6]. Despite an equal recommendation by EULAR recommendations after GCs plus IS failure in TAK, our approach is to prefer a TNF inhibitor as the first-line biologic in our Vasculitis Clinic due to larger experience with TNF inhibitors. Also both our clinical experience and mentioned retrospective study confirm better drug survival with TNF inhibitors in TAK.

References

1. Maksimowicz-McKinnon K, Clark TM, Hoffman GS. Limitations of therapy and a guarded prognosis in an American cohort of Takayasu arteritis patients. Arthritis Rheum. 2007;56:1000–9.
2. Proven A, Gabriel SE, Orces C, O'Fallon WM, Hunder GG. Glucocorticoid therapy in giant cell arteritis: duration and adverse outcomes. Arthritis Rheum. 2003;49:703–8.
3. Mazlumzadeh M, Hunder GG, Easley KA, Calamia KT, Matteson EL, Griffing WL, et al. Treatment of giantell arteritis using induction therapy with high-dose glucocorticoids: a double-blind, placebo-controlled, randomized prospective clinical trial. Arthritis Rheum. 2006;54:3310–8.
4. Park MC, Lee SW, Park YB, Chung NS, Lee SK. Clinical characteristics and outcomes of Takayasu's arteritis: analysis of 108 patients using standardized criteria for diagnosis, activity assessment, and angiographic classification. Scand J Rheumatol. 2005;34:284–92.
5. Keser G, Direskeneli H, Aksu K. Management of Takayasu arteritis: a systematic review. Rheumatology (Oxford). 2013;53:793–801.
6. Nakaoka Y, Isobe M, Takei S, Tanaka Y, Ishii T, Yokota S, et al. Efficacy and safety of tocilizumab in patients with refractory Takayasu arteritis: results from a randomised, double-blind, placebo-controlled, phase 3 trial in Japan (the TAKT study). Ann Rheum Dis. 2018;77(3):348–54.
7. Langford CA, Cuthbertson D, Ytterberg SR, Khalidi N, Monach PA, Carette S, et al. A randomized, double-blind trial of abatacept (CTLA-4Ig) for the treatment of Takayasu arteritis. Arthritis Rheumatol. 2017;69:846–53.
8. Hellmich B, Agueda A, Monti S, Buttgereit F, de Boysson H, Brouwer E, et al. 2018 Update of the EULAR recommendations for the management of large vessel vasculitis. Ann Rheum Dis. 2020;79(1):19–30.
9. Mevorach D, Leibowitz G, Brezis M, Raz E. Induction of remission in a patient with Takayasu's arteritis by low dose pulses of methotrexate. Ann Rheum Dis. 1992;51:904.
10. Shetty A, Stopa A, Gedalia A. Low-dose methotrexate as an steroid-sparing agent in a child with Takayasu's arteritis. Clin Exp Rheumatol. 1998;16:335–6.
11. Liang G, Nemickas R, Madayag M. Multiple percutaneous transluminal angioplasties and low dose pulse methotrexate for Takayasu's arteritis. J Rheumatol. 1989;16:1370–3.
12. Hoffman GS, Leavitt RY, Kerr GS, Rottem M, Sneller MC, Fauci AS. Treatment of glucocorticoid-resistant or relapsing Takayasu arteritis with methotrexate. Arthritis Rheum. 1994;37:578–82.
13. Liang P, Hoffman GS. Advances in the medical and surgical treatment of Takayasu arteritis. Curr Opin Rheumatol. 2005;17(1):16–24.
14. Goel R, Danda D, Joseph G, Ravindran R, Kumar S, Jayaseelan V, et al. Long-term outcome of 251 patients with Takayasu arteritis on combination immunosuppressant therapy: single centre experience from a large tertiary care teaching hospital in Southern India. Semin Arthritis Rheum. 2018;47(5):718–26.

15. Haberhauer G, Kittl EM, Dunky A, Feyertag J, Bauer K. Beneficial effects of leflunomide in glucocorticoid- and methotrexate-resistant Takayasu's arteritis. Clin Exp Rheumatol. 2001;19(4):477–8.
16. Unizony S, Stone JH, Stone JR. New treatment strategies in large-vessel vasculitis. Curr Opin Rheumatol. 2013;25(1):3–9.
17. de Souza A, da Silva M, Machado L, Oliveira A, Pinheiro F, Sato E. Short-term effect of leflunomide in patients with Takayasu arteritis: an observational study. Scand J Rheumatol. 2012;41(3):227–30. Epub 2012 Mar 9.
18. de Souza AW, de Almeida Agustinelli R, de Cinque Almeida H, Oliveira PB, Pinheiro FA, Oliveira AC, et al. Leflunomide in Takayasu arteritis—a long term observational study. Rev Bras Reumatol. 2016. pii: S0482-5004(16)00005-X.
19. Cui X, Dai X, Ma L, Yang C, Tan W, Zhang L, et al. East China Takayasu Arteritis (ECTA) Collaboration Group. Efficacy and safety of leflunomide treatment in Takayasu arteritis: case series from the East China cohort. Semin Arthritis Rheum. 2020;50(1):59–65.
20. Daina E, Schieppati A, Remuzzi G. Mycophenolate mofetil for the treatment of Takayasu arteritis: report of three cases. Ann Intern Med. 1999;130:422–6.
21. Shinjo SK, Pereira RM, Tizziani VA, Radu AS, Levy-Neto M. Mycophenolate mofetil reduces disease activity and steroid dosage in Takayasu arteritis. Clin Rheumatol. 2007;26:1871–5.
22. Goel R, Danda D, Mathew J, Edwin N. Mycophenolate mofetil in Takayasu's arteritis. Clin Rheumatol. 2010;29(3):329–32.
23. Li J, Yang Y, Zhao J, Li M, Tian X, Zeng X. The efficacy of Mycophenolate mofetil for the treatment of Chinese Takayasu's arteritis. Sci Rep. 2016;6:38687.
24. Shelhamer JH, Volkman DJ, Parrillo JE, Lawley TJ, Johnston MR, Fauci AS. Takayasu's arteritis and its therapy. Ann Intern Med. 1985;103:121–6.
25. Edwards K, Lindsley H, Lai C, Van Veldhuizen P. Takayasu arteritis presenting as retinal and vertebrobasilar ischemia. J Rheumatol. 1989;16:1000–2.
26. Cash J, Engelbrecht J. Takayasu's arteritis in western South Dakota. S D J Med. 1990;43:5–9.
27. Rodriguez-Hurtado F, Sabio J, Lucena J, Jimenez-Alonso J. Ocular involvement in Takayasu's arteritis: response to cyclophosphamide therapy. Eur J Med Res. 2002;7:128–30.
28. Talwar K, Chopra P, Narula J, Shrivastava S, Singh S, Sharma S, Saxena A, Rajani M, Bhatia M. Myocardial involvement and its response to immunosuppressive therapy in nonspecific aortoarteritis (Takayasu's disease)—a study by endomyocardial biopsy. Int J Cardiol. 1988;21:323–34.
29. Sun Y, Ma L, Ma L, Kong X, Chen H, Lv P, et al. Cyclophosphamide could be a better choice than methotrexate as induction treatment for patients with more severe Takayasu's arteritis. Rheumatol Int. 2017;37(12):2019–26.
30. Yokoe I, Haraoka H, Harashima H. A patient with Takayasu's arteritis and rheumatoid arthritis who responded to tacrolimus hydrate. Intern Med. 2007;46:1873–7.
31. Yamazaki H, Nanki T, Harigai M, Miyasaka N. Successful treatment of refractory Takayasu arteritis with tacrolimus. J Rheumatol. 2012;39(7):1487–8.
32. Fearfield L, Ross J, Farrell A, Costello C, Bunker C, Staughton R. Pyoderma gangrenosum associated with Takayasu's arteritis responding to cyclosporin. Br J Dermatol. 1999;141:339–43.
33. Fullerton SH, Abel EA, Getz K, El-Ramahi K. Cyclosporine treatment of severe recalcitrant pyoderma gangrenosum in a patient with Takayasu's arteritis. Arch Dermatol. 1991;127:1731–2.
34. Horigome H, Kamoda T, Matsui A. Treatment of glucocorticoiddependent Takayasu's arteritis with cyclosporin. Med J Aust. 1999;170:566.
35. Shimizu M, Ueno K, Ishikawa S, Tokuhisa Y, Inoue N, Yachie A. Successful multitarget therapy using mizoribine and tacrolimus for refractory Takayasu arteritis. Rheumatology (Oxford). 2014;53(8):1530–2.
36. Sato S, Matsumoto H, Temmoku J, Fujita Y, Matsuoka N, Furuya M, et al. A case of Takayasu arteritis complicated by refractory ulcerative colitis successfully treated with tofacitinib. Rheumatology (Oxford). 2019. pii: kez580.

37. Yamamura Y, Matsumoto Y, Asano Y, Katayama Y, Hayashi K, Ohashi K, et al. Refractory Takayasu arteritis responding to the oral Janus kinase inhibitor, tofacitinib. Rheumatol Adv Pract. 2019;4(1):rkz050.
38. Hoffman GS, Merkel PA, Brasington RD, et al. Antitumor necrosis factor therapy in patients with difficult to treat Takayasu arteritis. Arthritis Rheum. 2004;50:2296–304.
39. Novikov PI, Smitienko IO, Moiseev SV. Tumor necrosis factor alpha inhibitors in patients with Takayasu's arteritis refractory to standard immunosuppressive treatment: cases series and review of the literature. Clin Rheumatol. 2013;32:1827–32.
40. Schmidt J, Kermani TA, Bacani AK, Crowson CS, Matteson EL, Warrington KJ. Tumor necrosis factor inhibitors in patients with Takayasu arteritis: experience from a referral center with long-term followup. Arthritis Care Res. 2012;64:1079–83.
41. Molloy ES, Langford CA, Clark TM, Gota CE, Hoffman GS. Anti-tumour necrosis factor therapy in patients with refractory Takayasu arteritis: longterm follow-up. Ann Rheum Dis. 2008;67:1567–9.
42. Quartuccio L, Schiavon F, Zuliani F, Carraro V, Catarsi E, Tavoni AG, et al. Long-term efficacy and improvement of health-related quality of life in patients with Takayasu's arteritis treated with infliximab. Clin Exp Rheumatol. 2012;30:922–8.
43. Mekinian A, Neel A, Sibilia J, Cohen P, Connault J, Lambert M, et al. Club Rhumatismes et Inflammation, French Vasculitis Study Group and Société Nationale Française de Médecine Interne. Efficacy and tolerance of infliximab in refractory Takayasu arteritis: French multicentre study. Rheumatology. 2012;51:882–6.
44. Karageorgaki ZT, Mavragani CP, Papathanasiou MA, Skopouli FN. Infliximab in Takayasu arteritis: a safe alternative? Clin Rheumatol. 2007;26:984–7.
45. Clifford A, Hoffman GS. Recent advances in the medical management of Takayasu arteritis: an update on use of biologic therapies. Curr Opin Rheumatol. 2014;26:7–15.
46. Novikov PI, Smitienko IO, Sokolova MV, Alibaz-Oner F, Kaymaz-Tahra S, Direskeneli H, et al. Certolizumab pegol in the treatment of Takayasu arteritis. Rheumatology (Oxford). 2018;57(12):2101–5.
47. Ataş N, Varan Ö, Babaoğlu H, Satiş H, Bilici Salman R, Tufan A. Certolizumab pegol treatment in three patients with Takayasu arteritis. Arch Rheumatol. 2019;34(3):357–62.
48. Suematsu R, Tashiro S, Ono N, Koarada S, Ohta A, Tada Y. Successful golimumab therapy in four patients with refractory Takayasu's arteritis. Mod Rheumatol. 2018;28(4):712–5.
49. Gudbrandsson B, Molberg Ø, Palm Ø. TNF inhibitors appear to inhibit disease progression and improve outcome in Takayasu arteritis; an observational, population-based time trend study. Arthritis Res Ther. 2017;19(1):99.
50. Arnaud L, Kahn J-E, Girszyn N, Piette A-M, Bletry O. Takayasu's arteritis: an update on physiopathology. Eur J Intern Med. 2006;17(4):241–6.
51. Nishimoto N, Nakahara H, Yoshio-Hoshino N, Mima T. Successful treatment of a patient with Takayasu arteritis using a humanized anti-interleukin-6 receptor antibody. Arthritis Rheum. 2008;58:1197–200.
52. Decker P, Olivier P, Risse J, Zuily S, Wahl D. Tocilizumab and refractory Takayasu diease: four case reports and systematic review. Autoimmun Rev. 2018;17(4):353–60.
53. Nakaoka Y, Isobe M, Tanaka Y, Ishii T, Ooka S, Niiro H, et al. Long-term efficacy and safety of tocilizumab in refractory takayasu arteritis: final results of the randomized controlled phase 3 TAKT study. Rheumatology (Oxford). 2020;59(9):2427–34.
54. Hoyer BF, Mumtaz IM, Loddenkemper K, Bruns A, Sengler C, Hermann KG, et al. Takayasu arteritis is characterised by disturbances of B cell homeostasis and responds to B cell depletion therapy with rituximab. Ann Rheum Dis. 2012;71(1):75–9. Epub 2011 Sep 27.
55. Mutoh T, Shirai T, Ishii T, Shirota Y, Fujishima F, Takahashi F, et al. Identification of two major autoantigens negatively regulating endothelial activation in Takayasu arteritis. Nat Commun. 2020;11(1):1253.
56. Caltran E, Di Colo G, Ghigliotti G. Two Takayasu arteritis patients successfully treated with rituximab. Clin Rheumatol. 2014;33:11834.

57. Galarza C, Valencia D, Tobón GJ, Zurita L, Mantilla RD, Pineda-Tamayo R, et al. Should rituximab be considered as the first-choice treatment for severe autoimmune rheumatic diseases? Clin Rev Allergy Immunol. 2008;34:1248.
58. Ernst D, Greer M, Stoll M, Meyer-Olson D, Schmidt RE, Witte T. Remission achieved in refractory advanced Takayasu arteritis using rituximab. Case Rep Rheumatol. 2012;2012:406963.
59. O'Connor MB, O'Donovan N, Bond U, Phelan MJ. Successful treatment of Takayasu arteritis with rituximab as a first-line immunosuppressant. BMJ Case Rep. 2017;10:2017.
60. Mutoh T, Ishii T, Shirai T, Akita K, Kamogawa Y. Refractory Takayasu arteritis successfully treated with rituximab: case-based review. Rheumatol Int. 2009;39(11):1989–94.
61. Pazzola G, Muratore F, Pipitone N, Crescentini F, Cacoub P, Boiardi L, et al. Rituximab therapy for Takayasu arteritis: a seven patients experience and a review of the literature. Rheumatology (Oxford). 2018;57(7):1151–5.
62. Terao C, Yoshifuji H, Kimura A, Matsumura T, Ohmura K, Takahashi M, et al. Two susceptibility loci to Takayasu arteritis reveal a synergistic role of the IL12B and HLA-B regions in a Japanese population. Am J Hum Genet. 2013;93:289–97.
63. Saruhan-Direskeneli G, Hughes T, Aksu K, Keser G, Coit P, Aydin SZ, et al. Identification of multiple genetic susceptibility Loci in Takayasu arteritis. Am J Hum Genet. 2013;93:298–305.
64. Terao C, Yoshifuji H, Nakajima T, Yukawa N, Matsuda F, Mimori T. Ustekinumab as a therapeutic option for Takayasu arteritis: from genetic findings to clinical application. Scand J Rheumatol. 2016;45(1):80–2.
65. Yachoui R, Kreidy M, Siorek M, Sehgal R. Successful treatment with ustekinumab for corticosteroid- and immunosuppressant-resistant Takayasu's arteritis. Scand J Rheumatol. 2018;47(3):246–7.
66. Langford CA, Cuthbertson D, Ytterberg SR, Khalidi N, Monach PA, Carette S, et al. Vasculitis clinical research consortium. A randomized, double-blind trial of abatacept (CTLA-4Ig) for the treatment of Takayasu arteritis. Arthritis Rheumatol. 2017;69(4):846–53.
67. Campochiaro C, Tomelleri A, Sartorelli S, Cavalli G, De Luca G, Baldissera E, et al. Drug retention and discontinuation reasons between seven biologics in patients with Takayasu arteritis. Semin Arthritis Rheum. 2020. pii: S0049-0172(20)30005-6.
68. Liang P, Tan-Ong M, Hoffman GS. Takayasu's arteritis: vascular interventions and outcomes. J Rheumatol. 2004;31:102–6.
69. Mason JC. Surgical intervention and its role in Takayasu arteritis. Best Pract Res Clin Rheumatol. 2018;32(1):112–24.
70. Risse J, Mandry D, Settembre N, Vigouroux C, Claudin M, Tsintzila G, et al. Dramatic response to Tocilizumab before emergency surgery in severe active Takayasu disease. Circ Cardiovasc Imaging. 2016;9(7). pii: e004819.
71. Rosa Neto NS, Shinjo SK, Levy-Neto M, Pereira RMR. Vascular surgery: the main risk factor for mortality in 146 Takayasu arteritis patients. Rheumatol Int. 2017;37:1065–73.
72. Fields CE, Bower TC, Cooper LT, Hoskin T, Noel AA, Panneton JM, et al. Takayasu's arteritis: operative results and influence of disease activity. J Vasc Surg. 2006;43(1):64–71.
73. Labarca C, Makol A, Crowson CS, Kermani TA, Matteson EL, Warrington KJ. Retrospective comparison of open versus endovascular procedures for Takayasu arteritis. J Rheumatol. 2016;43:427–32.
74. Perera AH, Mason JC, Wolfe JH. Takayasu arteritis: criteria for surgical intervention should not be ignored. Int J Vasc Med. 2013;2013:618910.
75. Perera AH, Youngstein T, Gibbs RG, Jackson JE, Wolfe JH, Mason JC. Optimizing the outcome of vascular intervention for Takayasu arteritis. Br J Surg. 2014;101:43–50.
76. Saadoun D, Lambert M, Mirault T, Resche-Rigon M, Koskas F, Cluzel P, et al. Retrospective analysis of surgery versus endovascular intervention in Takayasu arteritis: a multicenter experience. Circulation. 2012;125:813–9.
77. Yang L, Zhang H, Jiang X, Zou Y, Qin F, Song L, et al. Clinical manifestations and longterm outcome for patients with Takayasu arteritis in China. J Rheumatol. 2014;41:2439–46.

78. Wrotniak L, Kabłak-Ziembińska A, Przewłodzki T, Pieniążek P, Podolec J, Musiałek P, et al. Longterm experience in patients undergoing endovascular revascularization procedures for symptomatic Takayasu arteritis (RCD code: I-3A.1). J Rare Cardiovasc Dis. 2013;1:8–13.
79. Kazibudzki M, Tekieli Ł, Trystuła M, Paluszek P, Moczulski Z, Pieniążek P. New endovascular techniques for treatment of life-threatening Takayasu arteritis. Adv Interv Cardiol. 2016;12:171–4.
80. Min PK, Park S, Jung JH, Ko YG, Choi D, Jang Y, et al. Endovascular therapy combined with immunosuppressive treatment for occlusive arterial disease in patients with Takayasu's arteritis. J Endovasc Ther. 2005;12:28–34.
81. Sharma BK, Jain S, Bali HK, Jain A, Kumari S. A follow-up study of balloon angioplasty and de-novo stenting in Takayasu arteritis. Int J Cardiol. 2000;75(Suppl 1):S147–52.
82. Jeong HS, Jung JH, Song GG, Choi SJ, Hong SJ. Endovascular balloon angioplasty versus stenting in patients with Takayasu arteritis: a meta-analysis. Medicine (Baltimore). 2017;96(29):e7558.
83. Jung JH, Lee YH, Song GG, Jeong HS, Kim JH, Choi SJ. Endovascular versus open surgical intervention in patients with Takayasu's arteritis: a meta-analysis. Eur J Vasc Endovasc Surg. 2018;2:S1078-5884(18)30128.
84. Horie N, Hayashi K, Morikawa M, So G, Takahata H, Suyama K, Nagata I. Restenosis after endovascular PTA/stenting for supra-aortic branches in Takayasu aortitis: report of three cases and review of the literature. Acta Neurochir. 2011;153:1135–9.
85. Spacek M, Zimolova P, Veselka J. Takayasu arteritis: use of drug-eluting stent and balloon to treat recurring carotid restenosis. J Invasive Cardiol. 2012;24:E190–2.
86. Visona A, Tonello D, Zalunardo B, Irsara S, Liessi G, Marigo L, et al. Antithrombotic treatment before and after peripheral artery percutaneous angioplasty. Blood Transfus. 2009;7:18–23.
87. Mekinian A, Comarmond C, Resche-Rigon M, Mirault T, Kahn JE, Lambert M, et al. French Takayasu Network. Efficacy of biological-targeted treatments in Takayasu arteritis: multicenter, retrospective study of 49 patients. Circulation. 2015;132(18):1693–700.

Part III

Polyarteritis Nodosa

Cutaneous Polyarteritis Nodosa

13

Matthew J. Koster and Julio C. Sartori Valinotti

Abstract

Cutaneous involvement of medium vessel vasculitis most commonly presents with features of inflammatory subcutaneous nodules, purpura, livedo reticularis, and ulceration. The clinical and histopathologic features of isolated cutaneous polyarteritis nodosa (c-PAN) are indistinguishable from the cutaneous involvement of systemic polyarteritis nodosa; however, these conditions differ in their prognosis and treatment. An approach to distinguish between these clinical entities is herein described. In addition, conditions commonly mimicking cutaneous polyarteritis nodosa are reviewed.

Keywords

Cutaneous · Polyarteritis nodosa · Livedo reticularis

M. J. Koster (✉)
Division of Rheumatology, Department of Internal Medicine,
Mayo Clinic College of Medicine and Science, Rochester, MN, USA
e-mail: koster.matthew@mayo.edu

J. C. Sartori Valinotti
Department of Dermatology, Mayo Clinic College of Medicine and Science,
Rochester, MN, USA
e-mail: sartorivalinotti.julio@mayo.edu

© Springer Nature Switzerland AG 2021
C. Salvarani et al. (eds.), *Large and Medium Size Vessel and Single Organ Vasculitis*, Rare Diseases of the Immune System,
https://doi.org/10.1007/978-3-030-67175-4_13

13.1 Introduction

Cutaneous polyarteritis nodosa (c-PAN) is a form of vasculitis that predominantly affects the medium-sized arteries of the dermis and the subcutaneous tissue without evidence of systemic involvement. Historically, it has been considered a subset of classical (systemic) polyarteritis nodosa (PAN). More recent nomenclature has suggested revised terminology classifying c-PAN as a single organ vasculitis (SOV) and recommended use of the term "cutaneous arteritis" [1]. However, given this entity has distinct clinical and histopathologic characteristics that differ from cutaneous small-vessel vasculitis, another subgroup of SOV, but analogous pathologic arterial findings indistinguishable from patients with systemic PAN that have cutaneous involvement, the term c-PAN remains in frequent use and will be utilized herein.

13.2 Epidemiology, Genetics, Pathogenesis

While the first descriptions of systemic PAN were reported in 1866 by Kussmaul and Maier (originally termed periarteritis nodosa) [2], it was not until 1931 that Lindberg described a separate cutaneous-limited form [3]. The true incidence and prevalence of c-PAN is unknown due to the combination of its rarity and lack of population-based studies. It is considered rarer than systemic PAN and accounts for less than 5% of described PAN variants [4]. The average age of presentation of c-PAN is in the fourth decade of life but can range from newborn (3–5 days old) to 81 years [5–8]. A female predominance has been reported with a male-to-female ratio ranging from 1:1.7 to 1:3.4 [5, 6]. Ethnic and geographic distribution has been less well-studied. Of reported cases, Caucasians appear to have a higher frequency of diagnosis, but c-PAN has also been observed in patients of African-American, Asian, and Middle-Eastern descent [5, 6, 9–11].

The etiology and pathogenesis of c-PAN remain unknown. Deposition of complement C3 and immunoglobulin M in the arterial walls has been observed through direct immunofluorescence and suggests the possibility of an immune-complex-mediated disease [12, 13]. Elevated levels of circulating antibodies, including anti-phosphatidylserine-prothrombin complex, have been noted with increased frequency in some series of c-PAN but have not been validated in all cases [14]. Although only three descriptions have been reported, c-PAN present in newborns of mothers with historical or active c-PAN at the time of delivery further supports a possible mechanism of transferred circulating antibodies resulting in arterial inflammation [7, 8, 15]. Mutations in the *CERC1* gene which encodes for adenosine deaminase 2, a plasma protein involved in the differentiation of leukocytes and endothelial cells have been observed in a small subset of patients with childhood-onset, refractory c-PAN suggesting genetic predisposition may also play a role [16, 17].

The majority of cases of c-PAN are considered idiopathic, but an associated medical condition or potential inciting event may be described in 30–40%. Inflammatory bowel disease has been observed in up to 6% of patients with c-PAN in one series [5]. Antecedent or active infections have also been demonstrated among patients developing c-PAN. The most common, particularly in childhood-onset c-PAN, is Group A β hemolytic *Streptococcus* [18, 19]. Hepatitis B and C, parvovirus B19, as well as *Mycobacterium tuberculosis* have also been reported, but with notably lower frequency [6, 20–22]. Drug-induced c-PAN is notably uncommon; however, prolonged use of minocycline for treatment of moderate–severe acne vulgaris is a well-established culprit [23–26].

13.3 Clinical Manifestations and Laboratory Markers

13.3.1 Clinical Manifestations

The definitions of the commonly occurring skin findings observed in c-PAN are listed in Table 13.1. The most frequent early manifestation of c-PAN is small (0.5–3.0 cm), tender, palpable subcutaneous nodules which are present in 80–100% of patients [5, 6, 9]. The lower extremities are preferentially affected (95–100%), but nodules can also be located on the upper extremities (16–45%) and trunk (13%) [5, 9]. Head and neck involvement has been reported in 39% of c-PAN in one series [27] but has not been demonstrated with regularity in larger cohorts [5, 28]. Subcutaneous nodules are typically present concomitantly with ulceration or may precede sites of ulcer formation by several weeks to months; however, painful ulceration may be the only finding on initial examination in up to 10% of patients (Fig. 13.1) [5]. Ulcers may be superficial or deep and often have a punched-out appearance with a necrotic center (Fig. 13.2). Distribution is similar to subcutaneous nodules with lower extremity predilection (100%) and less commonly concomitant ulceration on the upper extremities (20%) and trunk (3–5%) [5, 6, 9].

Table 13.1 Definitions of skin findings in cutaneous polyarteritis nodosa

Term	Definition/description
Subcutaneous nodules	Abnormal skin tissue growth resulting from inflammation of the vessels with muscular walls present in the deep dermis and subcutis, commonly tender and erythematous
Retiform purpura	Non-blanchable hemorrhagic skin lesions resulting from the leakage of red blood cells into the skin due to vascular damage or occlusion following an angulated or branched distribution
Livedo reticularis/ racemosa	Mottled reticulated vascular pattern appearing as a net-like or lace-like purplish discoloration of the skin
Atrophie blanche	Ivory-colored stellate or angular scar, predominantly on the lower extremity, occurring after skin injury for which the presence of impaired blood supply resulted in poor or delayed healing
Ulceration	Disruption of the skin accompanied by disintegration of tissue which can result in complete loss of the epidermis and portions of the dermis and subcutaneous fat, resulting from reduced vascular perfusion. When present in the phalanges, this can lead to digital necrosis and gangrene

Fig. 13.1 Inflammatory retiform purpura with small subcutaneous nodules overlying cutaneous erosion involving the posterior elbow in patient with cutaneous polyarteritis nodosa

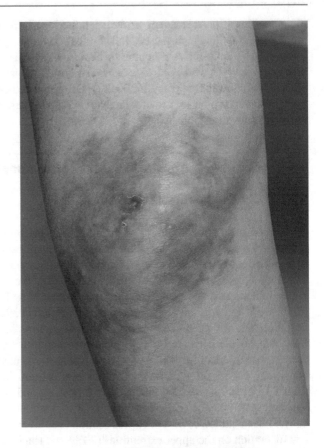

Fig. 13.2 Inflammatory retiform purpura and healing "punch out" ulcers of medial right ankle

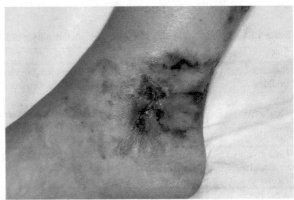

Livedo reticularis and livedo racemosa are observed in 55–78% of patients and is noted in areas of dependency or points of pressure such as the legs, feet, buttock, and scapulae (Fig. 13.3) [5, 6, 9, 27]. Atrophie blanche is isolated to the lower extremities [6] and if present in a patient without evidence of venous insufficiency or thrombophilic state is strongly suggestive of an underlying necrotizing

Fig. 13.3 Livedo racemosa involving the lower extremities in a young patient with cutaneous polyarteritis nodosa

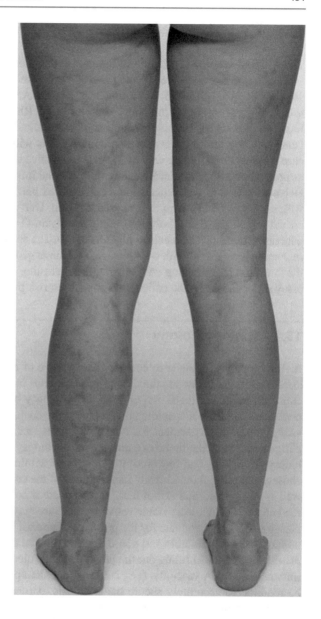

medium-sized vessel vasculitis within the reticular dermis and subcutis [29]. Digital arterial involvement due to fibrinoid necrosis and thrombotic occlusion is exceptional but can lead to gangrene [30].

Localized symptoms resulting from sequelae of cutaneous inflammation are frequently seen and include edema, pain, and paresthesias. Myalgia and arthralgia may also occur but are typically mild–moderate and transient. Constitutional symptoms of fever, weight loss, and fatigue are observed in approximately one-third of patients.

13.3.2 Laboratory Markers

There are no specific or diagnostic laboratory parameters for c-PAN. Erythrocyte sedimentation rate and C-reactive protein elevation are observed in 60% of patients and mild anemia in 33% [5, 9]. Antinuclear antigen (ANA) has been observed in up to 28% of patients but is commonly low-titer [5, 6]. Rheumatoid factor, cryoglobulins, and antineutrophilic cytoplasmic antibodies should be negative although the latter may be present in low levels among patients with minocycline-induced disease. Urinalysis should be void of features suggestive of glomerular irritation, such as proteinuria or hematuria. Evaluation of potential infectious triggers is suggested. Hepatitis B and C serologies should be obtained but are less strongly associated with c-PAN in comparison to the systemic form. Due to associations with streptococcal infections, throat culture or antistreptolysin-O titers may be considered in patients with current or recent symptomatology. The association of *Mycobacterium tuberculosis* exposure with c-PAN appears to have geographic variance; therefore, the threshold for screening with tuberculin skin testing or interferon gamma release assay is dependent on the patient and population risk profile.

13.4 Histopathology

A skin biopsy is requisite to confirm the presence of c-PAN. Cutaneous medium-sized vessels are located at the dermal-subcutaneous junction, deep dermis, or subcutis. Therefore, an incisional or deep punch biopsy of adequate depth should be performed to obtain a specimen that includes the deep dermis and subcutis to provide appropriate assessment for c-PAN. Biopsies lacking sufficient subcutis sampling increase the likelihood of a non-diagnostic biopsy [31]. Preferred locations for biopsy are lesions that have recently developed within 24–48 h. If an ulcer site is chosen, sampling should ideally include parts of the central and peripheral ulcer as well as adjacent normal skin if feasible [31]. Care should be given to avoid areas of marked necrotic tissue as viable vessel architecture may not be present in such samples to sufficiently evaluate for the presence of arterial inflammation. Direct immunofluorescence is variable and non-diagnostic for the diagnosis of c-PAN but may provide assistance in ruling out the presence of the ulcerative or bullous variants of immunoglobulin A vasculitis (i.e., Henoch Schönlein purpura). Repeat biopsy may be required to accurately secure the diagnosis, particularly if initial samples are negative despite a high clinical suspicion.

The histopathologic features of c-PAN are dependent on the stage at which the sample is obtained. Early lesions show evidence of fibrinoid necrosis with vessel wall thickening due to infiltration of neutrophils, lymphocytes, and to a lesser extent eosinophils (Figs. 13.4 and 13.5). Later stage vessels demonstrate intimal proliferation resulting in luminal narrowing or occlusion. Chronic changes include vessel wall fibrosis with associated neovascularization around the occluded arteriole lesions [5].

Fig. 13.4 Necrotizing vasculitis of medium-size vessel in the subcutaneous fat

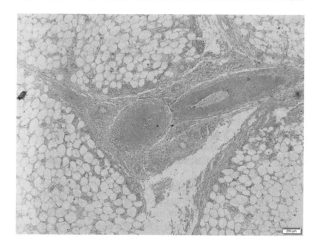

Fig. 13.5 Full-thickness inflammation and fibrinoid change of a medium-sized vessel with associated perivascular mixed inflammatory infiltrate

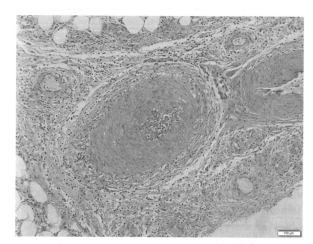

13.5   Diagnosis and Differential Diagnosis

The histopathological findings of c-PAN are indistinguishable from cutaneous involvement in patients with systemic PAN. While there are classification criteria for systemic PAN, currently there are no accepted classification or diagnostic criteria for c-PAN. Diagnostic criteria for c-PAN have been proposed by Nakamura and colleagues [9] but have not been formerly tested or prospectively validated (Table 13.2). Therefore, diagnosis of c-PAN is based on the presence of characteristic histopathological findings on skin biopsy in the appropriate clinical context in combination with exclusion of systemic involvement.

Although patients with c-PAN may have regional paresthesia and neuropathy due to localized cutaneous swelling, features of motor deficit (i.e., foot drop) should

Table 13.2 Nakamura drafted diagnostic criteria for cutaneous polyarteritis nodosa

1. Cutaneous manifestations—Subcutaneous nodules or Livedo or Purpura or Ulcers
2. Histopathological findings—Fibrinoid necrotizing vasculitis of small- and medium-sized arteries
3. Exclusion manifestations
    (a) Fever ≥38 °C for ≥2 weeks)
    (b) Weight loss (≥6 kg in 6 months)
    (c) Hypertension
    (d) Rapidly progressive renal failure, renal infarction
    (e) Cerebral hemorrhage or infarction
    (f) Myocardial infarction, ischemic heart disease, pericarditis, heart failure
    (g) Pleuritis
    (h) Intestinal hemorrhage or infarction
    (i) Peripheral neuropathy outside of the affected skin lesion area(s)
    (j) Arthralgia (arthritis) or myalgia (myositis) outside of the affected skin lesion area(s)
    (k) Abnormal arteriography (multiple microaneurysms, stenosis, occlusion)
4. Decision—A patient can be diagnosed with cutaneous polyarteritis nodosa if they fulfill both the cutaneous manifestations (1) and the histopathological findings (2) without the presence of any exclusion manifestations (3)

Adapted from Nakamura T. et al. Arch Dermatol Res 2009;301:117–121

raise the suspicion of systemic involvement with vasculitic neuropathy. In these circumstances, electromyogram and neurology consultation should be obtained to assist in determining if nerve biopsy is warranted. Abdominal pain is uncommon in patients with c-PAN and if present should prompt further investigation with advanced imaging such as an abdomino-pelvic computed tomography (CT) with angiography may assist in ruling out systemic PAN. Blood pressures should be obtained in all patients with c-PAN and if elevated evaluation of renal artery stenosis via ultrasonography or CT angiography should take place, given renal artery stenosis is a feature commonly observed in patients with systemic PAN. Due to an observed association of minocycline-induced disease, all patients presenting with c-PAN should be screened for current or recent long-term (>1 month) use of this medication.

In addition to systemic PAN, the differential diagnosis for c-PAN includes other disease entities that can involve inflammation of the subcutaneous fat as well as other vasculitides affecting the small- to medium-sized blood vessels. A summary of conditions that must be considered as well as their clinical features, laboratory parameters, and biopsy findings are listed in Table 13.3.

13.6 Treatment

To date there have been no controlled clinical trials evaluating treatment in patients with c-PAN. As such, therapeutic suggestions are based on limited retrospective studies, case series, and expert consensus. Agents chosen for therapeutic intervention in c-PAN depend on the severity of the cutaneous manifestations. Localized disease with limited, superficial inflammation may respond favorably to high

Table 13.3 Conditions considered in differential diagnosis of cutaneous polyarteritis nodosa

Condition	Common clinical features	Laboratory markers	Histopathology
Vasculitides			
Systemic polyarteritis nodosa	*Skin:* tender nodules, ulcers, livedo reticularis *Systemic:* hypertension, constitutional symptoms, visceral infarcts/aneurysm, testicular pain, mononeuritis multiplex	Elevated ESR, CRP	Identical to cutaneous polyarteritis nodosa
Granulomatosis with polyangiitis (formerly Wegener's granulomatosis)	*Skin:* palpable purpura *Systemic:* sinonasal inflammation, pulmonary nodules, hemoptysis, glomerulonephritis	c-ANCA > p-ANCA PR3 > MPO Detectable in 80–90% Hematuria	Leukocytoclastic vasculitis
Eosinophilic granulomatosis with polyangiitis (formerly Churg–Strauss syndrome)	*Skin:* tender nodules on extensor surfaces, palpable purpura *Systemic:* sinusitis, asthma, pericarditis, myocarditis, eosinophilic gastroenteritis, mononeuritis multiplex	p-ANCA > c-ANCA MPO > PR3 Detectable in 30–60% Peripheral eosinophilia	Purpuric lesions with leukocytoclastic vasculitis Nodules with eosinophilic-rich granulomas
Microscopic polyangiitis	*Skin:* palpable purpura *Systemic:* glomerulonephritis, alveolar hemorrhage	p-ANCA > c-ANCA MPO > PR3 Detectable in 60–80% Hematuria	Leukocytoclastic vasculitis
IgA vasculitis (formerly known as Henoch–Schönlein purpura)	*Skin:* leukocytoclastic vasculitis more common; ulceration, bullous lesions less common *Systemic:* arthralgia, abdominal pain, hematochezia	Hematuria Serum IgA not reliable	Leukocytoclastic vasculitis with IgA (predominant) deposition on direct immunofluorescence
Behcet's syndrome	*Skin:* oral/genital ulceration, nodules, pseudofolliculitis erythema nodosum *Systemic:* intestinal ulceration, uveitis		Septal panniculitis with medium vessel vasculitis (in 50%)

(continued)

Table 13.3 (continued)

Condition	Common clinical features	Laboratory markers	Histopathology
Vaso-occlusive disease			
Livedoid vasculopathy	*Skin:* deep livedoid changes with reticular or angular pattern. Atrophie blanche and stellate ulceration may be present		Blood vessel thickening and focal thrombosis with endothelial proliferation and hyaline degeneration of the subintimal layer. Elastic laminae and vascular wall should be preserved. Vasculitis is absent
Antiphospholipid antibody syndrome	*Skin:* Livedo reticularis, livedo racemosa *Systemic:* recurrent venous > arterial clots, multiple miscarriages	Lupus anticoagulant Anti-cardiolipin Anti-β2 glycoprotein Anti-phosphatidylserine prothrombin complex	Fibrin thrombi in dermal vessels ± necrosis of overlying epidermis, dermal hemorrhage. No evidence of vasculitis
Inflammatory skin disease			
Pyoderma gangrenosum	*Skin:* Papule or pustule that expand into erosion/ulcer *Systemic:* fever variable		Perifollicular inflammation and intradermal abscess formation. Lymphocytic and/or leukocytoclastic vasculitis may be present. Palisading granulomas in vegetative variant
Erythema nodosum	*Skin:* tender, erythematous, non-ulcerated nodules, typically on the anterior lower leg (shin)		Septal panniculitis without vasculitis
Erythema induratum (nodular vasculitis, Bazin's disease)	*Skin:* tender, erythematous nodules, typically on the posterior lower leg (calf)		Lobular panniculitis with mixed infiltrate (lymphocytes, plasma cells, histiocytes, neutrophils, eosinophils); extravascular fibrinoid necrosis; vasculitis may involve the arteries, arterioles, veins, and venules in the subcutaneous septa or lobules

ANCA anti-neutrophil cytoplasmic antibody, *c-ANCA* cytoplasmic-ANCA, *CRP* C-reactive protein, *ESR* erythrocyte sedimentation rate, *IgA* immunoglobulin A, *MPO* myeloperoxidase, *p-ANCA* perinuclear-ANCA PR3, proteinase-3 potency topical glucocorticoids [32]. Non-steroidal anti-inflammatory medications appear to have marginal benefit and are typically insufficient for control of cutaneous disease but may be of use as an adjunct for mild to moderate pain control from swelling. Colchicine (0.6 mg twice daily) and dapsone (50–150 mg daily) have been suggested by some experts, but supportive data is limited and mostly extrapolated from use of these therapies in other cutaneous forms of vasculitis [33]. For patients with nodules, livedo, and particularly those with ulceration or features of ischemia, glucocorticoids are requisite with doses of 0.5–1.0 mg/kg/day initially, followed by slow taper over 2–6 months. Patients with refractory or recurring symptoms on steroid therapy or during tapering require additional steroid-sparing immunosuppressive agents. Among these, the most commonly used are low- to moderate-dose methotrexate (7.5–20 mg/week) and azathioprine (1.5–2.0 mg/kg/day) [5, 34–37]. Limited case reports have shown potential benefit among patients using anti-tumor necrosis factor alpha agents such as etanercept [38–40] and infliximab [41]. Cyclophosphamide is reserved for patients with severe ischemia, gangrene, or failure to respond to lower level immunosuppression [5, 37, 42, 43]. Use of prophylactic penicillin and tonsillectomy remain controversial [44, 45]. For patients with confirmed streptococcal infections at the time of c-PAN diagnosis or with recurrent infections corresponding with cutaneous relapses, an antibiotic trial can be considered but insufficient data is available to recommend routinely [42, 46, 47]. Intravenous immunoglobulin (1 g/kg/day for 2 days, monthly) has been used in rare recalcitrant cases but results are variable [48–50].

13.7   Prognosis and Disease Activity

While some patients may have a monophasic course, relapses and recurrences are common and disease duration may range from several months to greater than 20 years [5]. Patients with ulcers present at initial diagnosis tend to have a more chronic course [5, 37]. The greatest concern for patients and providers is whether c-PAN will subsequently convert into systemic PAN, the latter heralding a poorer prognosis. For patients with isolated c-PAN without features or findings of systemic PAN at the time of diagnosis, this transition is notably rare. Indeed, among combined cohorts of c-PAN with long-term follow-up, the frequency of isolated cutaneous to systemic PAN transition was only observed in 3 of 92 (3%) cases [6, 9, 28, 51].

References

1. Jennette JC, Falk RJ, Bacon PA, Basu N, Cid MC, Ferrario F, et al. 2012 revised International Chapel Hill Consensus Conference Nomenclature of Vasculitides. Arthritis Rheum. 2013;65(1):1–11.
2. Kussmaul A, Maier K. Ueber eine nicht bisher beschriebene eigenhümliche Arterienerkrankung (Periarteritis Nodosa), die mit Morbus Brightii und rapid fortschreitender allgemeiner Muskellähmung einhergeht. Dtsch Arch Klin Med. 1866;1:484–518.

3. Lindberg K. Ein beitrag zur kenntnis der periarteritis nodosa. Acta Med Scand. 1931;76:183.
4. Pagnoux C, Seror R, Henegar C, Mahr A, Cohen P, Le Guern V, et al. Clinical features and outcomes in 348 patients with polyarteritis nodosa: a systematic retrospective study of patients diagnosed between 1963 and 2005 and entered into the French Vasculitis Study Group Database. Arthritis Rheum. 2010;62(2):616–26.
5. Daoud MS, Hutton KP, Gibson LE. Cutaneous periarteritis nodosa: a clinicopathological study of 79 cases. Br J Dermatol. 1997;136(5):706–13.
6. Criado PR, Marques GF, Morita TC, de Carvalho JF. Epidemiological, clinical and laboratory profiles of cutaneous polyarteritis nodosa patients: report of 22 cases and literature review. Autoimmun Rev. 2016;15(6):558–63.
7. Boren RJ, Everett MA. Cutaneous vasculitis in mother and infant. Arch Dermatol. 1965;92(5):568–70.
8. Stone MS, Olson RR, Weismann DN, Giller RH, Goeken JA. Cutaneous vasculitis in the newborn of a mother with cutaneous polyarteritis nodosa. J Am Acad Dermatol. 1993;28(1):101–5.
9. Nakamura T, Kanazawa N, Ikeda T, Yamamoto Y, Nakabayashi K, Ozaki S, et al. Cutaneous polyarteritis nodosa: revisiting its definition and diagnostic criteria. Arch Dermatol Res. 2009;301(1):117–21.
10. Karadag O, Erden A, Bilginer Y, Gopaluni S, Sari A, Armagan B, et al. A retrospective study comparing the phenotype and outcomes of patients with polyarteritis nodosa between UK and Turkish cohorts. Rheumatol Int. 2018;38(10):1833–40.
11. Mao Y, Yin L, Xia H, Huang H, Zhou Z, Chen T, et al. Incidence and clinical features of paediatric vasculitis in Eastern China: 14-year retrospective study, 1999-2013. J Int Med Res. 2016;44(3):710–7.
12. Diaz-Perez JL, Schroeter AL, Winkelmann RK. Cutaneous periarteritis nodosa: immunofluorescence studies. Arch Dermatol. 1980;116(1):56–8.
13. Okano T, Takeuchi S, Soma Y, Suzuki K, Tsukita S, Ishizu A, et al. Presence of anti-phosphatidylserine-prothrombin complex antibodies and anti-moesin antibodies in patients with polyarteritis nodosa. J Dermatol. 2017;44(1):18–22.
14. Kawakami T, Yamazaki M, Mizoguchi M, Soma Y. High titer of anti-phosphatidylserine-prothrombin complex antibodies in patients with cutaneous polyarteritis nodosa. Arthritis Rheum. 2007;57(8):1507–13.
15. Miller JJ 3rd, Fries JF. Simultaneous vasculitis in a mother and newborn infant. J Pediatr. 1975;87(3):443–5.
16. Navon Elkan P, Pierce SB, Segel R, Walsh T, Barash J, Padeh S, et al. Mutant adenosine deaminase 2 in a polyarteritis nodosa vasculopathy. N Engl J Med. 2014;370(10):921–31.
17. Gonzalez Santiago TM, Zavialov A, Saarela J, Seppanen M, Reed AM, Abraham RS, et al. Dermatologic features of ADA2 deficiency in cutaneous polyarteritis nodosa. JAMA Dermatol. 2015;151(11):1230–4.
18. Sheth AP, Olson JC, Esterly NB. Cutaneous polyarteritis nodosa of childhood. J Am Acad Dermatol. 1994;31(4):561–6.
19. Albornoz MA, Benedetto AV, Korman M, McFall S, Tourtellotte CD, Myers AR. Relapsing cutaneous polyarteritis nodosa associated with streptococcal infections. Int J Dermatol. 1998;37(9):664–6.
20. Minkowitz G, Smoller BR, McNutt NS. Benign cutaneous polyarteritis nodosa. Relationship to systemic polyarteritis nodosa and to hepatitis B infection. Arch Dermatol. 1991;127(10):1520–3.
21. Naouri M, Bacq Y, Machet MC, Rogez C, Machet L. [Interferon-alpha and ribavirin treatment in a patient with hepatitis C virus-associated cutaneous periarteritis nodosa]. Ann Dermatol Venereol. 2006;133(8–9 Pt 1):679–82.
22. Durst R, Goldschmidt N, Ben Yehuda A. Parvovirus B19 infection associated with myelosuppression and cutaneous polyarteritis nodosa. Rheumatology (Oxford). 2002;41(10):1210–2.
23. Tehrani R, Nash-Goelitz A, Adams E, Dahiya M, Eilers D. Minocycline-induced cutaneous polyarteritis nodosa. J Clin Rheumatol. 2007;13(3):146–9.

24. Pelletier F, Puzenat E, Blanc D, Faivre B, Humbert P, Aubin F. Minocycline-induced cutaneous polyarteritis nodosa with antineutrophil cytoplasmic antibodies. Eur J Dermatol. 2003;13(4):396–8.
25. Odhav A, Odhav C, Dayal NA. Rare adverse effect of treatment with minocycline. Minocycline-induced cutaneous polyarteritis nodosa. JAMA Pediatr. 2014;168(3):287–8.
26. Culver B, Itkin A, Pischel K. Case report and review of minocycline-induced cutaneous polyarteritis nodosa. Arthritis Rheum. 2005;53(3):468–70.
27. Diaz-Perez JL, Winkelmann RK. Cutaneous periarteritis nodosa. Arch Dermatol. 1974;110(3):407–14.
28. Alibaz-Oner F, Koster MJ, Crowson CS, Makol A, Ytterberg SR, Salvarani C, et al. Clinical spectrum of medium-sized vessel vasculitis. Arthritis Care Res (Hoboken). 2017;69(6):884–91.
29. Mimouni D, Ng PP, Rencic A, Nikolskaia OV, Bernstein BD, Nousari HC. Cutaneous polyarteritis nodosa in patients presenting with atrophie blanche. Br J Dermatol. 2003;148(4):789–94.
30. Choi SW, Lew S, Cho SD, Cha HJ, Eum EA, Jung HC, et al. Cutaneous polyarteritis nodosa presented with digital gangrene: a case report. J Korean Med Sci. 2006;21(2):371–3.
31. Ricotti C, Kowalczyk JP, Ghersi M, Nousari CH. The diagnostic yield of histopathologic sampling techniques in PAN-associated cutaneous ulcers. Arch Dermatol. 2007;143(10):1334–6.
32. Rogalski C, Sticherling M. Panarteritis cutanea benigna—an entity limited to the skin or cutaneous presentation of a systemic necrotizing vasculitis? Report of seven cases and review of the literature. Int J Dermatol. 2007;46(8):817–21.
33. Morgan AJ, Schwartz RA. Cutaneous polyarteritis nodosa: a comprehensive review. Int J Dermatol. 2010;49(7):750–6.
34. Jorizzo JL, White WL, Wise CM, Zanolli MD, Sherertz EF. Low-dose weekly methotrexate for unusual neutrophilic vascular reactions: cutaneous polyarteritis nodosa and Behcet's disease. J Am Acad Dermatol. 1991;24(6 Pt 1):973–8.
35. Schartz NE, Alaoui S, Vignon-Pennamen MD, Cordoliani F, Fermand JP, Morel P, et al. Successful treatment in two cases of steroid-dependent cutaneous polyarteritis nodosa with low-dose methotrexate. Dermatology. 2001;203(4):336–8.
36. Boehm I, Bauer R. Low-dose methotrexate controls a severe form of polyarteritis nodosa. Arch Dermatol. 2000;136(2):167–9.
37. Kato A, Hamada T, Miyake T, Morizane S, Hirai Y, Yamasaki O, et al. Clinical and laboratory markers associated with relapse in cutaneous polyarteritis nodosa. JAMA Dermatol. 2018;154(8):922–6.
38. Inoue N, Shimizu M, Mizuta M, Ikawa Y, Yachie A. Refractory cutaneous polyarteritis nodosa: successful treatment with etanercept. Pediatr Int. 2017;59(6):751–2.
39. Valor L, Monteagudo I, de la Torre I, Fernandez CG, Montoro M, Longo JL, et al. Young male patient diagnosed with cutaneous polyarteritis nodosa successfully treated with etanercept. Mod Rheumatol. 2014;24(4):688–9.
40. Zoshima T, Matsumura M, Suzuki Y, Kakuchi Y, Mizushima I, Fujii H, et al. A case of refractory cutaneous polyarteritis nodosa in a patient with hepatitis B carrier status successfully treated with tumor necrosis factor alpha blockade. Mod Rheumatol. 2013;23(5):1029–33.
41. Vega Gutierrez J, Rodriguez Prieto MA, Garcia Ruiz JM. Successful treatment of childhood cutaneous polyarteritis nodosa with infliximab. J Eur Acad Dermatol Venereol. 2007;21(4):570–1.
42. Bauza A, Espana A, Idoate M. Cutaneous polyarteritis nodosa. Br J Dermatol. 2002;146(4):694–9.
43. Kawakami T, Okano T, Takeuchi S, Kimura S, Soma Y. Complete resolution of refractory cutaneous arteritis by intravenous cyclophosphamide pulse therapy. Int J Dermatol. 2015;54(8):e323–5.
44. Misago N, Mochizuki Y, Sekiyama-Kodera H, Shirotani M, Suzuki K, Inokuchi A, et al. Cutaneous polyarteritis nodosa: therapy and clinical course in four cases. J Dermatol. 2001;28(12):719–27.

45. Yamamoto T, Inoue Y, Tomiita M, Oikawa M, Kambe N, Arima T, et al. Successful treatment of Group A beta-hemolytic Streptococcus infection-associated juvenile cutaneous polyarteritis nodosa with tonsillectomy. Mod Rheumatol. 2015;25(6):967–9.
46. Fink CW. The role of the streptococcus in poststreptococcal reactive arthritis and childhood polyarteritis nodosa. J Rheumatol Suppl. 1991;29:14–20.
47. Fathalla BM, Miller L, Brady S, Schaller JG. Cutaneous polyarteritis nodosa in children. J Am Acad Dermatol. 2005;53(4):724–8.
48. Marie I, Miranda S, Girszyn N, Soubrane JC, Vandhuick T, Levesque H. Intravenous immunoglobulins as treatment of severe cutaneous polyarteritis nodosa. Intern Med J. 2012;42(4):459–62.
49. Kroiss M, Hohenleutner U, Gruss C, Glaessl A, Landthaler M, Stolz W. Transient and partial effect of high-dose intravenous immunoglobulin in polyarteritis nodosa. Dermatology. 2001;203(2):188–9.
50. Pego PM, Camara IA, Andrade JP, Costa JM. Intravenous immunoglobulin therapy in vasculitic ulcers: a case of polyarteritis nodosa. Auto Immun Highlights. 2013;4(3):95–9.
51. He Q, Shu J, Chen F, Zhen XF. Analysis of the clinical characteristics and follow-up study of children with cutaneous polyarteritis nodosa. Curr Neurovasc Res. 2019;16:208.

Systemic Polyarteritis Nodosa

14

Matthew J. Koster

Abstract

Polyarteritis nodosa (PAN) is a rare systemic necrotizing vasculitis predominantly affecting the medium-sized arteries with widely variable presenting features, disease course, and outcomes. Recent updates regarding the nomenclature of PAN have resulted in the description of several PAN sub-phenotypes. Herein discussed are idiopathic PAN, Hepatitis B-associated PAN and monogenic disorders such as adenosine deaminase-2 deficiency. The current understanding of the pathogenesis, histopathological features, and treatment of these conditions are reviewed.

Keywords

Autoimmunity · Vasculitis · Polyarteritis nodosa · Hepatitis B · Adenosine deaminase 2 deficiency

14.1 Introduction

The terminology associated with polyarteritis nodosa (PAN) has undergone significant changes over the last century, particularly in the last four decades. Therefore, a review of the evolving nomenclature is integral to understanding this condition and its associated subgroups. The term "periarteritis nodosa" was first used by Kussmaul and Maier in 1866 during their description of a 27-year-old male with multiple nodules along the length of medium and small arteries in the thorax and abdomen [1].

M. J. Koster (✉)

Division of Rheumatology, Department of Internal Medicine, Mayo Clinic College of Medicine and Science, Rochester, MN, USA

e-mail: koster.matthew@mayo.edu

© Springer Nature Switzerland AG 2021

C. Salvarani et al. (eds.), *Large and Medium Size Vessel and Single Organ Vasculitis*, Rare Diseases of the Immune System,

https://doi.org/10.1007/978-3-030-67175-4_14

Further histologic evaluation by Ferrari in 1903 revealed that the inflammatory process was not relegated to the adventitia, but rather was transmural, so use of "polyarteritis nodosa" was proposed [2]. Historically, the presence of necrotizing vasculitis on any biopsy was attributed to PAN. Little further distinction was made during the first half of the twentieth century until granulomatosis with polyangiitis (GPA, formerly Wegener's granulomatosis) was initially described [3] and then subsequently considered as a separate vasculitic entity [4].

Discovery of anti-neutrophil cytoplasmic antibodies (ANCA) allowed for further distinguishing polyarteritis nodosa from the ANCA-associated vasculitides [GPA, microscopic polyangiitis (MPA), and eosinophilic granulomatosis with polyangiitis (EGPA, formerly Churg–Strauss)] [5, 6]. A definitive distinction between PAN and MPA was outlined through the 1994 [7] and the revised 2012 International Chapel Hill Consensus Conference (CHCC) nomenclature of vasculitides [8] where PAN was defined as a necrotizing inflammation of medium-sized or small arteries without glomerulonephritis or vasculitis of the small vessels (i.e., arterioles, capillaries, and venules) and not associated with ANCA. MPA was defined as a necrotizing vasculitis with few or no immune deposits, predominantly affecting the small vessels and associated with myeloperoxidase (MPO) ANCA or proteinase 3 (PR3) ANCA.

Further distinction between PAN and PAN-like conditions has reduced the number of patients classified as having systemic idiopathic PAN. These subgroups now include vasculitis associated with probable etiology (i.e., drug, viral) and monogenic disease-related PAN-like conditions. Given the presentation of hepatitis B virus (HBV)-associated PAN and systemic idiopathic PAN have the same clinical features, the chapter herein will focus on both systemic idiopathic PAN and HBV-associated PAN but will additionally note distinguishing characteristics of the presentation and treatment of other less common PAN-like variants.

14.2 Epidemiology

PAN can affect any age but more commonly affects adults between their fourth and sixth decades of life. There is a slight male to female predominance (1.5:1), but ethnic predilection has not been observed [9]. Annual incidence of systemic idiopathic PAN has been estimated to be 1–5 per 1,000,000 with a prevalence of approximately 30 per 1,000,000 [9–11]. Incidence of HBV-associated PAN has been reported as high as 77 per 1,000,000 in endemic areas [12]. Following the institution of safer transfusion practices, hospital hygiene, and HBV vaccination, the rates of HBV-associated PAN have dramatically reduced from 35% to less than 5% of PAN cases [10].

14.3 Etiopathogenesis

According to more recent understanding, necrotizing vasculitis likely represents a range of diseases with varying etiopathogenesis [13]. In systemic idiopathic PAN, the underlying mechanisms are not well understood, but the predominance of dendritic cells and CD4+ lymphocytes in vascular lesions suggest the possibility of an antigen-specific T-cell-mediated response [14]. Several infections have been identified as potential triggers. Hepatitis B virus is the most well-documented but hepatitis C [15], human immunodeficiency virus [16], parvovirus B19 [17], Epstein–Barr virus [18], and cytomegalovirus [19] have also been observed. In contrast to systemic idiopathic PAN, viral replication [20] and circulating immune-complex deposition [21, 22] have been noted to result in direct vascular inflammation among patients with HBV-associated PAN. Drug-induced causes are uncommon; however, systemic PAN-like disease in the context of chronic use of minocycline for treatment of acne vulgaris has been reported [23, 24].

Limited information is known regarding genetic abnormalities and risk of PAN. However, a monogenic polyarteritis with similar clinical and histological characteristics to systemic idiopathic PAN has been recently observed. This predominantly childhood-onset PAN-like variant called deficiency of adenosine deaminase 2 (DADA2) is caused by an autosomal recessive mutation in the Adenosine Deaminase 2 (*ADA2*) gene [formerly known as the Cat Eye Syndrome Chromosome Region 1 (*CECR1*) gene] [25], which encodes for the adenosine deaminase 2 enzyme (ADA2). ADA2 has been hypothesized to be a key growth factor for endothelial cells and a regulator in the differentiation of monocytes. Deficiency of ADA2 results in endothelial damages and skewing of monocytes to a pro-inflammatory macrophage subset [26]. Preliminary findings from evaluation of 117 adult-onset, HBV-negative systemic idiopathic PAN patients have also shown the presence of heterozygous or biallelic missense variants in *ADA2* among 8 (7%) patients resulting in reduced ADA2 activity. These findings suggest a potential genetic basis among a subset of systemic idiopathic PAN patients [27].

14.4 Clinical Manifestations and Laboratory Markers

14.4.1 Clinical Manifestations

Because medium- and small-sized arteries are involved in PAN, a wide spectrum of clinical manifestations has been reported (Table 14.1). Constitutional symptoms of fever, weight loss, myalgia, and arthralgia are common and are present in 30–70% [28–30]. Cutaneous findings are lower extremity predominant and occur in up to 50–60% of patients as demonstrated by purpura, livedo reticularis/racemosa, nodules, and ulcers [28]. Digital infarction resulting in gangrene can also occur (6%) but limb ischemia is rare [29, 31] (Fig. 14.1). Peripheral nerve involvement results from arteriolar occlusion of the vasa nervosum [32]. Mononeuritis multiplex, typically presenting as wrist drop or foot drop, is the most common neurologic feature. Patients will often note pain or change in sensation (hypo/hyper/dysesthesia) prior to the onset of a motor deficit, but palsy can develop suddenly without sensory prodrome. Symmetric sensorimotor peripheral neuropathy and pure sensory neuropathy are also seen; among which, the sciatic, peroneal, tibial, ulnar, median, and radial nerves appear to have a higher likelihood of involvement [33]. Cranial nerve palsies have been reported but are infrequent and affect less than 2% of patients

Table 14.1 Clinical features of polyarteritis nodosa [28–30, 36]

Symptoms	Frequency
Constitutional	**71–93%**
Fever	25–69%
Weight loss	46–70%
Myalgia	34–69%
Arthralgia	32–59%
Neurologic	**38–79%**
Peripheral neuropathy	27–74%
Mononeuritis multiplex	17–70%
Central nervous system	5–13%
Cutaneous	**28–58%**
Purpura	22–27%
Nodules	17–23%
Livedo	17–27%
Ulcers	13%
Digital gangrene	6–7%
Gastrointestinal	**14–53%**
Abdominal pain	36–38%
Bleeding	3–10%
GI manifestation requiring surgery	13–14%
Cardiac manifestations	**10–30%**
Cardiomyopathy	8%
Pericarditis	6%
Genitourinary	**37–51%**
Hematuria	2–15%
Proteinuria (>0.4 g/day)	11–21%
Hypertension	10–35%
Orchitis	17–38%

Fig. 14.1 Dry gangrene of the distal second and fourth phalanx on a background of livedo reticularis and acrocyanosis

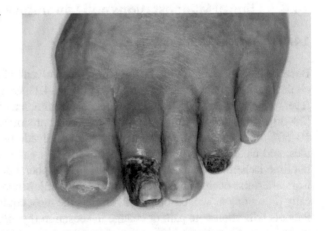

[33]. Stroke can occur in systemic idiopathic PAN but is rare. If present, particularly in a child or young adult, DADA2 variant should be considered.

Abdominal pain is the most frequent gastrointestinal feature but is nonspecific. If associated with or exacerbated by meals, this raises concern for intestinal angina secondary to mesenteric arteritis. Ischemia appears to be more common in the small intestine compared to the colon and can result in nausea, vomiting, diarrhea, melena, or hematochezia. Vasculitic involvement of visceral organs such as the gallbladder and appendix can be seen and mimic cholecystitis and appendicitis, respectively. Upon surgical removal, histologic evaluation confirms arteritic involvement if present. Both ischemic bowel perforation and rupture of a visceral artery aneurysm can manifest as a surgical abdomen; a presentation which carries high morbidity and mortality [34].

Renal abnormalities in PAN differ from ANCA-associated vasculitis as the former does not cause glomerulonephritis [8]. Renal infarcts (Fig. 14.2), resulting from either occlusion of intrarenal arteries or rupture of microaneurysms (Fig. 14.3), can produce micro- or macroscopic hematuria, but dysmorphia is generally absent. Proteinuria, if detected, is typically sub-nephrotic [28]. Renal insufficiency is uncommon but may develop as a consequence of significant renal parenchymal loss due to infarction or as a result of severe renovascular hypertension from renal artery stenosis. Urologic involvement has been noted in 17% of cases and is rarely the initial manifestation; nevertheless, non-infectious orchitis secondary to testicular arteritis is a characteristic feature of PAN [28, 29].

Fig. 14.2 Renal infarct, right inferior pole (CT, coronal view)

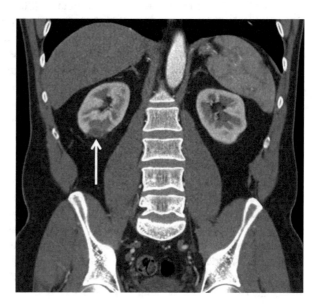

Fig. 14.3 Selective conventional right renal angiogram demonstrating multiple segmental microaneurysms

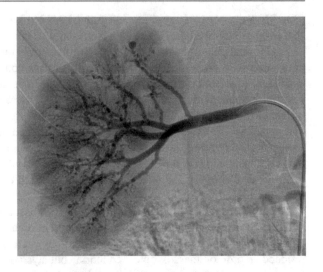

Cardiac involvement has been noted since the index description of PAN in 1866 but is an underreported finding as many patients may be asymptomatic. Indeed, only 2–10% of patients have clinically diagnosed cardiac findings [28, 29], whereas histologic evidence has been reported in up to 78% of patients in autopsy studies [35]. Left ventricular heart failure is the most frequently observed abnormality, and the etiology is likely multifactorial with coronary arteritis, myocardial infarction, and renovascular hypertension as potential contributors [36]. Coronary arteritis has been described in 50% of autopsy cases [35] but clinically symptomatic coronary angina (2–18%) and myocardial infarctions (1–12%) are less often reported [36]. Giant coronary aneurysms (Fig. 14.4) have been observed but are considered rare [37, 38]. These are likely sequelae of untreated disease and angiographically may be challenging to distinguish from patients with history of Kawasaki's Disease.

Myalgias occur in 60–70% [28, 29] of patients but inflammatory myopathy is rare [39]. Creatine kinase levels may be elevated but are generally less than 2000 IU/L. Pain can be present due to arterial insufficiency of the medium-sized muscular vessels. Thigh and calf muscle involvement is typical. Magnetic resonance imaging of the musculature can demonstrate diffuse or patchy hyperintensity of the affected muscle on T2-weighted imaging and contrast-enhanced images may demonstrate small fluffy enhancing lesions centered on the vessels ("cotton wool appearance") [40].

Overall, the clinical features of patients with classical PAN and HBV-associated PAN are similar. However, a few noted differences have been observed with HBV-associated PAN demonstrating a higher frequency of myalgia, neurologic manifestations, abdominal pain, and vasculitis-related cardiomyopathy but a lower frequency of livedo and nodular skin lesions [28].

Fig. 14.4 Conventional
coronary angiogram with
alternating stenotic and
aneurysmal segments of
the left anterior descending
(top) and giant aneurysm
of the left
circumflex (arrow)

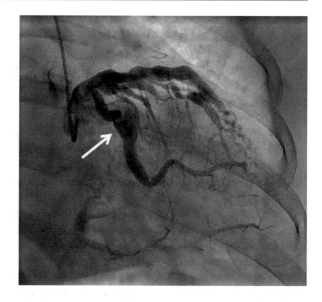

14.4.2 Laboratory Markers

There are no specific laboratory markers for PAN. An inflammatory state with normocytic anemia, thrombocytosis, and elevated erythrocyte sedimentation rate and/
or C-reactive protein is common. Leukocytosis may be seen. If peripheral eosinophilia is noted, particularly if >10%, then the possibility of eosinophilic granulomatosis with polyangiitis should be assessed. Renal insufficiency can be present, but is
not typically severe. Urinalysis may show sub-nephrotic proteinuria and non-
dysmorphic microscopic hematuria. ANCA serologies (cANCA/PR3, pANCA/
MPO) should be negative. Cryoglobulins, complements (C3, C4), and rheumatoid
factor should be evaluated to assess for possibility of cryoglobulinemia. The presence of HIV, hepatitis B, and hepatitis C should be investigated. Lactate levels may
be of assistance in patients presenting with severe abdominal pain or surgical abdomen to assess for tissue ischemia.

14.5   Histopathology

Cutaneous findings observed in classical systemic PAN are indistinguishable from
the isolated cutaneous variant (see histopathology 13.4). The vascular abnormalities
in PAN demonstrate a segmental pattern with a predilection for arterial branch points
of muscular arteries [41]. The cause for predisposition of branch points is unknown
but an increase in expression of adhesion molecules and intimal macrophages at
these locations has been proposed [42]. The vascular infiltrates observed vary

depending on the stage of the inflammatory process. In the early, active phase a transmural inflammatory infiltrate composed of an admixture of lymphocytes, macrophages, neutrophils and eosinophils are seen along with findings of fibrinoid necrosis of the vessel wall [41]. Subsequently, vascular remodeling occurs with dense vessel wall fibrosis as well as intimal hyperplasia. Thrombosis can lead to vascular occlusion whereas disruption of the elastic lamina results in aneurysmal dilation.

14.6 Diagnosis and Differential Diagnosis

There are no validated or approved diagnostic criteria for PAN. The American College of Rheumatology has developed classification criteria for PAN (Table 14.2) [43]. Unfortunately, these criteria are of limited utility for two reasons. First, these criteria are intended for research purposes to distinguish what subtype of vasculitis a patient has once they have a confirmed vasculitis diagnosis. As such they should not be used in the clinical setting to determine if a patient does or does not have vasculitis. Second, these criteria are not useful in differentiating patients with PAN from microscopic polyangiitis, given the latter was not considered a separate entity at the time of drafting. Because of these noted limitations, an ongoing international

Table 14.2 1990 American College of Rheumatology Classification criteria for polyarteritis nodosa [43][a]

Criterion	Description
1. Weight loss ≥4 kg	Loss of 4 kg or more since illness began, not due to dieting or other factors
2. Livedo reticularis	Mottled reticular pattern over the skin or portions of the extremities or torso
3. Testicular pain or tenderness	Pain or tenderness of the testicles, not due to infection, trauma, or other causes
4. Myalgias, weakness, or leg tenderness	Diffuse myalgias (excluding shoulder and hip girdle) or weakness of muscles or tenderness of leg muscles
5. Mononeuropathy or polyneuropathy	Development of mononeuropathy, multiple mononeuropathies, or polyneuropathy
6. Diastolic blood pressure >90 mmHg	Development of hypertension with diastolic blood pressure higher than 90 mmHg
7. Elevated blood urea nitrogen (BUN) or creatinine	Elevation of BUN >40 mg/dL or creatinine >1.5 mg/dL, not due to dehydration or obstruction
8. Hepatitis B virus	Presence of hepatitis B surface antigen or antibody in serum
9. Arteriographic abnormality	Arteriogram showing aneurysms or occlusions of the visceral arteries, not due to arteriosclerosis, fibromuscular dysplasia, or other noninflammatory causes
10. Biopsy of small- or medium-sized artery containing polymorphonuclear cells	Histologic changes showing the presence of granulocytes or granulocytes and mononuclear leukocytes in the artery wall

[a]For classification purposes, a patient shall be said to have polyarteritis nodosa if at least 3 of these 10 criteria are present. The presence of ≥3 criteria yields a sensitivity of 82.2% and a specificity of 86.8%

collaborative effort is currently underway to develop diagnostic and classification criteria for PAN [44].

Consequently, the diagnosis of PAN requires the combination of characteristic clinical manifestations, laboratory parameters, angiographic features, and histopathology in a suspected individual. Biopsy of an affected organ confirming the presence of focal, segmental, transmural, necrotizing inflammation of the medium- or small-sized arteries is considered the gold standard for diagnosis. If affected, the highest yield is typically observed in skin, nerve, muscle, and testicle [45]. Combined nerve and muscle biopsy appears to be superior to muscle biopsy alone for diagnosis. In a large series of patients with suspected PAN, vasculitis confirmation from dual nerve/muscle biopsy was obtained in 83% (90/108) of patients with peripheral neuropathy and 81% (17/21) of patients without peripheral neuropathy; compared with 68% (41/60) positive biopsy specimens in patients with peripheral neuropathy and 60% (24/40) without peripheral neuropathy among those with isolated muscle biopsy performed [28]. While this study highlights the potential utility of blind nerve and/or muscle biopsy even in asymptomatic patients, it is suggested that evaluation with electromyogram and/or muscle MRI be performed to identify if pathologic findings are present in order to guide biopsy location. Although confirmatory findings of PAN can be observed on kidney and liver biopsy specimens, these locations carry a high risk of post-procedure hemorrhage and therefore should not be considered as first-line targets.

Angiography provides additional diagnostic utility in patients with suspected PAN, particularly among those with abdominal or renal symptoms for which biopsy was not able to be obtained or was non-diagnostic. The typical angiographic features of PAN include saccular or fusiform microaneurysms (1–5 mm diameter) usually coinciding with stenotic lesions [46] (Fig. 14.5). Larger aneurysm may also be present within which dissections may occur (Figs. 14.6, 14.7, and 14.8). The most frequent arterial territories affected include the celiac, hepatic, renal, and mesenteric branches. Visceral organ infarcts, bowel wall thickening, and perinephric hematoma are commonly seen but are less specific for PAN and must be differentiated from

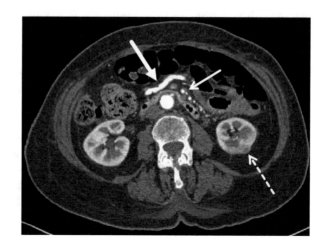

Fig. 14.5 Computed tomography angiography (axial view) demonstrating superior mesenteric artery branch with alternating stenotic and aneurysmal segments (thick arrow), mesenteric artery branches with arterial thickening (thin arrow), and mid-pole left renal infarct (dashed arrow)

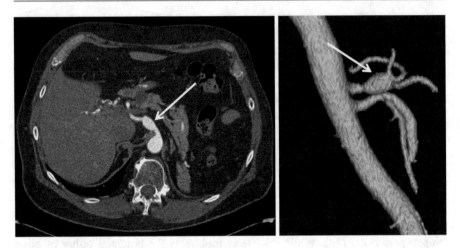

Fig. 14.6 Computed tomography angiography highlighting proximal celiac artery aneurysm (arrow) [Axial view, left pane; 3D formatted, right pane]

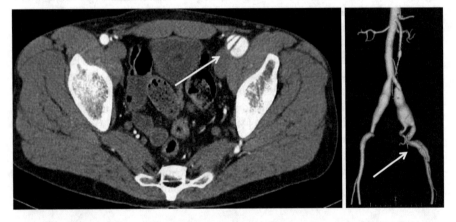

Fig. 14.7 Multiple aneurysms in the superior mesenteric artery, bilateral common iliac arteries, and common femoral arteries [computed tomography 3D formatted, right pane] with complex dissection of the left femoral artery (arrow) [axial view, left pane]

diseases causing in situ thrombosis or thromboembolism [47]. With the advancements in noninvasive imaging, computed tomography angiography (CTA) is a reasonable initial screening modality given it has spatial resolution detail that is sufficient to evaluate for the majority of findings suggestive of PAN including stenosis/occlusion, infarcts, and aneurysms >2 mm diameter. However, if CTA is negative or equivocal and suspicion remains, then conventional angiography is required. If characteristic angiographic findings are identified by an experienced radiologist the diagnosis may be confirmed, even without biopsy, provided there is appropriate clinical context and mimicking conditions (Table 14.3) have been ruled out.

Fig. 14.8 Selective
superior mesenteric artery
conventional angiogram
with long segment
proximal
dissection (arrow)

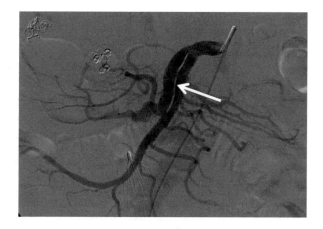

Table 14.3 Conditions to consider during evaluation of polyarteritis nodosa

Disease	Common clinical features	Common lab/imaging features
Rheumatic disease		
Granulomatosis with polyangiitis (Wegener's)	Sinusitis, upper airway inflammation, pulmonary nodules, glomerulonephritis	cANCA/PR3 > pANCA/MPO
Eosinophilic granulomatosis with polyangiitis (Churg–Strauss)	Asthma, nasal polyposis, upper airway inflammation, neuropathy	Eosinophilia (>10% peripheral) pANCA/MPO (40–60%)
Microscopic polyangiitis	Alveolar hemorrhage, glomerulonephritis	pANCA/MPO > cANCA/PR3
Behcet's Disease	Oral/genital/gastrointestinal ulcers	–
Infectious disease		
Infective endocarditis	Multifocal infarcts, splinter hemorrhages, subcutaneous nodules, fever	Echocardiography with vegetation +/− positive blood cultures
Mycotic aneurysm	Fever. Painful, pulsatile, enlarging aneurysm (if superficial). Gastrointestinal bleeding (if visceral)	CT angiography: saccular, eccentric aneurysm or multilobulated aneurysm. Perivascular fluid collection Intramural or perivascular air
Viral infection (HIV, HepB, HepC)	Fever, weight loss, arthralgia, myalgia	Positive viral studies
Vascular disease		
Antiphospholipid syndrome	Recurrent thromboses (arterial or venous)	Positive lupus anticoagulant and/or anticardiolipin ab (IgG/IgM) and/or Beta2 glycoprotein ab (IgG/IgM) times two draws separated by ≥12 weeks

(continued)

Table 14.3 (continued)

Disease	Common clinical features	Common lab/imaging features
Cholesterol emboli	Livedo, blue toe syndrome, renal insufficiency/infarct, gastrointestinal infarct typically following an endovascular procedure	Eosinophiluria Biopsy with cholesterol clefts within arterioles
Fibromuscular dysplasia (FMD)	Medium artery stenosis, spontaneous dissection, aneurysm. Female > Male Renal ≫ carotids > vertebrals > iliac > mesenteric	Normal inflammatory markers Multifocal FMD: vessel stenosis with intervening dilations causing "string of beads" pattern where diameter of beading is larger than the diameter of the artery
Segmental arterial mediolysis	Spontaneous intra-abdominal hemorrhage, more common at 50–80 years of age	Normal inflammatory markers Dissecting aneurysm

14.7 Prognosis

If left untreated, systemic PAN carries a high mortality with a 5-year survival of 13% [48]. Conversely, those receiving treatment have a notably improved outcome with 5-year survival nearing 80–90% [28, 49]. The overall outcome is largely dependent on the severity of disease at time of diagnosis. A prognostic scoring system called the Five-Factor Score (FFS) was devised by the French Vasculitis Study Group from evaluation of a prospective study of 342 patients with polyarteritis nodosa, microscopic polyangiitis, and eosinophilic granulomatosis with polyangiitis (Table 14.4) [50]. For patients with an FFS = 0, 5-year mortality was 12%, whereas the mortality rate for FFS = 1 was 26% and FFS ≥ 2 was 46% [50]. The same group re-evaluated this scoring system evaluating 1108 total patients with systemic necrotizing vasculitis, this time including granulomatosis with polyangiitis [51]. The updated 2009 FFS (Table 14.4) added age > 65 year at diagnosis as a poor prognostic factor but no longer includes CNS involvement among these parameters. Given patients with ANCA-vasculitis were included, ENT symptoms were evaluated and the absence of such findings were considered to carry a poorer prognosis; however, this is not applicable to patients with PAN. The updated rates are similar to the original FFS prediction model, demonstrating reliability of this prognostic tool [51]. Death in the first year is more commonly due to poorly controlled vasculitis, whereas subsequent mortality is more often attributable to complications resulting from sequelae of vasculitis-associated organ damage, cardiovascular disease, or consequences of immunosuppressive treatments, particularly infection [52, 53].

PAN has been noted to have a more frequent monophasic pattern when compared to other systemic necrotizing vasculitides; nevertheless, a proportion of patients will undergo a relapsing course. Among a cohort of 348 patients with PAN, 76 (22%) relapsed within 5 years of follow-up [28]. Patients with HBV-associated PAN have

Table 14.4 Prognostic scoring systems for polyarteritis nodosa

1996 Five-factor score [50]			2009 Revised five-factor score [51]		
Factor	Description	Score	Factor	Description	Score
Creatinine >1.58 mg/dL	At time of diagnosis	+1	Age > 65 years	Age at time of diagnosis	+1
Proteinuria >1 g/24 h	At time of diagnosis	+1	Renal insufficiency	Creatinine ≥150 μmol/L (1.70 mg/dL) measured at its stabilized peak level	+1
Cardiac insufficiency	Based on the presence of clinical symptoms (e.g., heart failure, pulmonary edema) and not on laboratory parameters (i.e., brain natriuretic peptide) or asymptomatic echocardiography abnormalities	+1	Cardiac insufficiency	Same as 1996 FFS	+1
Gastrointestinal involvement	Bowel perforation, bleeding, pancreatitis	+1	Gastrointestinal involvement	Same as 1996 FFS	+1
Central nervous system involvement	Not further defined	+1	*Absence* of ENT symptoms[a]	Clinical symptoms confirmed by examination of ENT specialist	+1
Five-year mortality rate FFS = 0—12% FFS = 1—26% FFS ≥ 2—46%			**Five-year mortality rate** FFS = 0—9% FFS = 1—21% FFS ≥ 2—40%		

[a]Pertinent only for patients with granulomatosis with polyangiitis and eosinophilic granulomatosis with polyangiitis; *ENT* ear/nose/throat, *FFS* Five-factor score

been observed to have less frequent relapse than those with non-HBV-associated disease with 5-year relapse-free survival rates being seen in 59.4% of patients with non-HBV-associated PAN, compared to 67% in those with HBV-associated disease [28]. Childhood-onset PAN has been reported to have a more benign course when compared to adults with less renal and neurologic involvement noted and shorter duration of induction treatment required [54].

Patients with PAN require long-term follow-up with specialists that are familiar with the disease process and its multi-system clinical manifestations, as well as clinicians that are comfortable with the immunosuppressive therapies required for induction and maintenance. During the active phase, patients should be closely observed with visits every 2–4 weeks for the first 3–6 months. Once stabilized, visits can occur at less frequent intervals of every 2–6 months for the 2 years following diagnosis. Because of possible late-stage relapse as well as potential development of comorbidities due to sequelae from vascular damage or immunosuppressive therapy, patients should be followed life-long at intervals of every 6–12 months, even during remission. At each visit, patients should (at a minimum) have a blood pressure evaluation, comprehensive multi-system physical examination, creatinine and urinalysis with microscopy. Additional labs may be needed for immunosuppressive drug monitoring. In asymptomatic patients, routine repeat angiography is not requisite but should be considered if there are new or progressive symptoms of abdominal or cardiac pain or if there are known arterial dilatations/aneurysms that require routine monitoring.

14.8   Treatment

The level of clinical trial evidence guiding the therapeutic decisions in the management of PAN is low [55]. In addition, trials evaluating this condition must be interpreted carefully as they commonly include an admixture of other systemic necrotizing vasculitides such as EGPA and MPA [49, 56–59]. In general, treatment for systemic PAN is determined based on the severity of disease at time of presentation as well as the presence or absence of HBV. Patients with systemic idiopathic PAN with mild disease (FFS = 0) may be treated with glucocorticoid monotherapy with initial doses of 1 mg/kg/day (up to 60 mg) with subsequent tapering over 6–8 months [28, 49]. For patients with glucocorticoid-resistant disease and in those that develop major relapse despite the use of adequate glucocorticoid doses, the addition of an adjunct disease-modifying agent may be required. Among patients with mild PAN, cyclophosphamide is generally avoided and medications such as azathioprine (up to 2 mg/kg/day) have shown similar efficacy to pulse dose cyclophosphamide but with lower risk of side effects [49]. While often used, the overall long-term benefit of azathioprine is debated. In a recent study evaluating 95 systemic necrotizing vasculitis patients (51, EGPA, 25 MPA, 19 PAN) with FFS = 0, the addition of azathioprine to a glucocorticoid remission-induction regimen did not significantly improve the rates of remission and failed to reduce the risk of relapse or overall steroid exposure [57]. Methotrexate (up to 25 mg/week) and mycophenolate (up to 1500 mg twice daily) have also been used in the management of glucocorticoid-resistant disease, but supportive data for these agents is limited to observational studies [29, 60] and largely extrapolated from their use in the treatment of other systemic necrotizing vasculitidies such as ANCA-associated vasculitis.

The treatment of patients with poor prognostic factors (FFS ≥1) requires more aggressive management. In such circumstances, cyclophosphamide is advocated in addition to high-dose glucocorticoids. Both oral (target 2 mg/kg/day) and intravenous pulse (600 mg/m^2 monthly) regimens have shown efficacy, but the latter has demonstrated a more tolerable side effect profile [59]. The duration of cyclophosphamide treatment is less well understood and has only been evaluated in the context of a single clinical trial evaluating 47 patients with MPA and 18 patients with PAN [58]. The results of this study suggest that 6 months of cyclophosphamide was less effective than 12 months of therapy; however, remission maintenance therapies were not utilized. Conventionally, patients with severe PAN are treated with cyclophosphamide for a minimum of 6 months, after which if they are in remission are transitioned to a lower level immunosuppression agent such as azathioprine, methotrexate, or mycophenolate for ongoing remission maintenance. The therapeutics options for patients with severe systemic idiopathic PAN failing to respond to cyclophosphamide are limited. Rituximab [61, 62] and tocilizumab [63] have been used with reported success, but results are limited to case reports and small case series and are considered currently experimental. Inhibitors of tumor necrosis factor alpha (infliximab, adalimumab, etanercept) have also shown preliminary benefit in systemic PAN [64–67] and appear to have a greater observed role in managing patients with the PAN-like DADA2 variant [68].

In patients with a potential precipitant for the development of PAN or PAN-like illness control or removal of the offending agent is imperative. For example, in patients with minocycline-induced PAN-like illness, cessation of minocycline may be sufficient to result in disease remission. However, in severe cases additional immunosuppressive therapy may be required [24].

Management of patients with HBV-associated PAN is focused on initial control of severe life-threatening manifestations (if present) followed by removal of immune complexes and subsequent clearance of viremia. Although prolonged use of glucocorticoids is contraindicated due to an increased risk of viral replication, short-term use of glucocorticoids (1 mg/kg/day for 1 week then tapered off over 1 additional week) has been safely utilized [69, 70]. Plasma exchange has not demonstrated improvement in outcomes among patients with systemic idiopathic PAN [71] but is considered integral in the treatment of HBV-associated PAN because clearance of immune complexes attenuates vessel inflammation [69, 70]. Suggestions for plasma exchange frequency are 3/week for 3 weeks, 2/week for 2 weeks, then weekly until hepatitis B e antigen to hepatitis B e antibody seroconversion is observed, or until 2–3 months of sustained clinical recovery has been obtained [69]. Antiviral therapy should be initiated at the time of diagnosis. Selection of the antiviral agent and determination of duration should be guided through coordination with hepatology. Interferon alpha2b and lamivudine have shown efficacy in prospective open-label trials [69, 72]. While newer nucleos(t)ide analogs (entecavir and tenofovir) have not been formally evaluated in patients with HBV-associated PAN their efficacy in patients with chronic hepatitis B viral infections is well established [73] and may be considered for assistance with viral clearance. Prolonged vasculitis control occurs in 90–100% of patients for which viral replication has ceased and seroconversion has occurred [69, 70].

References

1. Kussmaul A, Maier K. Ueber eine nicht bisher beschriebene eigenhümliche Arterienerkrankung (Periarteritis Nodosa), die mit Morbus Brightii und rapid fortschreitender allgemeiner Muskellähmung einhergeht. Dtsch Arch Klin Med. 1866;1:484–518.
2. Ferrari E. Uber polyarteritis acuta nodosa (sogenannte periarteritis nodosa) und ihre Beziehungen zur Polymyositis und Polyneuritis acuta. Zieglers Beitr. 1930;34:350–86.

3. Wegener F. Über eine eigenartige rhinogene Granulomatose mit besonderer Beteilgung des Arteriensystems und der Nieren. Beitr Path Anat. 1939;102:36–8.
4. Godman GC, Churg J. Wegener's granulomatosis: pathology and review of the literature. AMA Arch Pathol. 1954;58(6):533–53.
5. Davies DJ, Moran JE, Niall JF, Ryan GB. Segmental necrotising glomerulonephritis with antineutrophil antibody: possible arbovirus aetiology? Br Med J (Clin Res Ed). 1982;285(6342):606.
6. van der Woude FJ, Rasmussen N, Lobatto S, Wiik A, Permin H, van Es LA, et al. Autoantibodies against neutrophils and monocytes: tool for diagnosis and marker of disease activity in Wegener's granulomatosis. Lancet. 1985;1(8426):425–9.
7. Jennette JC, Falk RJ, Andrassy K, Bacon PA, Churg J, Gross WL, et al. Nomenclature of systemic vasculitides. Proposal of an international consensus conference. Arthritis Rheum. 1994;37(2):187–92.
8. Jennette JC, Falk RJ, Bacon PA, Basu N, Cid MC, Ferrario F, et al. 2012 revised International Chapel Hill Consensus Conference Nomenclature of Vasculitides. Arthritis Rheum. 2013;65(1):1–11.
9. Watts RA, Lane SE, Scott DG, Koldingsnes W, Nossent H, Gonzalez-Gay MA, et al. Epidemiology of vasculitis in Europe. Ann Rheum Dis. 2001;60(12):1156–7.
10. Mahr A, Guillevin L, Poissonnet M, Ayme S. Prevalences of polyarteritis nodosa, microscopic polyangiitis, Wegener's granulomatosis, and Churg-Strauss syndrome in a French urban multiethnic population in 2000: a capture-recapture estimate. Arthritis Rheum. 2004;51(1):92–9.
11. Mohammad AJ, Jacobsson LT, Mahr AD, Sturfelt G, Segelmark M. Prevalence of Wegener's granulomatosis, microscopic polyangiitis, polyarteritis nodosa and Churg-Strauss syndrome within a defined population in southern Sweden. Rheumatology (Oxford). 2007;46(8):1329–37.
12. McMahon BJ, Bender TR, Templin DW, Maynard JE, Barrett DH, Berquist KR, et al. Vasculitis in Eskimos living in an area hyperendemic for hepatitis B. JAMA. 1980;244(19):2180–2.
13. Ozen S. The changing face of polyarteritis nodosa and necrotizing vasculitis. Nat Rev Rheumatol. 2017;13(6):381–6.
14. Cid MC, Grau JM, Casademont J, Campo E, Coll-Vinent B, Lopez-Soto A, et al. Immunohistochemical characterization of inflammatory cells and immunologic activation markers in muscle and nerve biopsy specimens from patients with systemic polyarteritis nodosa. Arthritis Rheum. 1994;37(7):1055–61.
15. Saadoun D, Terrier B, Semoun O, Sene D, Maisonobe T, Musset L, et al. Hepatitis C virus-associated polyarteritis nodosa. Arthritis Care Res (Hoboken). 2011;63(3):427–35.
16. Font C, Miro O, Pedrol E, Masanes F, Coll-Vinent B, Casademont J, et al. Polyarteritis nodosa in human immunodeficiency virus infection: report of four cases and review of the literature. Br J Rheumatol. 1996;35(8):796–9.
17. Corman LC, Dolson DJ. Polyarteritis nodosa and parvovirus B19 infection. Lancet. 1992;339(8791):491.
18. Caldeira T, Meireles C, Cunha F, Valbuena C, Aparicio J, Ribeiro A. Systemic polyarteritis nodosa associated with acute Epstein-Barr virus infection. Clin Rheumatol. 2007;26(10):1733–5.
19. Kouchi M, Sato S, Kamono M, Taoda A, Iijima K, Mizuma A, et al. A case of polyarteritis nodosa associated with cytomegalovirus infection. Case Rep Rheumatol. 2014;2014:604874.
20. Trepo C, Guillevin L. Polyarteritis nodosa and extrahepatic manifestations of HBV infection: the case against autoimmune intervention in pathogenesis. J Autoimmun. 2001;16(3):269–74.
21. Guillevin L, Ronco P, Verroust P. Circulating immune complexes in systemic necrotizing vasculitis of the polyarteritis nodosa group. Comparison of HBV-related polyarteritis nodosa and Churg Strauss Angiitis. J Autoimmun. 1990;3(6):789–92.
22. Michalak T. Immune complexes of hepatitis B surface antigen in the pathogenesis of periarteritis nodosa. A study of seven necropsy cases. Am J Pathol. 1978;90(3):619–32.
23. Katada Y, Harada Y, Azuma N, Matsumoto K, Terada H, Kudo E, et al. Minocycline-induced vasculitis fulfilling the criteria of polyarteritis nodosa. Mod Rheumatol. 2006;16(4):256–9.

24. Kermani TA, Ham EK, Camilleri MJ, Warrington KJ. Polyarteritis nodosa-like vasculitis in association with minocycline use: a single-center case series. Semin Arthritis Rheum. 2012;42(2):213–21.
25. Zhou Q, Yang D, Ombrello AK, Zavialov AV, Toro C, Zavialov AV, et al. Early-onset stroke and vasculopathy associated with mutations in ADA2. N Engl J Med. 2014;370(10):911–20.
26. Fayand A, Sarrabay G, Belot A, Hentgen V, Kone-Paut I, Grateau G, et al. [Multiple facets of ADA2 deficiency: vasculitis, auto-inflammatory disease and immunodeficiency: a literature review of 135 cases from literature]. Rev Med Interne. 2018;39(4):297–306.
27. Schnappauf O, Stoffels M, Aksentijevich I, Kastner D, Grayson P, Cuthbertson D, et al. Screening of patients with adult-onset idiopathic polyarteritis nodosa for deficiency of adenosine deaminase 2. Arthritis Rheumatol. 2018;70.
28. Pagnoux C, Seror R, Henegar C, Mahr A, Cohen P, Le Guern V, et al. Clinical features and outcomes in 348 patients with polyarteritis nodosa: a systematic retrospective study of patients diagnosed between 1963 and 2005 and entered into the French Vasculitis Study Group Database. Arthritis Rheum. 2010;62(2):616–26.
29. Alibaz-Oner F, Koster MJ, Crowson CS, Makol A, Ytterberg SR, Salvarani C, et al. Clinical spectrum of medium-sized vessel vasculitis. Arthritis Care Res (Hoboken). 2017;69(6):884–91.
30. Lhote F, Cohen P, Guillevin L. Polyarteritis nodosa, microscopic polyangiitis and Churg-Strauss syndrome. Lupus. 1998;7(4):238–58.
31. Merlin E, Mouy R, Pereira B, Mouthon L, Bourmaud A, Piette JC, et al. Long-term outcome of children with pediatric-onset cutaneous and visceral polyarteritis nodosa. Joint Bone Spine. 2015;82(4):251–7.
32. Minagar A, Fowler M, Harris MK, Jaffe SL. Neurologic presentations of systemic vasculitides. Neurol Clin. 2010;28(1):171–84.
33. de Boysson H, Guillevin L. Polyarteritis nodosa neurologic manifestations. Neurol Clin. 2019;37(2):345–57.
34. Levine SM, Hellmann DB, Stone JH. Gastrointestinal involvement in polyarteritis nodosa (1986-2000): presentation and outcomes in 24 patients. Am J Med. 2002;112(5):386–91.
35. Schrader ML, Hochman JS, Bulkley BH. The heart in polyarteritis nodosa: a clinicopathologic study. Am Heart J. 1985;109(6):1353–9.
36. Pagnoux C, Guillevin L. Cardiac involvement in small and medium-sized vessel vasculitides. Lupus. 2005;14(9):718–22.
37. Ebersberger U, Rieber J, Wellmann P, Goebel C, Gansera B. Polyarteritis nodosa causing a vast coronary artery aneurysm. J Am Coll Cardiol. 2015;65(5):e1–2.
38. Wi J, Choi HH, Lee CJ, Kim T, Shin S, Ko YG, et al. Acute myocardial infarction due to polyarteritis nodosa in a young female patient. Korean Circ J. 2010;40(4):197–200.
39. Calvo R, Negri M, Ortiz A, Roverano S, Paira S. Myositis as the initial presentation of panarteritis nodosa. Reumatol Clin. 2019;15(5):e24–6.
40. Kang Y, Hong SH, Yoo HJ, Choi JY, Park JK, Park J, et al. Muscle involvement in polyarteritis nodosa: report of eight cases with characteristic contrast enhancement pattern on MRI. AJR Am J Roentgenol. 2016;206(2):378–84.
41. Lie JT. Systemic and isolated vasculitis. A rational approach to classification and pathologic diagnosis. Pathol Annu. 1989;24(Pt 1):25–114.
42. Jennette JC. Implications for pathogenesis of patterns of injury in small- and medium-sized-vessel vasculitis. Cleve Clin J Med. 2002;69(Suppl 2):SII33–8.
43. Lightfoot RW Jr, Michel BA, Bloch DA, Hunder GG, Zvaifler NJ, McShane DJ, et al. The American College of Rheumatology 1990 criteria for the classification of polyarteritis nodosa. Arthritis Rheum. 1990;33(8):1088–93.
44. Craven A, Robson J, Ponte C, Grayson PC, Suppiah R, Judge A, et al. ACR/EULAR-endorsed study to develop Diagnostic and Classification Criteria for Vasculitis (DCVAS). Clin Exp Nephrol. 2013;17(5):619–21.
45. Hernandez-Rodriguez J, Alba MA, Prieto-Gonzalez S, Cid MC. Diagnosis and classification of polyarteritis nodosa. J Autoimmun. 2014;48–49:84–9.

46. Jee KN, Ha HK, Lee IJ, Kim JK, Sung KB, Cho KS, et al. Radiologic findings of abdominal polyarteritis nodosa. AJR Am J Roentgenol. 2000;174(6):1675–9.
47. Singhal M, Gupta P, Sharma A, Lal A, Rathi M, Khandelwal N. Role of multidetector abdominal CT in the evaluation of abnormalities in polyarteritis nodosa. Clin Radiol. 2016;71(3):222–7.
48. Frohnert PP, Sheps SG. Long-term follow-up study of periarteritis nodosa. Am J Med. 1967;43(1):8–14.
49. Ribi C, Cohen P, Pagnoux C, Mahr A, Arene JP, Puechal X, et al. Treatment of polyarteritis nodosa and microscopic polyangiitis without poor-prognosis factors: a prospective random-ized study of one hundred twenty-four patients. Arthritis Rheum. 2010;62(4):1186–97.
50. Guillevin L, Lhote F, Gayraud M, Cohen P, Jarrousse B, Lortholary O, et al. Prognostic fac-tors in polyarteritis nodosa and Churg-Strauss syndrome. A prospective study in 342 patients. Medicine (Baltimore). 1996;75(1):17–28.
51. Guillevin L, Pagnoux C, Seror R, Mahr A, Mouthon L, Le Toumelin P, et al. The Five-Factor Score revisited: assessment of prognoses of systemic necrotizing vasculitides based on the French Vasculitis Study Group (FVSG) cohort. Medicine (Baltimore). 2011;90(1):19–27.
52. Bourgarit A, Le Toumelin P, Pagnoux C, Cohen P, Mahr A, Le Guern V, et al. Deaths occurring during the first year after treatment onset for polyarteritis nodosa, microscopic polyangiitis, and Churg-Strauss syndrome: a retrospective analysis of causes and factors predictive of mor-tality based on 595 patients. Medicine (Baltimore). 2005;84(5):323–30.
53. Jardel S, Puechal X, Le Quellec A, Pagnoux C, Hamidou M, Maurier F, et al. Mortality in sys-temic necrotizing vasculitides: a retrospective analysis of the French Vasculitis Study Group registry. Autoimmun Rev. 2018;17(7):653–9.
54. Erden A, Batu ED, Sonmez HE, Sari A, Armagan B, Arici ZS, et al. Comparing polyarteritis nodosa in children and adults: a single center study. Int J Rheum Dis. 2017;20(8):1016–22.
55. Mukhtyar C, Guillevin L, Cid MC, Dasgupta B, de Groot K, Gross W, et al. EULAR recom-mendations for the management of primary small and medium vessel vasculitis. Ann Rheum Dis. 2009;68(3):310–7.
56. Pagnoux C, Quemeneur T, Ninet J, Diot E, Kyndt X, de Wazieres B, et al. Treatment of sys-temic necrotizing vasculitides in patients aged sixty-five years or older: results of a multi-center, open-label, randomized controlled trial of corticosteroid and cyclophosphamide-based induction therapy. Arthritis Rheumatol. 2015;67(4):1117–27.
57. Puechal X, Pagnoux C, Baron G, Quemeneur T, Neel A, Agard C, et al. Adding azathioprine to remission-induction glucocorticoids for eosinophilic granulomatosis with polyangiitis (Churg-Strauss), microscopic polyangiitis, or polyarteritis nodosa without poor prognosis factors: a randomized, controlled trial. Arthritis Rheumatol. 2017;69(11):2175–86.
58. Guillevin L, Cohen P, Mahr A, Arene JP, Mouthon L, Puechal X, et al. Treatment of polyar-teritis nodosa and microscopic polyangiitis with poor prognosis factors: a prospective trial comparing glucocorticoids and six or twelve cyclophosphamide pulses in sixty-five patients. Arthritis Rheum. 2003;49(1):93–100.
59. Gayraud M, Guillevin L, Cohen P, Lhote F, Cacoub P, Deblois P, et al. Treatment of good-prognosis polyarteritis nodosa and Churg-Strauss syndrome: comparison of steroids and oral or pulse cyclophosphamide in 25 patients. French Cooperative Study Group for Vasculitides. Br J Rheumatol. 1997;36(12):1290–7.
60. Eleftheriou D, Dillon MJ, Tullus K, Marks SD, Pilkington CA, Roebuck DJ, et al. Systemic polyarteritis nodosa in the young: a single-center experience over thirty-two years. Arthritis Rheum. 2013;65(9):2476–85.
61. Ribeiro E, Cressend T, Duffau P, Grenouillet-Delacre M, Rouanet-Lariviere M, Vital A, et al. Rituximab efficacy during a refractory polyarteritis nodosa flare. Case Rep Med. 2009;2009:738293.
62. Neel A, Masseau A, Hervier B, Bossard C, Cacoub P, Pagnoux C, et al. Life-threatening hepati-tis C virus-associated polyarteritis nodosa successfully treated by rituximab. J Clin Rheumatol. 2011;17(8):439–41.
63. Krusche M, Ruffer N, Kotter I. Tocilizumab treatment in refractory polyarteritis nodosa: a case report and review of the literature. Rheumatol Int. 2019;39(2):337–44.

64. Capuozzo M, Ottaiano A, Nava E, Cascone S, Fico R, Iaffaioli RV, et al. Etanercept induces remission of polyarteritis nodosa: a case report. Front Pharmacol. 2014;5:122.
65. Wang CR, Yang CC. Adalimumab therapy in hepatitis B virus-negative polyarteritis nodosa: a case report. Medicine (Baltimore). 2018;97(25):e11053.
66. Lerkvaleekul B, Treepongkaruna S, Ruangwattanapaisarn N, Treesit T, Vilaiyuk S. Recurrent ruptured abdominal aneurysms in polyarteritis nodosa successfully treated with infliximab. Biologics. 2019;13:111–6.
67. Ginsberg S, Rosner I, Slobodin G, Rozenbaum M, Kaly L, Jiries N, et al. Infliximab for the treatment of refractory polyarteritis nodosa. Clin Rheumatol. 2019;38:2825.
68. Ombrello AK, Qin J, Hoffmann PM, Kumar P, Stone D, Jones A, et al. Treatment strategies for deficiency of adenosine deaminase 2. N Engl J Med. 2019;380(16):1582–4.
69. Guillevin L, Mahr A, Cohen P, Larroche C, Queyrel V, Loustaud-Ratti V, et al. Short-term corticosteroids then lamivudine and plasma exchanges to treat hepatitis B virus-related polyarteritis nodosa. Arthritis Rheum. 2004;51(3):482–7.
70. Guillevin L, Lhote F, Leon A, Fauvelle F, Vivitski L, Trepo C. Treatment of polyarteritis nodosa related to hepatitis B virus with short term steroid therapy associated with antiviral agents and plasma exchanges. A prospective trial in 33 patients. J Rheumatol. 1993;20(2):289–98.
71. Guillevin L, Lhote F, Cohen P, Jarrousse B, Lortholary O, Genereau T, et al. Corticosteroids plus pulse cyclophosphamide and plasma exchanges versus corticosteroids plus pulse cyclophosphamide alone in the treatment of polyarteritis nodosa and Churg-Strauss syndrome patients with factors predicting poor prognosis. A prospective, randomized trial in sixty-two patients. Arthritis Rheum. 1995;38(11):1638–45.
72. Guillevin L, Lhote F, Sauvaget F, Deblois P, Rossi F, Levallois D, et al. Treatment of polyarteritis nodosa related to hepatitis B virus with interferon-alpha and plasma exchanges. Ann Rheum Dis. 1994;53(5):334–7.
73. Lok AS, McMahon BJ, Brown RS Jr, Wong JB, Ahmed AT, Farah W, et al. Antiviral therapy for chronic hepatitis B viral infection in adults: a systematic review and meta-analysis. Hepatology. 2016;63(1):284–306.

Part IV

Single Organ Vasculitis

Carlo Salvarani, Robert D. Brown Jr, Caterina Giannini, and Gene G. Hunder

Abstract

Primary CNS vasculitis is an uncommon disorder of unknown cause that is restricted to brain and spinal cord. The median age of onset is 50 years. The neurological manifestations are diverse, but generally consist of headache, altered cognition, focal weakness, or stroke. Serological markers of inflammation are usually normal. Cerebrospinal fluid is abnormal in about 80–90% of patients. Diagnosis is unlikely in the presence of a normal MRI of the brain. Biopsy of CNS tissue showing vasculitis is the only definitive test; however, angiography has often been used for diagnosis even though it has only moderate sensitivity and specificity. Granulomatous vasculitis is the most common pattern of vasculitis (around 60% of cases), and β-amyloid deposition is present in almost 50% of these patients. Several subsets of PCNSV have been identified, which differ in terms of outcomes and optimal management. The size of the affected vessels varies and determines outcome and response to treatment. Early recognition is important because treatment with corticosteroi15

C. Salvarani (✉)
Rheumatology Unit, Azienda Unita' Sanitaria Locale IRCCS di Reggio Emilia, Reggio Emilia, Italy

Rheumatology Unit, Università di Modena e Reggio Emilia, Reggio Emilia, Italy
e-mail: carlo.salvarani@ausl.re.it; salvarani.carlo@ausl.re.it

R. D. Brown Jr · C. Giannini · G. G. Hunder
Department of Neurology (R.D.B.), the Division of Anatomic Pathology (C.G.), and Division of Rheumatology (GGH, Emeritus Member), Mayo Clinic, Rochester, MN, USA
e-mail: brown@mayo.edu; caterina.giannini@mayo.edu; ghunder@mayo.edu

© Springer Nature Switzerland AG 2021
C. Salvarani et al. (eds.), *Large and Medium Size Vessel and Single Organ Vasculitis*, Rare Diseases of the Immune System,
https://doi.org/10.1007/978-3-030-67175-4_15

ds with or without cytotoxic drugs can often prevent serious outcomes. Cyclophosphamide (CYC) and mycophenolate mofetil appear to be effective for the induction of remission. Rituximab may be helpful in patients who are intolerant or respond poorly to CYC. The differential diagnosis includes reversible cerebral vasoconstriction syndromes and secondary cerebral vasculitis.

Keywords

Vasculitis · Central nervous system · Cerebral biopsy · Angiography · Magnetic resonance imaging · Glucocorticoids · Cyclophosphamide

15.1   Introduction

Primary central nervous system vasculitis (PCNSV) is an uncommon and poorly understood form of vasculitis that it is limited to the brain and spinal cord [1–5]. PCNSV represents the most frequent vasculitis involving the central nervous system (CNS) [6]. The neurological manifestations are diverse and nonspecific. Serological markers of inflammation are usually normal. Cerebrospinal fluid (CSF) is abnormal in approximately 80–90% of the cases. The diagnosis is unlikely in the presence of a normal brain MRI. Biopsy of CNS tissue showing vasculitis is the only definitive test; however, angiography is often used to confirm the diagnosis. Early recognition is important because treatment with glucocorticoids (GCs) with or without cytotoxic drugs may prevent serious or even lethal outcomes. The differential diagnosis is broad and includes the reversible cerebral vasoconstriction syndromes (RCVS), secondary cerebral vasculitis, malignancy, and infections. Modern recognition of PCNSV as a separate entity is generally dated to the mid-1950s when Cravioto and Feigin [7] described several cases with a "noninfectious granulomatous angiitis" with a predilection for the nervous system. The term "granulomatous angiitis of the nervous system" was applied because of the histopathologic findings observed in the arteries from initial cases. Since then, primary CNS vasculitis has been referred to as granulomatous angiitis of the CNS, or more specifically, noninfectious or idiopathic granulomatous angiitis of the CNS, and giant-cell arteritis of the CNS, isolated angiitis of the CNS, primary angiitis of the CNS, and benign angiopathy of the CNS [1, 8]. Outcome in early reports was frequently fatal, and diagnosis was often made at autopsy [1, 2, 4]. By contrast, in later studies outcomes were more favorable, and biopsy and angiography were used for diagnosis [9–11]. Recently, major advances have been made in the field of PCNSV. Studies of larger numbers of cases have revealed a more varied histopathologic inflammatory picture and an association with amyloid angiopathy [12–16]. It has also become recognized that PCNSV is more heterogeneous than previously thought, encompassing clinical subsets that differ in terms of prognosis and therapy [17–23]. Finally, over the past few years, childhood PCNSV (cPCNSV) has been recognized as a possible cause of vascular strokes in children [24]. This review aimed to provide an update on the major advances made in adult PCNSV.

15.2   Diagnosis and Diagnostic Criteria

Diagnostic criteria for PCNSV were proposed by Calabrese and Mallek [10] in 1988 on the basis of their clinical experience and of published evidence (Table 15.1). These criteria included angiographic changes indicating a high probability of vasculitis, that is, areas of smooth vessel wall narrowing or occlusions alternating with dilated cerebral arteries affecting multiple cerebral arteries in the absence of proximal vessel atherosclerosis or other recognized abnormalities. A single abnormality in multiple arteries or multiple abnormalities in a single vessel were considered to be less consistent with PCNSV [1, 3]. Because of the more invasive nature of CNS biopsy, angiography has become the most used method of confirming the diagnosis in patients with suggestive clinical findings. However, angiographic changes typical of vasculitis may be seen in nonvasculitic conditions such as vasospasm, CNS infections, lymphomas, cerebral arterial emboli, and also atherosclerosis [1, 2]. Furthermore, among pathologically documented cases, cerebral angiography may be normal, reflecting vascular involvement in small vessels below the resolution of angiography [17]. Overall, the sensitivity of angiography varies between 40 and 90%, whereas its specificity has shown to be as low as 30% [1, 25–27]. Magnetic resonance angiography (MRA) is a reasonable initial approach to investigate patients with suspected PCNSV. However, MRA is less sensitive than conventional angiography in detecting structural lesions involving the posterior circulation and distal vessels [1, 28]. Therefore, if the clinical suspicion is high but MRA is normal, a standard cerebral angiography is warranted. It is important to emphasize that the diagnosis of PCNSV should not be based on the findings of a positive angiography alone, and that angiography results should always be interpreted in conjunction with

Table 15.1 Diagnostic criteria for adult primary central nervous system vasculitis

Diagnostic criteria for PCNSV proposed by Calabrese and Mallek [10]
A history or clinical findings of an acquired neurologic deficit, which remained unexplained after a thorough initial basic evaluation
Either classic angiographic or histopathologic features of vasculitis within the central nervous system
No evidence of systemic vasculitis or of any other condition to which the angiographic or pathologic features could be secondary
A diagnosis of primary central nervous system vasculitis is made if all the above criteria are satisfied.
Diagnostic criteria for PCNSV proposed by Birnbaum and Hellmann [29]
Definite diagnosis: confirmation of vasculitis on analysis of a tissue biopsy specimen
Probable diagnosis: in the absence of tissue confirmation, if there are high probability findings on an angiogram with abnormal findings on MRI and a CSF profile consistent with PCNSV

clinical, laboratory, and MRI findings. Recently, to prevent misdiagnosis, particularly with the RCVS, Birnbaum and Hellman [29] have proposed new criteria based on the levels of certainty of the diagnosis (Table 15.1). These criteria may prevent patients with RCVS from being treated with cytotoxic therapy. However, they are not able to categorize patients with high-probability angiographic findings, but normal CSF analysis who may have either RCVS or PCNSV. The presence of precipitating factors, the type of onset and the neurological findings may be useful distinguishing features. Onset in the postpartum or following exposure to vasoactive substances would point to RCVS [30]. RCVS has an acute onset followed by a monophasic course, usually without any new complications after 4 weeks, whereas in PCNSV, the onset is more insidious and the course is progressive with frequent appearance of cerebral infarcts. Headache is of the thunderclap type in RCVS, whereas it is subacute and progressive in PCNSV. MRI is often normal in RCVS, whereas PCNSV is extremely unlikely in the presence of a normal MRI. Several studies have indeed reported a sensitivity of MRI for PCNSV close to 100% [1, 2, 26]. Abnormal findings on MRI are nonspecific and include cortical and subcortical infarction, parenchymal and leptomeningeal enhancement, intracranial hemorrhage, tumor-like mass lesions, and nonspecific areas of increased signal intensity on fluid-attenuated inversion recovery or T2-weighted images. Advances in the neuroimaging techniques visualizing the wall of intracranial blood vessels could in the future improve the capacity to distinguish inflammatory from non-inflammatory lesions and, thus, the performance of the criteria [31]. Vessel wall thickening and intramural contrast enhancement are quite specific findings in patients with active cerebral vasculitis affecting large arteries. Occasionally, enhancement may be marked and extend into the adjacent leptomeningeal tissue (perivascular enhancement) [32–34]. High-resolution, high-field contrast-enhanced MRI may be able to differentiate enhancement patterns of intracranial atherosclerotic plaques (eccentric), inflammation (concentric), and other wall pathologies. However, the sensitivity and specificity of MRI in this regard remain to be determined [35]. Cerebral and meningeal biopsy remains the gold standard for the diagnosis of PCNSV [1, 9, 12, 15]. The procedure in expert hands is well tolerated. Small intraparenchymal hematomas at the biopsy site are the most frequent complication (4.9%); however, permanent neurological sequelae are rare (only about 1% of cases) [36, 37]. A positive biopsy confirms vasculitis and excludes its mimickers.

An optimal biopsy should include samples of dura, leptomeninges, cortex, and white matter. Diagnostic histopathological features include transmural vascular inflammation affecting small and medium-sized leptomeningeal and parenchymal arterial vessels. Vasculitis is characterized by skip and segmental vascular lesions. Therefore, because of sampling error, a negative biopsy does not entirely rule out the diagnosis of vasculitis. In fact, there is evidence that biopsy has a sensitivity of 53–63% in diagnosing PCNSV [12, 26]. Biopsy of a radiographically abnormal area is preferable to random sampling of the nondominant frontal lobe or temporal tip. Miller et al. [12] showed that 78% of the targeted biopsies were diagnostic, whereas none of the blind biopsies demonstrated vasculitis. Inclusion of leptomeninges may increase the diagnostic yield when PCNSV is suspected. Stereotactic guidance may be used for deeper lesions, but is usually unnecessary for more super-ficial lesions.

15.3 Histopathology

Three main histopathological patterns are seen in PCNSV [12, 15]. Granulomatous vasculitis is the most common pattern of vasculitis (around 60% of cases). It is characterized by vasculocentric mononuclear inflammation associated with well-formed granulomas and multinucleated cells (Fig. 15.1a). β-amyloid deposition is present in almost 50% of these patients (Fig. 15.1b). Amyloid angiopathy is usually associated with granulomatous vasculitis and occasionally with necrotizing vascu-litis. The inflammatory response to vascular amyloid observed in a transgenic mouse model that develops prominent cerebral amyloid angiopathy (CAA) and the pres-ence of anti-amyloid β (Aβ) autoantibodies in the acute phase of CAA-related inflammation (CAA-ri) support a role for amyloid deposition in triggering vascular inflammation [38, 39]. Lymphocytic vasculitis is the second most predominant pat-tern (around 25% of cases). It is characterized by predominantly lymphocytic inflammation with occasional plasma cells extending through the vessel wall with features of vascular distortion and destruction (Fig. 15.1c). Lymphocytic vasculitis is a form more benign of vasculitis compared to granulomatous and necrotizing vasculitides with less mortality and less disability at last follow-up [40]. Necrotizing vasculitis is the least frequently seen pattern (14% of cases). It is characterized by acute necrotizing vasculitis similar to polyarteritis nodosa with transmural fibrinoid necrosis (Fig. 15.1d). This process involves predominantly the small muscular arter-ies with disruption of the internal elastic lamina. Necrotizing vasculitis is signifi-cantly associated with intracranial hemorrhage [20]. The destructive vasculitic process with fibrinoid necrosis may cause severe vessel wall weakening, thus, pre-disposing to blood vessels rupture and aneurysm formation. This mechanism may account for the association between necrotizing vasculitis and intracranial hemorrhage.

15.4 Clinical Manifestations and Laboratory Findings

Clinical manifestations at diagnosis are nonspecific, and many symptoms are usu-ally present [3, 41]. The onset of disease can be acute, but it is more frequently insidious and slowly progressive. Diagnosis is made in 75% of patients within 6 months of the onset of symptoms. Headache, the most common symptom, can be generalized or localized, it often slowly worsens, can spontaneously remit for peri-ods, and varies in severity. Cognitive impairment is also often insidious in onset, and is the second most frequent manifestation. Focal neurological manifestations

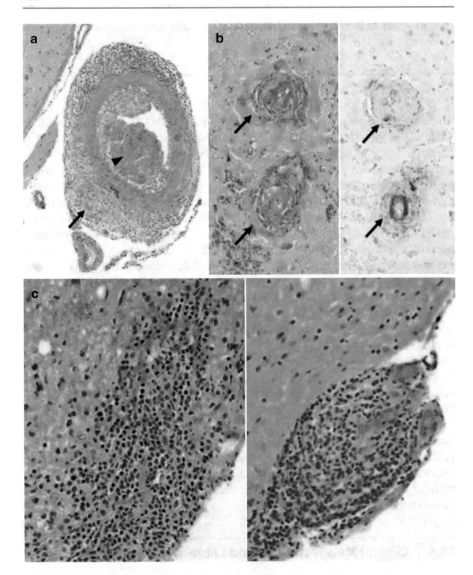

Fig. 15.1 Histopathologic patterns of primary central nervous system vasculitis. (**a**) Granulomatous pattern. Transmural inflammation involving an artery of the leptomeninges with prominent mononuclear and granulomatous (arrow) adventitial inflammation; focal fibrin thrombus formation is also present (arrow head; Hematoxylin and eosin ×20). (**b**) Granulomatous pattern with β-A4 amyloid deposition. Left panel: two intraparenchymal arterioles showing transmural inflammation with vessel wall destruction (upper) and granulomas (lower; arrows; Hematoxylin and eosin, ×20). Right panel: both vessels show amyloid deposition (arrows; immunoperoxidase staining for β-A4 amyloid, ×20). (**c**) Lymphocytic pattern. Several leptomeningeal vessels show marked transmural lymphocytic inflammation, devoid of granulomas and histiocytes (Hematoxylin and eosin, ×40). (**d**) Necrotizing pattern. Left panel: a segment of intraparenchymal muscular artery shows extensive mural necrosis with karyorrhectic debris and acute neutrophilic inflammation (arrows; Hematoxylin and eosin, ×10). Right panel: the lumen is completely obliterated and clumped aggregates of fibrin are seen (Hematoxylin and eosin, ×20). *Reproduced from Salvarani et al. Adult primary central nervous system vasculitis: an update. Curr Opin Rheumatol 2012; 24:46–52* [2]

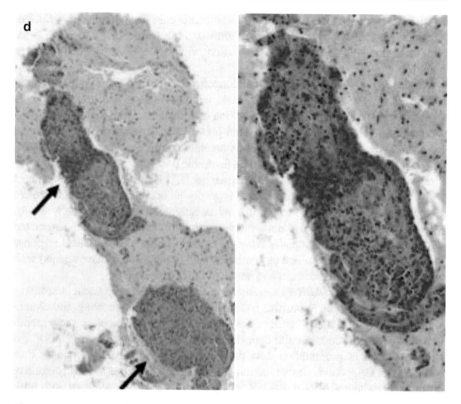

Fig. 15.1 (continued)

with or without distinct cerebral infarction are present in many patients. Other features such as ataxia, seizure, and intracerebral hemorrhage are less frequent. By contrast with other systemic vasculitides, constitutional symptoms such as fever and weight loss are uncommon.

Results of blood tests in patients with primary CNS vasculitis are usually normal and consist of tests for acute-phase reactants, antinuclear antibodies, antineutrophil cytoplasm antibodies, and antiphospholipid antibodies [1–3]. CSF analysis is abnormal in 80–90% of patients [3, 41]. Changes consist of a mildly increased leucocyte count and total protein concentration. Patients with angiography-negative primary CNS vasculitis often have greatly raised protein concentrations [17]. CSF analysis should be composed of appropriate stains, cultures, serological and molecular tests, and flow cytometry studies to exclude infection or malignancy.

15.5   PCNSV Subsets

Several subsets of PCNSV have been identified, which differ in terms of outcomes and optimal management.

Spinal cord involvement has been documented in 5% of patients, but it is rarely the only manifestation [5]. Most patients have concurrent or subsequent brain involvement during the disease course. The thoracic cord is predominantly affected. A careful medical evaluation must be performed to confirm the diagnosis of PCNSV and to exclude other conditions associated with acute or subacute transverse myelitis.

Angiography-negative PCNSV is characterized by normal angiograms but brain biopsies positive for vasculitis [17]. These findings suggest that the vasculitis is limited to small vessels below the resolution of conventional angiography. Patients with angiography-negative PCNSV often present with cognitive dysfunction and have markedly elevated CSF protein, meningeal or parenchymal enhancing lesions on MRI, good response to therapy, and a favorable outcome.

Prominent leptomeningeal enhancement on MRI identifies a subset of patients with PCNSV [18]. These patients have typically an acute clinical onset, frequent cognitive dysfunction at presentation, and negative cerebral angiography and/or MRA. CNS biopsies show a granulomatous vascular inflammation, often associated with vascular amyloid angiopathy. Almost all patients have a good clinical response to corticosteroid therapy (alone or combined with immunosuppressive agents) with resolution of MRI enhancement and an overall favorable course.

Aβ-related angiitis (ABRA). Cerebral amyloid angiopathy is present in around a quarter of PCNSV biopsy-positive patients and half of those showing granulomatous vasculitis associate evidence of CAA [12, 15, 34]. Brain biopsies show granulomatous vasculitis and vascular deposits of amyloid-β. Patients with PCNSV and CAA are older at presentation than those with PCNSV only, but younger than patients with CAA and no inflammation [14, 16]. They often present with cognitive dysfunction, whereas MRI shows enhancing meningeal lesions alone or with infiltrative white matter hyperintensity lesions [34]. In these patients, the symptoms related to the vasculitic component respond well to immunosuppressive treatment, but in the long-term follow-up the clinical manifestations related to CAA prevail with increased disability and mortality. The inflammatory reaction related to the presence of amyloid β-peptide is defined CAA-ri and varies from little or no inflammation, to perivascular infiltrates, and to frank granulomatous vasculitis. Patients with CAA-related perivascular inflammation have characteristics similar to those of patients associating CAA and granulomatous vasculitis [16]. Recently, clinicoradiological criteria for the diagnosis of CAA-ri have been proposed [42].

Rapidly progressive PCNSV represents the worst end of the clinical spectrum of this vasculitis [19]. These patients have a rapidly advancing course with often-fatal outcome. They are characterized by bilateral, multiple, large cerebral vessel lesions on angiograms, and multiple bilateral cerebral infarctions on MRI. The predominant histopathological pattern is of granulomatous and/or necrotizing vasculitis. These patients respond poorly to traditional immunosuppressive treatment and need to be treated aggressively from the beginning.

Solitary tumor-like mass lesion is an underrecognized subset of PCNSV, which is found in approximately 7% of the patients [23]. An association with CAA and granulomatous vasculitis was observed. Excision of the lesion may be curative; however, in some patients aggressive immunosuppressive therapy has led to a favorable outcome obviating the need of surgery.

Intracranial hemorrhage is a not infrequent presentation of PCNSV, having been reported in 11–12.2% of patients [4, 20]. Intracerebral hemorrhage is the most common presentation, followed by subarachnoid hemorrhage. These patients have less frequently altered cognition, persistent neurologic deficit or stroke at presentation, as well as MRI evidence of cerebral infarctions. Necrotizing vasculitis is the predominant histopathologic pattern.

Association with lymphoma. Lymphoma is reported to occur in patients with PCNSV in a frequency of around 6% [43]. The two conditions usually occur and are diagnosed simultaneously, suggesting an immunologic paraneoplastic mechanism. PCNSV is prevalently associated with Hodgkin lymphoma. The predominant histopathologic pattern is granulomatous vasculitis and cerebral amyloid angiopathy may be associated. Patients associating lymphoma are more frequently male and more commonly have leptomeningeal enhancement at diagnosis. Furthermore, they have a more severe form of cerebral vasculitis with increased disability and mortality.

15.6 Differential Diagnosis

Primary CNS vasculitis should be differentiated from other similar disorders to avoid therapeutic and prognostic errors [1]. The most common mimicker of PCNSV is RCVS [30]. Other common causes of secondary CNS vasculitis are infection, systemic vasculitis, connective tissue diseases, and miscellaneous disorders (Table 15.2).

15.7 Treatment

No randomized clinical trials of medical management in PCNSV exist. Treatments for PCNSV have been similar to those first used in other vasculitides. In 1983, in a small series, Cupps et al. [11] first found cyclophosphamide (CYC) in combination with corticosteroids to be also effective in PCNSV. However, optimal management and treatment outcomes remained uncertain because of the lack of uniform diagnostic criteria and the small studies.

Two recent cohort studies [40, 44] have described the treatment and outcomes of patients with PCNSV. Although limited by the retrospective nature and by the low number of patients diagnosed using cerebral biopsy, these studies represent the two largest reported series of cases in adult PCNSV.

15.7.1 Mayo Clinic Cohort of Patients with Adult PCNSV

In the Mayo Clinic series, a favorable response was observed in most of the patients treated with prednisone alone or in combination with CYC [40]. Response rates were similar (about 83%) in both treatment groups with improvement of disability

Table 15.2 Causes of
secondary CNS vasculitis
*(Reproduced with permission
from Salvarani C et al. Adult
primary central nervous
system vasculitis. Lancet
2012; 380:767–77)* [1]

Viral infections
Varicella zoster virus
HIV
Hepatitis C virus
Cytomegalovirus
Parvovirus B19
Bacterial infections
Treponema pallidum
Borrelia Burgdorferi
Mycobacterium tuberculosis
Mycoplasma pneumoniae
Bartonella henselae
Rickettsia spp
Fungal infections
Aspergillosis
Mucormycosis
Coccidioidomycosis
Candidosis
Parasitic infections
Cysticercosis
Systemic vasculitides
Granulomatosis with polyangiitis (Wegener's granulomatosis)
Eosinophilic granulomatosis with polyangiitis (Churg–Strauss syndrome)
Behçet's disease
Polyarteritis nodosa
Henoch-Schönlein purpura
Kawasaki disease
Giant-cell arteritis
Takayasu arteritis
Connective tissue diseases
Systemic lupus erythematosus
Rheumatoid arthritis
Sjøgren's syndrome
Dermatomyositis
Mixed connective tissue disease
Miscellaneous
Antiphospholipid antibodies syndrome
Hodgkin and non-Hodgkin lymphomas
Neurosarcoidosis
Inflammatory bowel disease
Graft versus host disease
Bacterial endocarditis
Acute bacterial meningitis
Drug-induced CNS vasculitis (cocaine, amphetamine, ephedrine, phenylpropanolamine)

(Rankin scale scores) over time. Seventy-two percent of the patients achieved a sustained therapeutic response (no relapses) during follow-up. The median duration of all therapy was around 11 months in both treatment groups. No differences in outcomes (disability and mortality) were observed in the two treatment groups. Patients with relapses needed longer therapy compared with those without relapses, but relapses were not associated with increased mortality or worse disability (Rankin score) at the last follow-up visit.

This study also evaluated clinical characteristics by diagnosis associated with treatment response, relapses, and the inability to discontinue treatment at the last follow-up. Large-vessel involvement and cerebral infarcts on MRI at diagnosis were significantly associated with a poor response to treatment, whereas prominent gadolinium-enhanced cerebral lesions or meninges assessed by MRI were significantly associated with longer therapy, which was often being continued at the time of last follow-up. Some patients initially treated with an immunosuppressive agent different from CYC (mainly, azathioprine and mycophenolate mofetil) had a favorable response, suggesting in some patients the possible use of a less toxic alternative to CYC for the induction of remission.

We also evaluated the association of clinical findings at diagnosis with Rankin score outcomes at last follow-up and survival [40]. High disability scores at last follow-up and increased mortality were both significantly associated with increasing age and the presence of cerebral infarction observed on MRI at presentation, while patients with gadolinium-enhanced meninges or lesions on MRI had lower disability and less risk of death. Patients with amyloid angiopathy had lower disability at follow-up, while diagnosis by angiography alone compared with biopsy and the presence of large-vessel involvement on angiograms were significantly associated with an increased mortality. These differences were related to the different size of cerebral vessels involved in the inflammatory process. Patients with rapidly progressive PCNSV and often-fatal outcome were characterized by the angiographic presence of bilateral, multiple, large-vessel lesions, and MRI evidence of multiple cerebral infarctions. They represented the worst end of the clinical spectrum of PCNSV [19, 21]. A more benign course was observed with angiography-negative patients with involvement at biopsy of small cortical and leptomeningeal vessels often presenting with a cognitive disorder and MRI evidence of prominent leptomeningeal enhancement [17, 18]. Patients with Aβ-related angiitis defined by deposition of amyloid-β in the media and adventitia of small cortical and leptomeningeal vessels belong to this clinically less aggressive subset [14, 16]. In view of these findings, we proposed a treatment algorithm mainly based on the size of the vessels involved in the inflammation (Fig. 15.2) [41]. In patients with inflammation restricted to small cortical and leptomeningeal vessels who have a more benign disease, prednisone alone was recommended as initial therapy (initial dose of 1 mg/kg/day), whereas in patients with more severe large/proximal vessel disease and in those with a rapidly progressive course, high-dose intravenous methylprednisolone (1000 mg daily for 3–5 days) and CYC can be used to attempt to induce remission immediately after diagnosis.

There is insufficient reported experience to suggest replacing CYC by the less toxic azathioprine (AZA) or mycophenolate mofetil (MMF) for the induction of

Suggested Treatment Algorithm for Adult PCNSV

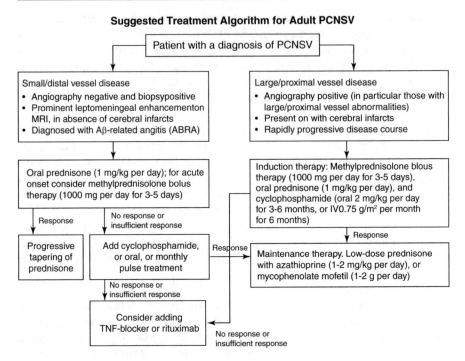

Fig. 15.2 Suggested treatment algorithm for primary central nervous system vasculitis. *Reproduced from Salvarani et al. An update of the Mayo Clinic cohort of patients with adult primary central nervous system vasculitis: description of 163 patients. Medicine (Baltimore) 2015; 94(21):e738* [41]

remission. However, these two immunosuppressors appear to be effective for the maintenance of remission [45–47]. A small number of case reports have shown the efficacy of tumor necrosis factor-a blockers [48]. Rituximab may be helpful in patients who are intolerant or respond poorly to CYC [49].

15.7.2 French Cohort of Patients with Primary Central Nervous System Vasculitis

In the initial French cohort [44], most patients received GCs and CYC: 61.5% responded to treatment with improved modified Rankin scale scores and 27% of patients had relapsing disease. Relapse was more common in patients with meningeal gadolinium enhancement on MRI and in those with seizures at diagnosis. Subsequently in an enlarged cohort, they evaluated in a long-term follow-up study the role of maintenance treatment with an immunosuppressant combined with GCs in improving survival and disability [45, 46]. They found that maintenance therapy is associated with better functional outcomes, lower relapse rates, and prolonged remission. Azathioprine, after induction of remission with CYC and GCs, was the most used drug for maintenance therapy. Mortality during the follow-up period was lower in the French cohort of PCNSV patients compared with the Mayo Clinic cohort (6% versus 15%). A better outcome in patients with lymphocytic vasculitis [44] that represented the prevalent histopathologic pattern in the French cohort may partially explain this difference.

15.7.3 Monitoring Disease Course

Serial MRI and MRA (4–6 weeks after the beginning of treatment, then every 3–4 months during the first year of treatment, or when a new neurological deficit arises), and repeat careful neurological examinations, are useful to monitor disease course. In patients with stable imaging but worsening clinical symptoms, repeat spinal fluid examination and repeat angiography might be necessary. For those patients without biopsy verification at the time of initial diagnosis who have worsening symptoms despite immunosuppressive therapy, a brain biopsy should be considered.

References

1. Salvarani C, Brown RD Jr, Hunder GG. Adult primary central nervous system vasculitis. Lancet. 2012;380:767–77.
2. Salvarani C, Brown RD Jr, Hunder GG. Adult primary central nervous system vasculitis: an update. Curr Opin Rheumatol. 2012;24:46–52.
3. Salvarani C, Brown RD Jr, Calamia KT, et al. Primary central nervous system vasculitis: analysis of 101 patients. Ann Neurol. 2007;62:442–51.
4. Calabrese LH, Duna GF, Lie JT. Vasculitis in the central nervous system. Arthritis Rheum. 1997;40:1189–201.
5. Salvarani C, Brown RD Jr, Calamia KT, et al. Primary CNS vasculitis with spinal cord involvement. Neurology. 2008;70:2394–400.
6. Salvarani C, Giannini C, Miller DV, Hunder G. Giant cell arteritis: involvement of intracranial arteries. Arthritis Rheum. 2006;55:985–9.
7. Cravioto H, Feigin I. Noninfectious granulomatous angiitis with a predilection for the nervous system. Neurology. 1959;9:599–609.
8. Calabrese LH, Gragg LA, Furlan AJ. Benign angiopathy: a distinct subset of angiographically defined primary angiitis of the central nervous system. J Rheumatol. 1993;20:2046–50.
9. Moore PM. Diagnosis and management of isolated angiitis of the central nervous system. Neurology. 1989;39:167–73.
10. Calabrese LH, Mallek JA. Primary angiitis of the central nervous system. Report of 8 new cases, review of the literature, and proposal for diagnostic criteria. Medicine (Baltimore). 1988;67:20–39.
11. Cupps TR, Moore PM, Fauci AS. Isolated angiitis of the central nervous system: prospective diagnostic and therapeutic experience. Am J Med. 1983;74:97–105.
12. Miller DV, Salvarani C, Hunder GG, et al. Biopsy findings in primary angiitis of the central nervous system. Am J Surg Pathol. 2009;33:35–43.
13. Scolding NJ, Joseph F, Kirby PA, et al. Abeta-related angiitis: primary angiitis of the central nervous system associated with cerebral amyloid angiopathy. Brain. 2005;128:500–15.

14. Salvarani C, Brown RD Jr, Calamia KT, et al. Primary central nervous system vasculitis: comparison of patients with and without cerebral amyloid angiopathy. Rheumatology (Oxford). 2008;47:1671–7.

15. Giannini C, Salvarani C, Hunder G, Brown RD. Primary central nervous system vasculitis: pathology and mechanisms. Acta Neuropathol. 2012;123:759–72.

16. Salvarani C, Hunder GG, Morris JM, et al. Aβ-related angiitis: comparison with CAA without inflammation and primary CNS vasculitis. Neurology. 2013;81:1596–603.

17. Salvarani C, Brown RD Jr, Calamia KT, et al. Angiography-negative primary central nervous system vasculitis: a syndrome involving small cerebral vessels. Medicine (Baltimore). 2008;87:264–71.

18. Salvarani C, Brown RD Jr, Calamia KT, et al. Primary central nervous system vasculitis with prominent leptomeningeal enhancement: a subset with a benign outcome. Arthritis Rheum. 2008;58:595–603.

19. Salvarani C, Brown RD Jr, Calamia KT, et al. Rapidly progressive primary central nervous system vasculitis. Rheumatology (Oxford). 2010;50:349–58.

20. Salvarani C, Brown RD Jr, Calamia KT, et al. Primary central nervous system vasculitis presenting with intracranial hemorrhage. Arthritis Rheum. 2011;63:3598–606.

21. Salvarani C, Brown RD Jr, Morris JM, et al. Catastrophic primary central nervous system vasculitis. Clin Exp Rheumatol. 2014;32(Suppl 82):S3–4.

22. Hunder GG, Salvarani C, Brown RD Jr. Primary central nervous system vasculitis: is it a single disease? Ann Neurol. 2010;68:573–4.

23. Salvarani C, Brown RD Jr, Christianson TJH, et al. Primary central nervous system vasculitis mimicking brain tumor: comprehensive analysis of 13 cases from a single institutional cohort of 191 cases. J Autoimmun. 2019;97:22–8.

24. Cellucci T, Benseler SM. Central nervous system vasculitis in children. Curr Opin Rheumatol. 2010;22:590–7.

25. Vollmer TL, Guarnaccia J, Harrington W, Pacia SV, Petroff OA. Idiopathic granulomatous angiitis of the central nervous system: diagnostic challenges. Arch Neurol. 1993;50:925–30.

26. Duna GF, Calabrese LH. Limitations of invasive modalities in the diagnosis of primary angiitis of the central nervous system. J Rheumatol. 1995;22:662–7.

27. Harris KG, Tran DD, Sickels WJ, et al. Diagnosing intracranial vasculitis: the roles of MR and angiography. AJNR Am J Neuroradiol. 1994;15:317–30.

28. Eleftheriou D, Cox T, Saunders D, et al. Investigation of childhood central nervous system vasculitis: magnetic resonance angiography versus catheter cerebral angiography. Dev Med Child Neurol. 2010;52:863–7.

29. Birnbaum J, Hellmann DB. Primary angiitis of the central nervous system. Arch Neurol. 2009;66:704–9.

30. Ducros A, Bousser MG. Reversible cerebral vasoconstriction syndrome. Pract Neurol. 2009;9:256–67.

31. Zuccoli G, Pipitone N, Haldipur A, et al. Imaging findings in primary central nervous system vasculitis. Clin Exp Rheumatol. 2011;29(Suppl 64):S104–9.

32. Küker W, Gaertner S, Nagele T, et al. Vessel wall contrast enhancement: a diagnostic sign of cerebral vasculitis. Cerebrovasc Dis. 2008;26:23–9.

33. Salvarani C, Brown RD Jr, Huston J 3rd, Hunder GG. Prominent perivascular enhancement in primary central nervous system vasculitis. Clin Exp Rheumatol. 2008;26(3 Suppl 49):S111.

34. Salvarani C, Morris JM, Giannini C, et al. Imaging findings of cerebral amyloid angiopathy, Aβ-related angiitis (ABRA), and cerebral amyloid angiopathy-related inflammation: a single-institution 25-year experience. Medicine (Baltimore). 2016;95:e3613.

35. Swartz RH, Bhuta SS, Farb RI, et al. Intracranial arterial wall imaging using high-resolution 3-tesla contrast-enhanced MRI. Neurology. 2009;72:627–34.

36. Alrawi A, Trobe JD, Blaivas M, Musch DC. Brain biopsy in primary angiitis of the central nervous system. Neurology. 1999;53:858–60.

37. Parisi JE, Moore PM. The role of biopsy in vasculitis of the central nervous system. Semin Neurol. 1994;14:341–8.

38. Winkler DT, Bondolfi L, Herzig MC, et al. Spontaneous hemorrhagic stroke in a mouse model of cerebral amyloid angiopathy. J Neurosci. 2001;21:1619–27.
39. Piazza F, Greenberg SM, Savoiardo M, et al. Anti-amyloid β autoantibodies in cerebral amyloid angiopathy-related inflammation: implications for amyloid-modifying therapies. Ann Neurol. 2013;73:449–58.
40. Salvarani C, Brown RD Jr, Christianson TJ, et al. Adult primary central nervous system vasculitis treatment and course: analysis of one hundred sixty-three patients. Arthritis Rheumatol. 2015;67:1637–45.
41. Salvarani C, Brown RD Jr, Christianson T, et al. An update of the Mayo Clinic cohort of patients with adult primary central nervous system vasculitis: description of 163 patients. Medicine (Baltimore). 2015;94(21):e738.
42. Auriel E, Charidimou A, Gurol ME, et al. Validation of clinicoradiological criteria for the diagnosis of cerebral amyloid angiopathy-related inflammation. JAMA Neurol. 2016;73:197–202.
43. Salvarani C, Brown RD Jr, Christianson TJH, et al. Primary central nervous system vasculitis associated with lymphoma. Neurology. 2018;90:e847–55.
44. de Boysson H, Zuber M, Naggara O, et al. French Vasculitis Study Group and the French NeuroVascular Society. Primary angiitis of the central nervous system: description of the first fifty-two adults enrolled in the French cohort of patients with primary vasculitis of the central nervous system. Arthritis Rheumatol. 2014;66:1315–26.
45. de Boysson H, Arquizan C, Touzé E, et al. Treatment and long-term outcomes of primary central nervous system vasculitis. Stroke. 2018;49:1946–52.
46. de Boysson H, Parienti JJ, Arquizan C, et al. Maintenance therapy is associated with better long-term outcomes in adult patients with primary angiitis of the central nervous system. Rheumatology (Oxford). 2017;56:1684–93.
47. Salvarani C, Brown RD Jr, Christianson TJ, et al. Mycophenolate mofetil in primary central nervous system vasculitis. Semin Arthritis Rheum. 2015;45:55–9.
48. Salvarani C, Brown RD Jr, Calamia KT, et al. Efficacy of tumor necrosis factor alpha blockade in primary central nervous system vasculitis resistant to immunosuppressive treatment. Arthritis Rheum. 2008;59:291–6.
49. Salvarani C, Brown RD Jr, Muratore F, et al. Rituximab therapy for primary central nervous system vasculitis: a 6 patient experience and review of the literature. Autoimmun Rev. 2019;18:399–405.

Isolated Aortitis and Periaortitis

16

Chiara Marvisi, Laura Fortunato, and Augusto Vaglio

Abstract

Isolated aortitis and periaortitis are inflammatory diseases of the aorta and its branches. They essentially differ in the extension of inflammation, which is confined to the aortic wall in aortitis and extends into the periaortic space in periaortitis. Isolated aortitis is classified as a single-organ vasculitis and occurs in the absence of other infectious or rheumatologic disorders. Periaortitis is either idiopathic or secondary to a wide array of etiologies (drugs, infections, malignancies, other proliferative diseases). Notably, both isolated aortitis and periaortitis may arise in the context of IgG4-related disease, a recently recognized fibro-inflammatory systemic disease. Prompt diagnosis and treatment are essential for both conditions in order to avoid life-threatening complications.

Keywords

Aortitis · Periaortitis · IgG4-related disease · Vasculitis · Fibrosis · CT ^{18}F-FDG-PET

C. Marvisi
Division of Rheumatology, University of Modena and Reggio Emilia, Modena, Italy

L. Fortunato · A. Vaglio (✉)
Division of Nephrology and Dialysis, Meyer Children's Hospital, Firenze, Italy

Department of Biomedical, Experimental and Clinical Sciences, University of Firenze, Firenze, Italy
e-mail: augusto.vaglio@unifi.it

© Springer Nature Switzerland AG 2021
C. Salvarani et al. (eds.), *Large and Medium Size Vessel and Single Organ Vasculitis*, Rare Diseases of the Immune System,
https://doi.org/10.1007/978-3-030-67175-4_16

Abbreviations

^{18}F-FDG-PET	^{18}F-fluorodeoxyglucose positron emission tomography
AAV	ANCA-associated vasculitis
ANCA	Anti-neutrophil cytoplasm antibody
CRP	C-reactive protein
CT	Computed tomography
ECD	Erdheim–Chester disease
ESR	Erythrocyte sedimentation rate;
GCA	Giant cell arteritis
HLA	Human leucocyte antigen
IAAA	Inflammatory abdominal aortic aneurysm
IgG4-RD	IgG4-related disease
LVV	Large-vessel vasculitis
MRI	Magnetic resonance imaging
RPF	Retroperitoneal fibrosis
SLE	Systemic lupus erythematosus
SUV	Standardized uptake value
TA	Takayasu arteritis
US	Ultrasonography

16.1 Introduction

Aortitis and periaortitis denote a spectrum of systemic inflammatory disorders characterized by chronic inflammation that is limited to the aortic wall in the former case or extends into the periaortic space in the latter [1]. They can both be idiopathic or a feature of other rheumatological, infectious, or neoplastic disorders. Both conditions may arise in the context of a recently recognized clinical–pathological entity known as IgG4-related disease (IgG4-RD), characterized by marked fibrosis, T-lymphocyte, and IgG4-positive plasma cell infiltration of various organs [2]. The diagnosis is quite challenging, with histological examination being the gold standard, but biopsy is not always feasible. Therefore, imaging studies often have a crucial diagnostic role, along with laboratory tests. In this chapter, we will review the nosology, clinical manifestations, diagnosis, and treatment of isolated aortitis and periaortitis.

16.2 Clinical Features and Diagnosis

16.2.1 Isolated Aortitis

The term isolated aortitis brings together all forms of inflammatory aortitis not related to autoimmune diseases, other rheumatologic disorders or infectious causes. It is therefore defined as a single-organ vasculitis and is frequently located in the ascending aorta. The epidemiology of isolated aortitis is not clearly established but its frequency is probably underestimated. The incidence of isolated aortitis in the population of patients undergoing thoracic aortic surgery ranges between 3.8 and 4.4%. Some studies show a higher incidence in women, others in men. The mean age at diagnosis ranges between 63 and 72 years [3–6].

Given the absence of systemic or organ-specific symptoms, isolated aortitis is often an incidental finding or is diagnosed when complications arise. Severe complication include thoracic aortic aneurysms, aortic dissection, or aortic valve regurgitation [3, 4]. The diagnosis may be pathological or radiological. Traditionally and most commonly, the disorder is diagnosed pathologically following surgical resection of an aortic segment for aneurysm or dissection, and the patient is clinically found to have no other signs or symptoms of vasculitis. In isolated forms, histological examination often shows a granulomatous/giant cell pattern of inflammation usually localized in the *media* layer. The inflammatory infiltrate comprises macrophages, lymphocytes, plasma cells, giant cells, and well-formed granulomas replacing irregular areas of medial destruction. Adventitial inflammation is minimal, usually mononuclear and without granulomas.

Isolated aortitis can also be identified radiologically, most often by computed tomography (CT) or magnetic resonance (MRI), as an isolated aneurysm or as wall thickening limited to one segment of the aorta [7]. The absence of a diffuse atherosclerotic disease or of common risk factors for atherosclerosis should heighten suspicion of isolated aortitis in patients showing the above abnormalities on CT or MRI.

The diagnostic work-up of isolated aortitis is also based on the exclusion of secondary forms of the disease. Thanks to the introduction of antibiotics, infectious aortitis is not so frequent as it was in the past; nevertheless, in immunocompromised subjects or in patients presenting with systemic symptoms of infection, it is mandatory to rule out particularly syphilis, tuberculosis, and other bacterial or fungal etiologies with laboratory tests. Although isolated aortitis may arise in the context of many rheumatologic disorders (e.g., ANCA-associated vasculitis, systemic lupus erythematosus, rheumatoid arthritis, HLA-B27 spondyloarthropathies, and Behçet disease [8–12]), the most common rheumatologic causes are giant cell arteritis (GCA) and Takayasu arteritis (TA). In the routine clinical practice, the diagnosis of GCA and TA is based on typical symptoms and on the age at onset of the disease, but sometimes they can occur in the absence of specific clinical manifestations and differentiating them from isolated aortitis can be quite challenging. The main clinical issue about isolated aortitis remains whether it tends to evolve to a systemic vasculitis and for this reason a careful follow-up is always required [6].

IgG4-related aortitis accounts for 75% of all cases of isolated aortitis [13], and it must be suspected when its histological pattern shows dense lymphoplasmacytic infiltrates. If biopsy is not available, serum IgG4 levels should be tested (see below).

16.2.2 Periaortitis

First described by Mitchinson et al. in 1980 [14], periaortitis is a rare disease and data about its epidemiology are limited to idiopathic retroperitoneal fibrosis (RPF) and inflammatory abdominal aortic aneurysms (IAAAs), which represent the two ends of the spectrum of periaortitis. The incidence of idiopathic RPF is 0.1–1.3 per 100,000 person/year and its prevalence is around 1.4/100,000 inhabitants [15, 16]. IAAAs represent 4–10% of all abdominal aortic aneurysms [17]. The mean age at onset of periaortitis is 50–60 years [18] although rarely cases have been reported in pediatric patients [19]. Men are affected two to three times more often than women, and this ratio is higher in the aneurysmal forms [15].

Pathologic changes in periaortitis involve both the aortic wall and the surrounding soft tissues. The typical macroscopic appearance of periaortitis is that of a whitish mass infiltrating the retroperitoneal tissue surrounding the abdominal aorta, the iliac arteries and, in most cases, the inferior vena cava and the ureters [20]. The perivascular mass usually develops between the origin of the renal arteries and the pelvic brim. In some instances, RPF shows atypical localizations, which might be peri-duodenal, peri-pancreatic, pelvic, presacral, peri-ureteral, or perirenal and not characterized by involvement of the periaortic space. These cases are thought to have a different pathogenesis as compared to the more typical periaortic RPF.

Microscopic examination reveals the presence of two components: a fibrous tissue and an inflammatory infiltrate [21]. The fibrous component comprises fibroblasts that show signs of activation and transition into myofibroblasts (α-smooth muscle actin expression) and produce an extracellular matrix composed of type I collagen fibers organized in thick irregular bundles. The inflammatory infiltrate consists of numerous lymphocytes, plasma cells, macrophages, and scattered eosinophils. The inflammatory cells are interspersed within the collagen bundles (diffuse pattern), but also organized in nodular aggregates, usually around small vessels (perivascular nodular pattern). These aggregates have a B-cell core surrounded by T cells, which are predominantly CD4+. In some cases, these lymphoid follicles have the structure of germinal centers, which is a sign of ectopic lymphoneogenesis, thus proving the presence of a highly structured immune-mediated/autoimmune response.

The aortic wall shows intimal atherosclerosis, medial thinning, and adventitial inflammation and fibrosis. The composition of the inflammatory infiltrate in the aortic adventitia is similar to the retroperitoneal one. When the pattern is arranged in nodular aggregates, these are usually centered on the adventitial *vasa vasorum* which can show signs of vasculitis [22].

The clinical presentation of periaortitis includes two types of manifestations: localized, due to the compressive effects of the retroperitoneal mass, and systemic, related to the inflammatory nature of the disease. The more frequent symptom, present in about 80% of the patients, is side, back or abdominal pain. It is usually described as persistent and dull; it transiently responds to nonsteroidal anti-inflammatory drugs and, in cases of ureteral involvement, it can be colic-like [23]. Ureteral involvement is the most frequent complication and can be unilateral or bilateral. In cases with unilateral involvement, ureteral obstruction can also be asymptomatic for a long time and, at diagnosis, these patients present with renal hypoplasia/atrophy, whose frequency is estimated to be up to 30%. However, most cases are symptomatic and bilateral involvement usually leads to acute renal failure. Other urologic manifestations are frequent: they range from testicular pain, often accompanied by hydrocele and/or varicocele due to spermatic vein encasement by periaortitis, to retrograde ejaculation and erectile dysfunction [21]. The extrinsic compression of retroperitoneal lymphatic vessels and veins can be the cause of lower extremity edema and deep vein thrombosis. Claudication and intestinal ischemia are less common. Systemic symptoms include fatigue, weight loss, anorexia, sleep disturbances, and low-grade fever [23].

Periaortitis can affect not only the lower abdominal aorta and the iliac arteries but also other vascular segments, in particular the thoracic aorta and its major branches [24].

In these cases, the symptoms may range from laryngeal nerve paralysis and dry cough to upper limb claudication and paresthesias; however, in about 85% of cases it is asymptomatic. Patients with thoracic involvement had a significantly higher female prevalence, a greater age at disease onset, a higher prevalence of systemic symptoms and of back or abdominal pain [24].

Periaortitis may be associated with a variety of autoimmune conditions. Hashimoto's thyroiditis is the most commonly associated autoimmune disorder [25]; but ANCA-associated vasculitis, systemic lupus erythematosus, rheumatoid arthritis, and psoriasis have been described in association with periaortitis [23].

The diagnosis of periaortitis is based on imaging studies, indeed laboratory tests are quite nonspecific and periaortic biopsy is not always feasible. However, histological examination remains the gold standard in all cases of difficult interpretation, especially when there is suspicion of malignancies or infections, in patients not responsive to treatment or in those undergoing surgical procedures (e.g., ureterolysis or aneurysmal repair).

Ultrasonography (US) is usually performed at onset: it may detect both aneurysmal aortic dilatation and also periaortitis as a hypoechoic periaortic halo. It also allows the detection of hydronephrosis; such US findings are crucial both at diagnosis and during the follow-up.

On CT, periaortitis appears as a homogeneous, plaque-like tissue, isodense to muscle which develops around the anterolateral sides of the abdominal aorta. In the retroperitoneum, it may encase the ureters, drawing them medially, and also cause inferior vena cava compression (Fig. 16.1) [20]. On MRI, the inflammatory aortic/periaortic thickening and the tissue surrounding the vessels are seen as hypointense on T1-weighted images, while they are hyperintense on T2-weighted images during active disease phases, due to the presence of edema and inflammatory infiltration. Contrast-enhancement, both on CT and MRI, is more pronounced during the early disease stages [26].

Imaging studies also allow the differentiation between idiopathic periaortitis and secondary forms. In particular, neoplasms appear to be inhomogeneous and lobulated, more adherent to surrounding organs with no clear cleavage site, and often extend above the origin of the renal arteries, unlike typical idiopathic periaortitis [27, 28]. In addition, they develop anterior to the spine and tend to displace the aorta anteriorly and may also infiltrate muscles and erode bones [27–29].

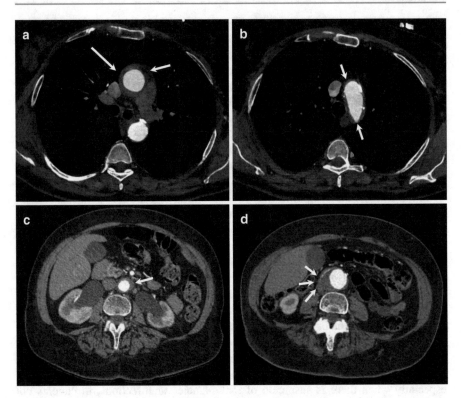

Fig. 16.1 Computed tomographic (CT) appearance of aortitis and periaortitis. (**a, b**) Show CT images of a case of isolated thoracic aortitis. The scans (axial view) show aortic wall thickening involving the ascending aorta (**a**, arrows) and the aortic arch (**b**, arrows). (**c, d**) Show CT images of a case of abdominal periaortitis. The scans (axial view) show a periaortic tissue (**c**, arrow) and bilateral hydronephrosis (caused by ureteral involvement by periaortitis); the abdominal aorta is of normal caliber. In (**d**), a case of aneurysmal periaortitis is shown, where the periaortic tissue (arrows) surrounds an aneurysmal abdominal aorta

In the diagnostic work-up of periaortitis, ^{18}F-fluorodeoxyglucose positron emission tomography (^{18}F-FDG PET) is increasingly used, although its specificity is low given that forms of periaortitis secondary to infections or neoplasms may also be hypermetabolic on PET (Fig. 16.2).

In the setting of periaortitis, ^{18}F-FDG PET recently proved able to predict response to therapy since metabolically inactive forms are less likely to respond to glucocorticoid treatment than highly active lesions. However, no significant differences in response to treatment were detected among patients with mild, moderate, or high degree of FDG uptake [30].

A rare cause of aortic wall and periaortic involvement is Erdheim–Chester disease (ECD), a non-Langerhans cell histiocytosis with predilection for long bones, cardiovascular system, central nervous system, and endocrine glands [31]. Interestingly, ECD can involve both the thoracic and abdominal aorta, giving rise to an aspect usually reported as "coated aorta." On CT or MRI, ECD should be

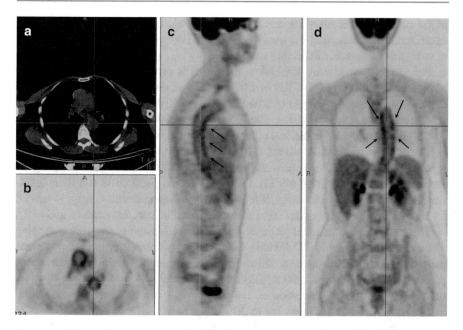

Fig. 16.2 FDG positron emission tomography (PET)-computed tomography-(CT) in a case of thoracic aortitis. (**a**) Shows a non-contrast-enhanced CT of the chest (axial view) and (**b**) the corresponding PET image, the latter showing hypermetabolism in both the ascending and descending aorta. In the same patient, whole-body PET images in (**c, d**) (sagittal and coronal views, respectively) show increased FDG uptake along the thoracic aorta (arrows)

suspected when the fibrous tissue surrounds not only the abdominal aorta but also the kidneys, showing the typical finding of "hairy kidneys" [32]. In these cases, biopsy is recommended, indeed morphological and immune staining features are very different in ECD versus idiopathic periaortitis. Typical findings in ECD include tissue infiltration by CD68+ CD1a- "foamy" histiocytes, along with diffuse lymphoplasmacytic infiltrates and abundant fibrosis [33].

16.2.3 IgG4-Related Aortitis and Periaortitis

Since the early 2000s, when IgG4-RD was first described, it has become evident how different clinical entities with no clear nosology could fall under the spectrum of this systemic fibro-inflammatory disease [34]. Among these are cases of aortitis and periaortitis, once classified as isolated or idiopathic.

IgG4-related aortitis preferentially affects the thoracic aorta and particularly the aortic arch [13, 35]. It has been reported to account for a significant proportion of all noninfectious thoracic aortitis cases and for approximately 75% of lymphoplasmacytic thoracic aortitis cases [13, 36]. The vasculitic process may also involve the abdominal aorta, along with medium-sized vessels originating from the aorta, such as the carotid and coronary arteries [2, 37]. Small-vessel involvement has also been described, thus supporting the idea that IgG4-RD may be included in the category of vasculitis of vessels of variable size [38].

Periaortitis (particularly the abdominal form) is reported among the most frequent manifestations of IgG4-RD in different studies, even if its prevalence remains quite variable, ranging from 11 to 30% [39–42]. Both IgG4-related aortitis and periaortitis are more frequent among elderly men (age > 60 years), in keeping with the epidemiology of the systemic and other organ-limited forms of IgG4-RD [36].

The inflammatory infiltrate affects predominantly the adventitia with a lesser involvement of the media. From a clinical standpoint, there are no substantial differences between IgG4-related aortitis and IgG4-related periaortitis and their IgG4-unrelated counterparts. However, it must always be remembered that IgG4-related forms are more commonly associated with extravascular manifestations of IgG4-RD.

The most frequent clinical pictures other than aortitis and periaortitis belonging to the spectrum of IgG4-RD include sclerosing pancreatitis (type 1 autoimmune pancreatitis), Mikulicz disease, diffuse lymphadenopathy, sclerosing cholangitis, pseudotumor of the orbit, and tubulo-interstitial nephritis. Involvement of other organs may not be present at onset, but may appear during the follow-up with a metachronous pattern [43], leading to difficulties to promptly recognize IgG4-RD.

In 2008, a set of diagnostic criteria was proposed for the diagnosis of IgG4-RD [44]. These criteria are widely used, even if their specificity and sensitivity still warrant validation. They include: (1) typical organ involvement (pseudotumoral lesions) with organ swelling and/or dysfunction; (2) histologically compatible features and immunohistochemical evidence of IgG4+/IgG+ plasma cells >40% together with >10 IgG4+ plasma cells/high power field (hpf); (3) serum IgG4 level >135 mg/dL. The diagnosis is considered to be "definite" when all three criteria are fulfilled, "probable" when (1) and (2) are met, and "possible" when (1) and (2) are met and histopathology is either unavailable or non-diagnostic. The last scenario is frequent, indeed biopsy is not always feasible; moreover, it has been reported that in aortic and periaortic tissue, immune staining findings might be inconsistent with a diagnosis of IgG4-RD, even on a background where the three main characteristics (storiform fibrosis, obliterative phlebitis, and lymphoplasmacytic infiltrate) are found [45]. In these cases, the diagnosis of IgG4-RD remains "possible."

Laboratory abnormalities, other than high IgG4 levels (>135 mg/dL), include elevation of acute-phase reactants, especially in cases with multifocal involvement, and polyclonal hypergammaglobulinemia. Peripheral eosinophilia and serum IgE increase may be encountered in about one third of the cases. Positive ANCA with specificity for either myeloperoxidase or proteinase 3 may also occur, indeed overlap forms of IgG4-RD and AAV have been recently described [46].

The same imaging studies used for the diagnosis and follow-up of aortitis and periaortitis not associated with other IgG4-related lesions are employed for cases arising in the context of IgG4-RD. Thus, US, CT, or MRI and ^{18}F-FDG PET may all be helpful both at diagnosis and during the follow-up to detect the main involved sites and to assess their metabolic activity although the FDG-avidity of the different IgG4-related lesions varies widely. It is important to emphasize that differences between idiopathic, IgG4-unrelated aortitis and periaortitis, and IgG4-related forms may be slight, leading to the concept that they might be part of the same disease process.

16.3 Treatment

The exclusion of neoplastic, infectious, and other proliferative (e.g., ECD) causes of aortic disease has obvious therapeutic implications since most of the idiopathic forms of aortitis and periaortitis are treated with glucocorticoids (GCs) and immunosuppressive therapies. It is also important to carefully differentiate aortitis/periaortitis occurring in the setting of either LVV, systemic connective tissue or small-vessel vasculitic syndromes, or fibro-inflammatory disorders including IgG4-RD.

Idiopathic aortitis and periaortitis, either isolated or in the context of IgG4-RD, are glucocorticoid-sensitive conditions and therefore GCs alone are considered first-line treatment. In relapsing or difficult-to-treat cases, rituximab has recently proved effective [47, 48]. Moreover, tocilizumab (an anti-interleukin-6 receptor antibody) has been already approved in the management of GCA and could be effective also in isolated aortitis [49].

In addition, it must be kept in mind that aortitis and periaortitis may lead to aneurysmal dilatation of both the abdominal and thoracic aorta; this requires evaluation by vascular surgeons because prompt treatment using endovascular or surgical techniques may prevent life-threatening complications.

The outcome of isolated forms is poorly known because they are certainly underdiagnosed since only cases in which complications occur may come to our attention. Moreover, not all the surgical specimens undergo pathologic examination, making the real frequency of these diseases difficult to assess.

16.4 Conclusions

Isolated aortitis and periaortitis are inflammatory diseases of varying etiology, and recognition of the underlying conditions is crucial for an appropriate management. Imaging studies such as CT, MRI, and ^{18}F-FDG-PET are widely used for their diagnosis and follow-up. Diagnostic biopsies are required in only a fraction of cases. Treatment significantly differs depending on their cause, and in isolated cases or in patients suffering from systemic immune-mediated conditions it is usually based on different combinations of glucocorticoids and immunosuppressive drugs. Surgical evaluation is also needed for cases presenting with significant aneurysmal dilatation or with less common complications such as dissection and rupture.

References

1. Stone JR, Bruneval P, Angelini A, et al. Consensus statement on surgical pathology of the aorta from the Society for Cardiovascular Pathology and the Association for European Cardiovascular Pathology: I. inflammatory diseases. Cardiovasc Pathol. 2015;24(5):267–78.
2. Perugino CA, Wallace ZS, Meyersohn N, Oliveira G, Stone JR, Stone JH. Large vessel involvement by IgG4-related disease. Medicine (Baltimore). 2016;95(28):e3344.
3. Rojo-Leyva F, Ratliff NB, Cosgrove DM, Hoffman GS. Study of 52 patients with idiopathic aortitis from a cohort of 1,204 surgical cases. Arthritis Rheum. 2000;43(4):901.
4. Miller DV, Isotalo PA, Weyand CM, Edwards WD, Aubry M-C, Tazelaar HD. Surgical pathology of noninfectious ascending aortitis: a study of 45 cases with emphasis on an isolated variant. Am J Surg Pathol. 2006;30(9):1150–8.
5. Schmidt J, Sunesen K, Kornum JB, Duhaut P, Thomsen RW. Predictors for pathologically confirmed aortitis after resection of the ascending aorta: a 12-year Danish nationwide population-based cross-sectional study. Arthritis Res Ther. 2011;13(3):R87.
6. Talarico R, Boiardi L, Pipitone N, et al. Isolated aortitis versus giant cell arteritis: are they really two sides of the same coin? Clin Exp Rheumatol. 32(3 Suppl 82):S55–8.
7. Cinar I, Wang H, Stone JR. Clinically isolated aortitis: pitfalls, progress, and possibilities. Cardiovasc Pathol. 2017;29:23–32.
8. Gravallese EM, Corson JM, Coblyn JS, Pinkus GS, Weinblatt ME. Rheumatoid aortitis: a rarely recognized but clinically significant entity. Medicine (Baltimore). 1989;68(2):95–106.
9. Hull RG, Asherson RA, Rennie JA. Ankylosing spondylitis and an aortic arch syndrome. Br Heart J. 1984;51(6):663–5.
10. Kurata A, Kawakami T, Sato J, Sakamoto A, Muramatsu T, Nakabayashi K. Aortic aneurysms in systemic lupus erythematosus: a meta-analysis of 35 cases in the literature and two different pathogeneses. Cardiovasc Pathol. 2011;20(1):e1–7.
11. Haynes BF, Kaiser-Kupfer MI, Mason P, Fauci AS. Cogan syndrome: studies in thirteen patients, long-term follow-up, and a review of the literature. Medicine (Baltimore). 1980;59(6):426–41.
12. Singer O. Cogan and Behcet syndromes. Rheum Dis Clin North Am. 2015;41(1):75–91, viii.
13. Stone JH, Khosroshahi A, Deshpande V, Stone JR. IgG4-related systemic disease accounts for a significant proportion of thoracic lymphoplasmacytic aortitis cases. Arthritis Care Res (Hoboken). 2010;62(3):316–22.
14. Mitchinson MJ. Chronic periaortitis and periarteritis. Histopathology. 1984;8(4):589–600.
15. Uibu T, Oksa P, Auvinen A, et al. Asbestos exposure as a risk factor for retroperitoneal fibrosis. Lancet (London, England). 2004;363(9419):1422–6.
16. van Bommel EFH, Jansen I, Hendriksz TR, Aarnoudse ALHJ. Idiopathic retroperitoneal fibrosis. Medicine (Baltimore). 2009;88(4):193–201.
17. von Fritschen U, Malzfeld E, Clasen A, Kortmann H. Inflammatory abdominal aortic aneurysm: a postoperative course of retroperitoneal fibrosis. J Vasc Surg. 1999;30(6):1090–8.
18. Vaglio A, Palmisano A, Alberici F, et al. Prednisone versus tamoxifen in patients with idiopathic retroperitoneal fibrosis: an open-label randomised controlled trial. Lancet (London, England). 2011;378(9788):338–46.
19. Miller OF, Smith LJ, Ferrara EX, McAleer IM, Kaplan GW. Presentation of idiopathic retroperitoneal fibrosis in the pediatric population. J Pediatr Surg. 2003;38(11):1685–8.
20. Corradi D, Maestri R, Palmisano A, et al. Idiopathic retroperitoneal fibrosis: clinicopathologic features and differential diagnosis. Kidney Int. 2007;72(6):742–53.
21. Vaglio A, Maritati F. Idiopathic retroperitoneal fibrosis. J Am Soc Nephrol. 2016;27(7):1880–9.
22. Vaglio A, Corradi D, Manenti L, Ferretti S, Garini G, Buzio C. Evidence of autoimmunity in chronic periaortitis: a prospective study. Am J Med. 2003;114(6):454–62.
23. Vaglio A, Salvarani C, Buzio C. Retroperitoneal fibrosis. Lancet (London, England). 2006;367(9506):241–51.
24. Palmisano A, Urban ML, Corradi D, et al. Chronic periaortitis with thoracic aorta and epiaortic artery involvement: a systemic large vessel vasculitis? Rheumatology. 2015;54(11):2004–9.

25. Ceresini G, Urban ML, Corradi D, et al. Association between idiopathic retroperitoneal fibrosis and autoimmune thyroiditis: a case–control study. Autoimmun Rev. 2015;14(1):16–22.
26. Pipitone N, Versari A, Salvarani C. Role of imaging studies in the diagnosis and follow-up of large-vessel vasculitis: an update. Rheumatology. 2007;47(4):403–8.
27. Cronin CG, Lohan DG, Blake MA, Roche C, McCarthy P, Murphy JM. Retroperitoneal fibrosis: a review of clinical features and imaging findings. Am J Roentgenol. 2008;191(2):423–31.
28. Urban ML, Palmisano A, Nicastro M, Corradi D, Buzio C, Vaglio A. Idiopathic and secondary forms of retroperitoneal fibrosis: a diagnostic approach. La Rev Méd Intern. 2015;36(1):15–21.
29. Mirault T, Lambert M, Puech P, et al. Malignant retroperitoneal fibrosis. Medicine (Baltimore). 2012;91(5):242–50.
30. Accorsi Buttini E, Maritati F, Vaglio A. [18 F]-Fluorodeoxyglucose positron emission tomography and response to therapy in idiopathic retroperitoneal fibrosis. Eur Urol. 2018;73(1):145–6.
31. Gianfreda D, Musetti C, Nicastro M, et al. Erdheim-Chester disease as a mimic of IgG4-related disease. Medicine (Baltimore). 2016;95(21):e3625.
32. Palmisano A, Vaglio A. Chronic periaortitis: a fibro-inflammatory disorder. Best Pract Res Clin Rheumatol. 2009;23(3):339–53.
33. Diamond EL, Dagna L, Hyman DM, et al. Consensus guidelines for the diagnosis and clinical management of Erdheim-Chester disease. Blood. 2014;124(4):483–92.
34. Hamano H, Kawa S, Horiuchi A, et al. High serum IgG4 concentrations in patients with sclerosing pancreatitis. N Engl J Med. 2001;344(10):732–8.
35. Stone JR. Aortitis, periaortitis, and retroperitoneal fibrosis, as manifestations of IgG4-related systemic disease. Curr Opin Rheumatol. 2011;23(1):88–94.
36. Koo BS, Koh YW, Hong S, et al. Frequency of immunoglobulin G4-related aortitis in cases with aortic resection and their clinical characteristics compared to other aortitises. Int J Rheum Dis. 2014;17(4):420–4.
37. Kasashima S, Zen Y, Kawashima A, et al. Inflammatory abdominal aortic aneurysm: close relationship to IgG4-related periaortitis. Am J Surg Pathol. 2008;32(2):197–204.
38. Alba MA, Milisenda J, Fernández S, et al. Small-vessel vasculitis with prominent IgG4 positive plasma cell infiltrates as potential part of the spectrum of IgG4-related disease: a case report. Clin Exp Rheumatol. 33(2 Suppl 89):S-138–41.
39. Campochiaro C, Ramirez GA, Bozzolo EP, et al. IgG4-related disease in Italy: clinical features and outcomes of a large cohort of patients. Scand J Rheumatol. 2015;9742:1–11.
40. Inoue D, Yoshida K, Yoneda N, et al. IgG4-related disease: dataset of 235 consecutive patients. Medicine (Baltimore). 2015;94(15):e680.
41. Wallace ZS, Deshpande V, Mattoo H, et al. IgG4-related disease: clinical and laboratory features in one hundred twenty-five patients. Arthritis Rheumatol (Hoboken, NJ). 2015;67(9):2466–75.
42. Zen Y, Nakanuma Y. IgG4-related disease. Am J Surg Pathol. 2010;34(12):1812–9.
43. Kamisawa T, Zenimoto M, Obayashi T. [IgG4-related sclerosing disease]. Rinsho Byori. 2009;57(11):1113–9.
44. Umehara H, Okazaki K, Nakamura T, et al. Current approach to the diagnosis of IgG4-related disease—combination of comprehensive diagnostic and organ-specific criteria. Mod Rheumatol. 2017;27(3):381–91.
45. Corradi D, Nicastro M, Vaglio A. Immunoglobulin G4-related disease: some missing pieces in a still unsolved complex puzzle. Cardiovasc Pathol. 2016;25(2):90–2.
46. Danlos FX, Rossi GM, Blockmans D, et al. ANCA-associated vasculitis and IgG4-related disease: a new overlap syndrome. Autoimmun Rev. 2017;16(10):1036–43.
47. Maritati F, Corradi D, Versari A, et al. Rituximab therapy for chronic periaortitis. Ann Rheum Dis. 2012;71(7):1262–4.
48. Carruthers MN, Topazian MD, Khosroshahi A, et al. Rituximab for IgG4-related disease: a prospective, open-label trial. Ann Rheum Dis. 2015;74(6):1171–7.
49. Huang IJ, Pugh T, Liew J. Early initiation of tocilizumab in clinically isolated aortitis. Cureus. 2019;11(4):e4479.

Isolated Gastrointestinal Vasculitis

17

Thomas D. Garvey and Kenneth J. Warrington

Abstract

Gastrointestinal single-organ vasculitis is a vasculitis restricted to one organ in the gastrointestinal system and without systemic manifestations. These diseases are rare and true incidence and prevalence are difficult to determine. Most patients will have predominantly gastrointestinal symptoms although some will be asymptomatic, and in these cases the diagnosis is incidental. The diagnosis typically relies on pathology and/or imaging studies. Systemic vasculitis must be excluded in all cases. Cases of limited single-organ vasculitis can sometimes be managed with surgery alone whereas cases of diffuse disease often require immunosuppressive therapy. The disease has been associated with significant morbidity and mortality, particularly in the first year after diagnosis. All cases should be monitored closely for the possible evolution to systemic vasculitis.

Keywords

Vasculitis · Single-organ vasculitis (SOV) · Gastrointestinal single-organ vasculitis (GI-SOV) · Gallbladder single-organ vasculitis (GB-SOV)

The original version of this chapter was revised, authorship has been updated. The correction to this chapter can be found at https://doi.org/10.1007/978-3-030-67175-4_21

T. D. Garvey
Mayo Clinic, Rochester, MN, USA

K. J. Warrington (✉)
Division of Rheumatology, Mayo Clinic, Rochester, MN, USA
e-mail: warrington.kenneth@mayo.edu

© Springer Nature Switzerland AG 2021, corrected publication 2021
C. Salvarani et al. (eds.), *Large and Medium Size Vessel and Single Organ Vasculitis*, Rare Diseases of the Immune System,
https://doi.org/10.1007/978-3-030-67175-4_17

17.1   Introduction

The vasculitides are a group of diseases characterized by inflammation of blood vessels. They may affect all types and sizes of vessels. While vascular inflammation is commonly part of a systemic disease process, it has also sometimes been found to be more restricted and on rare occasions has even been limited to a single organ. These forms of vasculitis were first formally named in the 2012 Chapel Hill Consensus Conference (CHCC) Guidelines as Single-Organ Vasculitis (SOV). In these guidelines, SOV was defined as a "vasculitis in arteries or veins of any size in a single organ that has no features that indicate that it is a limited expression of a systemic vasculitis [1]."

Single-organ vasculitis can be diffuse (multifocal) or limited (unifocal). In diffuse SOV, the lesions of vasculitis, while still affecting only one organ by definition, are spatially multifocal. As a consequence of being non-contiguous, these diseases can have manifestations that are remote from one another [2]. Examples of diffuse SOV have been reported in the skin, central nervous system, kidneys, peripheral nerves, calf muscles, coronary and pulmonary vessels, and the retina [3]. In contrast, the lesions of limited SOV are more circumscribed, having a spatial focus within a single organ. Limited SOV has been reported to occur in the breasts, aorta, genitourinary structures, and gastrointestinal (GI) structures [2].

When vasculitis affects the GI system, it can be due to systemic vasculitis (GI-SV) or to SOV of the GI tract (GI-SOV). This chapter focuses on the latter: GI-SOV. Gastrointestinal organs which have been reported to be affected by SOV are: the esophagus, the stomach, the omentum, the small intestine, the colon, the pancreas, the gallbladder, and the appendix [4, 5].

Of note, when reviewing the reports on GI-SOV it is critical to remember that our understanding—and nomenclature—of the disease has changed over time. As discussed, the term SOV was first formally added to the nomenclature for the vasculitides in the 2012 CHCC Guidelines. As one moves further back in time from these guidelines, it becomes increasingly important to review the published literature on GI-SOV with a mind to their definitions and descriptions of disease. For instance, one landmark case series on localized GI vasculitis excluded patients with systemic vasculitis at onset; however, it also noted that several patients later developed systemic disease during follow-up [6]. Furthermore, this series included patients with positive serum autoantibodies and with systemic diseases such as rheumatoid arthritis and systemic lupus erythematosus. Therefore, in several reported case series of GI-SOV, one cannot entirely exclude that select patients had GI involvement by systemic vasculitis or other systemic rheumatic disease.

17.2   Epidemiology

The rarity and heterogeneity of the vasculitides renders epidemiologic study difficult. This challenge only grows when looking at increasingly specific subtypes of vasculitis. In patients with systemic vasculitis, it has been estimated that approximately 20% have gastrointestinal system involvement [7]. Among these patients, far fewer have only gastrointestinal manifestations and true GI-SOV. At this time, the current body of literature on GI-SOV is limited primarily to case reports and small case series with no population-based epidemiologic studies ever performed. Consequently, the precise incidence and prevalence of GI-SOV is not known [4].

Studies have reported the frequency with which GI vasculitis was identified on pathology specimens. In some of these cases, the vasculitis was a limited expression of a systemic vasculitis such as polyarteritis nodosa or was likely secondary to an underlying disease such as systemic lupus erythematosus which was present or later found. Consequently, this would support that the frequency of disease might be even lower than was reported in these studies. Alternatively, one could argue that GI-SOV is under-reported. In many cases, the patients were minimally symptomatic or even asymptomatic and SOV was identified coincidentally. This suggests that there are subclinical cases which go unrecognized and that typically only the most severe cases are identified.

One study found 12 cases of necrotizing arteritis of the appendix from 4283 total histologically examined appendix samples [8]. Three of these cases were found to have systemic PAN thus 9 of the 4283 (0.21%) were potentially appendiceal SOV. This study included surgical (3686) and autopsy (597) specimens. They noted however that the appendix was not always examined microscopically during autopsy and that the 597 appendixes represented only about 8% of the total autopsies performed. In 1951, Dr. Plaut identified focal arteritis in 88 out of 6576 appendixes (1.34%) [9].

SOV of the gallbladder (GB-SOV) appears less common and was found in only five cases during a 10-year period at a community hospital performing approximately 12,000 cholecystectomies annually [10]. In another study of 2080 gallbladders obtained from cholecystectomy for treatment of cholecystitis or cholelithiasis over a period of 22 years, six cases of vasculitis were found (0.29%) [5]. Four of the six cases were GB-SOV and the remaining two were part of a systemic vasculitis (GB-SV). A third study found two cases of GB-SOV among over 4000 cholecystectomy specimens obtained over 10 years [11].

In a series of 248 tissue samples taken from the stomach during vertical sleeve gastrectomy, one was found incidentally to have necrotizing vasculitis (0.4%) and evaluation for systemic vasculitis was negative [12]. Vasculitis of the pancreas is exceedingly rare [13]. Review of data from one hospital identified 344 patients being managed between 1980 and 2001 with a systemic necrotizing vasculitis. While one of these patients had vasculitis of the pancreas, it was a case of hepatitis B-associated PAN and not pancreas SOV. SOV of the intestine has been reported to be the most common form of the GI-SOV, and the small intestine is thought to be more frequently involved than the large intestine [14].

Some studies have suggested that GI-SOV might have a slight predilection for female patients. In 1951, Dr. Plaut identified focal arteritis in 15 of 1930 (0.78%) specimens from males and 73 of 4646 (1.57%) specimens from females [9]. A case series noted that 67% of the patients with GI-SOV were female [15]. A follow-up study comparing GI-SV and GI-SOV at the same institution found that 40% of the patients with GI-SV were female versus 58% of the patients with GI-SOV. This was a statistically significant difference [16]. Another study looking specifically at gallbladder vasculitis found no difference in gender distribution between patients with systemic vasculitis affecting the gallbladder (GB-SV) and gallbladder single-organ vasculitis (GB-SOV) [5].

17.3   Clinical Manifestations

Symptoms of GI-SOV are nonspecific and, although sometimes absent entirely, are predominantly gastrointestinal in nature. Patients may complain of abdominal pain and abdominal angina, nausea, vomiting, loss of appetite, weight loss, constipation, and gastrointestinal bleeding [6, 15]. These symptoms are also present in many other conditions which are much more common and can lead to initial diagnoses of GI bleed, bowel obstruction, bowel infarction, bowel perforation, mesenteric ischemia, toxic megacolon, cholecystitis, appendicitis, pancreatitis, and esophagitis [6, 15, 17]. It is often only later in the clinical course when additional radiographic or histologic data becomes available that SOV is considered as the underlying etiology.

Ischemic abdominal pain has been reported to be the most common manifestation and present in 89% of patients in one case series [16]. A review suggests that two-thirds of patients present with acute abdomen [18]. The absence of abdominal pain has been suggested to nearly rule-out GI vasculitis in general; however, this is likely less true in GI-SOV since many cases are identified incidentally [13]. Systemic and non-GI manifestations may occur in GI-SOV and include fever, fatigue, myalgias, and hypertension [5, 16]. As a consequence of the reliance on pathological examination of tissue to diagnose most cases of SOV, the reported symptoms of disease might be skewed by only representing those cases severe enough to lead to a surgical intervention [18]. For instance, one study showed that 32% of patients diagnosed with GI-SOV had GI manifestations requiring surgery as compared with 13% of patients with PAN [16].

The presentations by organ affected have been reported as follows. SOV of the appendix can be identified either incidentally or after appendectomy for acute abdomen [6, 8, 9, 19]. Patients with GB-SOV can commonly have abdominal pain, cholecystitis, or be asymptomatic, and more rare presentations include jaundice, liver dysfunction, pancreatitis, and even pleural effusions [6, 10, 11, 19–24]. SOV of the stomach can be found incidentally or in patients with abdominal pain [6, 12, 25]. Pancreas SOV can be diagnosed during investigation of pancreatitis (acute or chronic), epigastric pain, and pancreatic masses [6, 22, 24, 26]. SOV of the intestines can present with acute abdomen, lower GI hemorrhage, small bowel obstruction, post-prandial diarrhea, nausea, vomiting, toxic megacolon, an abdominal mass, or be found incidentally [6, 17, 19, 27–31]. SOV of the omentum has been reported to cause severe abdominal pain and fever [6]. A patient with SOV of the esophagus presented with achalasia [6]. Common presentations have been summarized Table 17.1.

17.4   Diagnosis

GI-SOV is generally diagnosed by histopathology or radiographic studies as specific serum biomarkers are not available for this condition. When SOV is suspected, it must be approached as a diagnosis of exclusion: all such cases require that a thorough workup for systemic vasculitis be undertaken. Imaging of vessels and

Table 17.1 Common presenting features and treatment for GI-SOV organized by organ affected

	Presenting features	Treatment
GI-SOV generally	Abdominal pain Acute abdomen Nausea/vomiting Weight loss	Focal: surgical excision Diffuse: immunosuppression ± surgical excision
Esophagus	Achalasia	Surgical excision
Stomach	Abdominal pain	Surgical excision
Small intestine	Acute abdomen GI bleeding Small bowel obstruction	Immunosuppression ± surgical excision
Large intestine	Acute abdomen GI bleeding	Immunosuppression ± surgical excision
Pancreas	Chronic pancreatitis	Surgical excision
Gallbladder	Acalculous cholecystitis Asymptomatic	Surgical excision
Appendix	Acute abdomen Asymptomatic	Surgical excision
Omentum	Abdominal pain Fever	Surgical excision

pathology from affected organs can confirm vasculitis in one area; however, they cannot exclude it elsewhere. A review of symptoms, comprehensive physical examination, laboratory studies, and imaging must be used to assess for more widespread disease.

Several laboratory studies can be performed to aid in the investigation. Their utility is usually greatest in ruling out SOV by identifying systemic or coexisting diseases which might account for a case of vasculitis. Anti-neutrophil cytoplasmic antibodies (ANCA) should be performed and if positive suggest possible ANCA-vasculitis. Hepatitis B, hepatitis C, and human immunodeficiency virus serologies should be performed to assess for viral causes. One can interrogate for secondary vasculitis as might be seen in cases of rheumatoid arthritis (RA) or systemic lupus erythematosus (SLE). Rheumatoid factor, cyclic-citrullinated peptide antibodies, anti-nuclear antibodies, complement levels, antiphospholipid antibodies, and cryo-globulins can all be tested, depending on the clinical presentation, and are typically negative [15, 16]. Indeed, if these markers are positive in a case of suspected SOV, it would suggest that an underlying systemic vasculitis or connective tissue disease is more likely [6, 13].

Inflammatory markers have not been found to be reliably abnormal in GI-SOV. A study of 19 patients with GI vasculitis found a median C-reactive protein level of 23.2 mg/L with an interquartile range of 7.5–83 mg/L [16]. One case series found that a statistically significant difference in erythrocyte sedimentation rates between GB-SV and GB-SOV (80 ± 28 vs 37 ± 25 mm/h respectively; $p = 0.006$) [5]. In one case series, the ESR was elevated (>30 mm/h) in 50% of patients [15]. The median value was 30.5 with a range of 4–77 mm/h.

Fig. 17.1 CT Angiogram
of the abdomen and pelvis
demonstrating wall edema,
thickening, and irregularity
(white arrow) in the
proximal superior
mesenteric artery
consistent with vasculitis

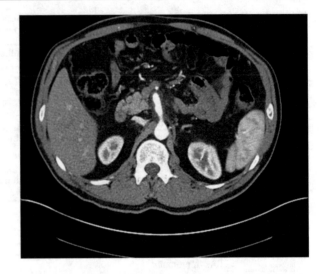

Advanced imaging studies such as abdominal angiography may reveal typical
features of vasculitis. Catheter-directed mesenteric angiography is able to detect
luminal changes such as stenosis, occlusion, or dilatation/aneurysm while CT and
MR angiography have the additional benefit of demonstrating vessel wall edema
and enhancement (Fig. 17.1). In one case series of 18 patients with GI-SOV, 15 of
the patients underwent abdominal angiography [15]. Changes of vasculitis were
seen in 14 of these 15 patients. The lesions noted were arterial stenosis (86.7%),
dilatation (53.3%), aneurysm (33.3%), obstruction (26.7%), and wall thickening
(13.3%) which is suggestive of vascular inflammation [15]. Vascular involvement
was noted in the superior mesenteric artery (73.3%), celiac artery (60%), hepatic
artery (53.3%), inferior mesenteric artery (46.7%), splenic artery (40%), and gastric
artery (6.7%). There is currently limited data regarding the utility of positron-
emission tomography to guide management of patients with GI-SOV. It may however help to pick up the presence of an inflammatory process in the GI tract
(Fig. 17.2).

SOV of the pancreas can be found after imaging reveals a pancreatic mass and
leads to additional workup [6, 26]. Computed tomography and ultrasound of
GB-SOV often reveals inflammatory changes suggestive of cholecystitis [21, 22].
SOV of the pancreas may sometimes produce a mass lesion visible on imaging studies and which can resemble a neoplasm [7, 26]. In SOV of the colon imaging studies
can mimic findings seen in inflammatory bowel disease. In one case, X-rays of the
abdomen showed tapering of the descending colon; a CT of the abdomen showed
bowel wall thickening in the left colon and rectum; and an MRI showed inflamma-
tory-appearing changes in the rectum and colon [30]. Marked dilation of the colon
has also been reported in a case of toxic megacolon from colon SOV [17]. In one
case of SOV of the cecum, a barium enema revealed an apple-core lesion of the
cecum concerning for carcinoma of the colon [27].

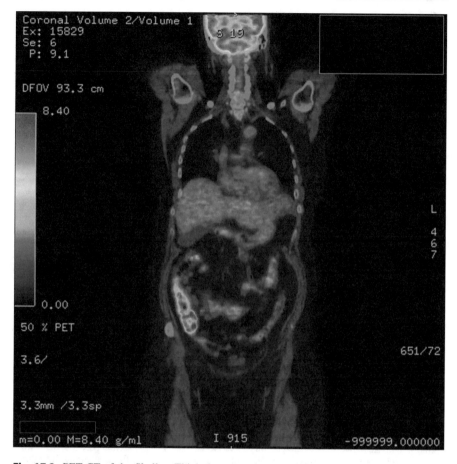

Fig. 17.2 PET CT of the Skull to Thigh demonstrating areas of moderate fluorodeoxyglucose (FDG) activity in the colon of a patient with a suspected malignancy. Resection of the colon revealed a marked lymphohistiocytic inflammatory infiltrate predominantly involving the subserosa and mesentery with associated fibrosis and small-vessel vasculitis (arteritis and phlebitis). No evidence of malignancy was found

Histologic examination generally shows non-granulomatous necrotizing arteritis involving medium-sized vessels and cannot be differentiated from systemic PAN [16]. One study comparing histology from SOV and systemic vasculitis cases noted that the pathologic processes were similar but more severe in the systemic cases [24]. A limitation in applying this study to GI-SOV is that only two of the seven cases of SOV were GI-SOV and the others were in non-GI organs. Examples of histology from GB-SOV and pancreas SOV are presented in Fig. 17.3.

A study of appendiceal SOV showed necrotizing arteritis in the submucosa, muscularis propria, and serosa with a perivascular inflammatory cell infiltrate [8]. In cases of GB-SOV, histology frequently revealed arteritis with fibrinoid necrosis of medium-sized arteries and inflammatory cell infiltration [10, 21, 22]. In a study of

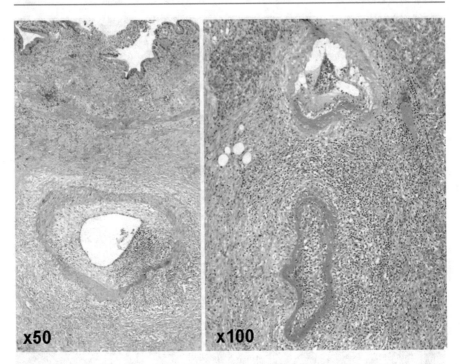

Fig. 17.3 Arteritis in the gallbladder and pancreas. (Left panel) Photomicrograph of the gallbladder showing inflamed mucosa toward the top with transmural inflammation involving a submucosal muscular artery. The artery shows focal fibrinoid necrosis (lower right) as well as diffuse intimal fibroplasia [hematoxylin and eosin (H&E), ×50]. (Right panel) Photomicrograph of the pancreas, removed as a Whipple specimen. Two muscular arteries are shown with segmental (middle) and complete (lower) necrotizing arteritis with fibrinoid degeneration of the arterial wall. Dense perivascular lymphoplasmacytic inflammation is seen. The pancreatic parenchyma toward the top is relatively well preserved (H&E, ×100). Salvarani, C., MD, Rheumatology, July 2010, Volume 47, Issue 7, 1326–1335 by permission of Oxford University Press

61 patients with gallbladder vasculitis, all 19 who had GB-SOV had involvement of medium-sized vessels. Of those 17 had non-granulomatous vasculitis and 3 had granulomatous vasculitis [5]. Pathology from a case report of pancreas SOV showed necrotizing arteritis in the pancreaticoduodenal artery and its penetrating branch [22]. Case reports of isolated leukocytoclastic vasculitis of the colon without systemic disease have been reported [28, 30]. Giant cells have rarely been found in pathology from GI vasculitis affecting the bowel and gallbladder [14]. While some of these reported cases represent GI-SOV, others occurred in the context of systemic vasculitis with documented temporal arteritis.

In one case report, a patient presented with abdominal pain and was found to have isolated vasculitis of the stomach [25]. Upper endoscopy revealed giant gastric folds with an antral ulcer and at laparotomy, the stomach had the appearance of a scirrhous gastric carcinoma leading to resection of most of the organ. Histology showed dense infiltrates of lymphocytes, plasma cells, and granulocytes in the large and small blood vessels with occasional fibrinoid necrosis, consistent with severe obliterative vasculitis of the stomach. At 22 months of follow-up, the patient remained well with no new symptoms or evidence for recurrence.

Because systemic vasculitis may initially have a limited presentation in a single organ, it has been suggested that all diagnoses of SOV be considered preliminary until disease in other organs has not been identified over at least 6 months of follow-up [3]. Even after careful monitoring during this period and the diagnosis of GI-SOV, subsequent monitoring has shown the development of systemic disease in up to 25% of patients within 5 years [18]. This has led to the suggestion that patients have close monitoring for a period of at least 5 years after diagnosis.

17.5   Differential Diagnosis

Systemic causes of GI vasculitis should be considered. While systemic symptoms are reported in studies of GI-SOV, they do appear to be statistically less common than in cases of GI-SV [5, 16]. Similarly having only GI symptoms cannot rule-out a systemic vasculitis. This is illustrated by a study showing that 13.5% of patients ultimately diagnosed with GB-SV initially had only GI symptoms [5]. While the absence or presence of systemic symptoms might help to distinguish systemic from single-organ disease, they are insufficient by themselves to make the distinction [5].

It is estimated that less than 10% of vascular disease of the GI tract is caused by vasculitis [32]. While ischemic abdominal pain is a frequent presentation of GI-SOV, mesenteric ischemia itself is usually caused by atherosclerosis [18]. Potential causes of GI-SV include IgA vasculitis, polyarteritis nodosa, Behcet's disease, eosinophilia with granulomatous polyangiitis, granulomatous polyangiitis, microscopic polyangiitis, systemic lupus erythematosus, systemic sclerosis, and mixed/undifferentiated connective tissue disease, as well as drug-induced vasculitis. Polyarteritis nodosa involves the GI system in roughly 25% of cases [6]. GI manifestations are part of the classic tetrad of IgA vasculitis; however, they are less common in patients of older ages who develop the disease [6].

Gallbladder vasculitis and appendix vasculitis may be manifestations of systemic vasculitis such as polyarteritis nodosa or ANCA-associated vasculitis [15]. Other systemic vasculitides causing gallbladder vasculitis include HBV-associated vasculitis, cryoglobulinemic vasculitis, IgA vasculitis, giant cell arteritis, and autoimmune disease such as rheumatoid arthritis, systemic lupus erythematosus, and systemic sclerosis [5, 33]. Cases of pancreas SOV have had features initially concerning for neoplasm; however, on histologic examination necrotizing arteritis has been found rather than neoplasm [7, 22, 26]. Similarly SOV of the stomach can resemble neoplasm [25]. Stomach SOV may also be a rare cause of gastric ulceration [6]. SOV of the colon can resemble other forms of colitis such as inflammatory bowel disease or infectious colitis [17, 30].

The changes in abdominal vasculature identified on imaging in cases of GI-SOV are not unique to the vasculitides. Fibromuscular dysplasia (FMD) and segmental arterial mediolysis (SAM) are two mimics of note. FMD is defined as an idiopathic, non-atherosclerotic, and non-inflammatory disease with abnormal cellular growth affecting the musculature of arterial walls [34, 35]. It primarily affects women (approximately 90% of cases) and usually involves more than one vascular territory [36]. Like vasculitis, it produces stenosis, aneurysm, and dissection of vessel walls; however, unlike vasculitis it does not cause wall thickening, edema, or uptake of contrast [36]. SAM is another disease commonly misdiagnosed as a vasculitis based on symptoms and imaging findings and was in fact previously labeled as a vasculitis [37]. SAM is a non-atherosclerotic, non-inflammatory arteriopathy primarily affecting medium-sized arteries in the abdomen [38]. Vacuolization in the outer portion of blood vessel media leads to dissecting aneurysms characterized by luminal stenosis and vessel dilatation [36]. Other imaging findings include aneurysms, stenosis, and occlusions [39, 40]. Differentiation from vasculitis is challenging but important as treatment differs based on the diagnosis: immunosuppression provides no benefit in the disease and might even worsen prognosis [40]. Arterial biopsy is often required for diagnosis and should lack inflammation [40].

Other potential conditions that mimic GI-SOV may include Ehlers–Danlos type IV, antiphospholipid antibody syndrome, thromboembolism, and IgG4-related disease [36].

17.6   Management

Many patients with GI-SOV have been reported to achieve cure through surgery only [5]. This is not possible in every case however as some cases of GI-SOV have ultimately required systemic immunosuppression for management. In general, limited (focal) SOV tends to be amenable to surgical intervention alone whereas diffuse (multifocal) SOV often requires systemic therapy [3].

In one case series of 18 patients with GI-SOV, 10 patients were treated medically [15]. All medically managed patients received prednisone and some also received additional immunosuppressive therapy such as cyclophosphamide, azathioprine, or methotrexate. Appendix SOV often resolves with appendectomy with no further symptoms or complications [8]. GB-SOV is usually cured with cholecystectomy alone although some patients have been treated with glucocorticoids [5, 21]. Cure of SOV of the pancreas has been reported with surgical excision [6, 22].

Small and large bowel vasculitides in particular often require immune suppression for management [3, 13, 15, 29]. A case of SOV of the colon reported disease control with IV steroids, a single bolus of IV cyclophosphamide, and then maintenance with azathioprine and a tapering dose of oral prednisone [30]. Another case was able to achieve control surgically via left colectomy with right colon end colostomy and rectal Hartman's pouch [17]. This patient was well 3 months later and the colostomy was reversed. In 1999, Raza reported two cases of SOV of the colon treated initially with surgical excision alone [29]. While the first case remained in remission after 30 months of follow-up the second case had a relapse after roughly 18 months. Treatment in a different case involved methylprednisolone with a transition to maintenance prednisone [28]. Common treatment strategies organized by affected organ are listed in Table 17.1.

Although rare, progression to systemic vasculitis may occur. As a consequence, proper management includes long-term medical follow-up. The patient should be educated on the disease, the possibility of later generalization, and instructed to remain vigilant for and report any new symptoms of concern. A study of localized vasculitis of the GI tract showed that 6 of 23 patients with localized polyarteritis and 4 of 5 patients with localized eosinophilic granulomatosis with polyangiitis developed systemic disease in follow-up [6]. In the same study, none of the five patients with small-vessel vasculitis had progression to systemic disease during follow-up.

17.7 Prognosis

The prognosis of patients with GI-SOV is highly variable and depends on the specific organ manifestations. Patients with localized disease frequently achieve surgical cure and have an excellent prognosis [5, 8]. That being said considerable damage is still possible from GI-SOV despite the fact that the disease process is limited to a single organ. A study of medium-sized vessel vasculitis showed similar Vasculitis Damage Indices (VDI)—a tool used to quantify vasculitis-induced damage—between patients with systemic polyarteritis nodosa and GI-SOV [16]. Furthermore, patients may have significant morbidity and mortality as illustrated in one study in which the survival of patients with GI-SOV was significantly reduced compared to an age-matched US White population [15]. In these patients, mortality was reported at 40% in the first year following diagnosis. Notably however in the years that followed no additional deaths or relapses were noted [15, 16]. This suggests the possibility that any possible additional mortality might be clustered around the time of initial diagnosis and treatment.

References

1. Jennette JC, Falk RJ, Bacon PA, Basu N, Cid MC, Ferrario F, et al. 2012 revised International Chapel Hill Consensus Conference Nomenclature of Vasculitides. Arthritis Rheum. 2013;65(1):1–11.
2. Mahr A, Battistella M, Bouaziz JD, Chaigne-Delalande S. L47. Single-organ vasculitis: conceptual and practical considerations. Presse Med. 2013;42(4 Pt 2):628–34.
3. Hernandez-Rodriguez J, Hoffman GS. Updating single-organ vasculitis. Curr Opin Rheumatol. 2012;24(1):38–45.
4. Koster MJ, Warrington KJ. Vasculitis of the mesenteric circulation. Best Pract Res Clin Gastroenterol. 2017;31(1):85–96.
5. Hernandez-Rodriguez J, Tan CD, Rodriguez ER, Hoffman GS. Single-organ gallbladder vasculitis: characterization and distinction from systemic vasculitis involving the gallbladder. An analysis of 61 patients. Medicine (Baltimore). 2014;93(24):405–13.
6. Burke AP, Sobin LH, Virmani R. Localized vasculitis of the gastrointestinal tract. Am J Surg Pathol. 1995;19(3):338–49.
7. Hernandez-Rodriguez J, Molloy ES, Hoffman GS. Single-organ vasculitis. Curr Opin Rheumatol. 2008;20(1):40–6.

8. Moyana TN. Necrotizing arteritis of the vermiform appendix. A clinicopathologic study of 12 cases. Arch Pathol Lab Med. 1988;112(7):738–41.
9. Plaut A. Asymptomatic focal arteritis of the appendix; 88 cases. Am J Pathol. 1951;27(2):247–63.
10. Chen KT. Gallbladder vasculitis. J Clin Gastroenterol. 1989;11(5):537–40.
11. Kumar B, Krishnani N, Misra R, Pandey R. Isolated necrotizing vasculitis of gallbladder: a report of two cases and review of literature. Indian J Pathol Microbiol. 2003;46(3):429–31.
12. Raess PW, Baird-Howell M, Aggarwal R, Williams NN, Furth EE. Vertical sleeve gastrectomy specimens have a high prevalence of unexpected histopathologic findings requiring additional clinical management. Surg Obes Relat Dis. 2015;11(5):1020–3.
13. Pagnoux C, Mahr A, Cohen P, Guillevin L. Presentation and outcome of gastrointestinal involvement in systemic necrotizing vasculitides: analysis of 62 patients with polyarteritis nodosa, microscopic polyangiitis, Wegener granulomatosis, Churg-Strauss syndrome, or rheumatoid arthritis-associated vasculitis. Medicine (Baltimore). 2005;84(2):115–28.
14. Quinet RJ, Zakem JM, McCain M. Localized versus systemic vasculitis: diagnosis and management. Curr Rheumatol Rep. 2003;5(2):93–9.
15. Salvarani C, Calamia KT, Crowson CS, Miller DV, Broadwell AW, Hunder GG, et al. Localized vasculitis of the gastrointestinal tract: a case series. Rheumatology (Oxford). 2010;49(7):1326–35.
16. Alibaz-Oner F, Koster MJ, Crowson CS, Makol A, Ytterberg SR, Salvarani C, et al. Clinical spectrum of medium-sized vessel vasculitis. Arthritis Care Res (Hoboken). 2017;69(6):884–91.
17. Vlahos K, Theodoropoulos GE, Lazaris A, Agapitos E, Christakopoulos A, Papatheodorou D, et al. Isolated colonic leukocytoclastic vasculitis causing segmental megacolon: report of a rare case. Dis Colon Rectum. 2005;48(1):167–71.
18. Soowamber M, Weizman AV, Pagnoux C. Gastrointestinal aspects of vasculitides. Nat Rev Gastroenterol Hepatol. 2016;14(3):185–94.
19. Daniels J, Deshpande V, Serra S, Chetty R. Incidental single-organ vasculitis of the gastrointestinal tract: an unusual form of single-organ vasculitis with coexistent pathology. Pathology. 2017;49(6):661–5.
20. Bohrod MG, Bodon GR. Isolated polyarteritis nodosa of the gallbladder. Am Surg. 1970;36(11):681–5.
21. Nohr M, Laustsen J, Falk E. Isolated necrotizing panarteritis of the gallbladder. Case report. Acta Chir Scand. 1989;155(9):485–7.
22. Ito M, Sano K, Inaba H, Hotchi M. Localized necrotizing arteritis. A report of two cases involving the gallbladder and pancreas. Arch Pathol Lab Med. 1991;115(8):780–3.
23. Tagoe C, Naghavi R, Faltz L, Rifkind K, Saw D. Localized polyarteritis nodosa of the gallbladder. Clin Exp Rheumatol. 2002;20(3):435–6.
24. Matsumoto T, Kobayashi S, Ogishima D, Aoki Y, Sonoue H, Abe H, et al. Isolated necrotizing arteritis (localized polyarteritis nodosa): examination of the histological process and disease entity based on the histological classification of stage and histological differences from polyarteritis nodosa. Cardiovasc Pathol. 2007;16(2):92–7.
25. Will U, Gerlach R, Wanzar I, Urban H, Manger T, Meyer F. Isolated vasculitis of the stomach: a novel or rare disease with a difficult differential diagnosis. Endoscopy. 2006;38(8):848–51.
26. Gonzalez-Gay MA, Vazquez-Rodriguez TR, Miranda-Filloy JA, Pazos-Ferro A, Garcia-Rodeja E. Localized vasculitis of the gastrointestinal tract: a case report and literature review. Clin Exp Rheumatol. 2008;26(3 Suppl 49):S101–4.
27. Meyer GW, Lichtenstein J. Isolated polyarteritis nodosa affecting the cecum. Dig Dis Sci. 1982;27(5):467–9.
28. Powers BJ, Brown G, Williams RW, Speers W. Leukocytoclastic vasculitis, not associated with Henoch-Schonlein purpura, causing recurrent massive painless gastrointestinal hemorrhage. Am J Gastroenterol. 1992;87(9):1191–3.
29. Raza K, Exley AR, Carruthers DM, Buckley C, Hammond LA, Bacon PA. Localized bowel vasculitis: postoperative cyclophosphamide or not? Arthritis Rheum. 1999;42(1):182–5.

30. Garcia-Porrua C, Gutierrez-Duque O, Soto S, Garcia-Rodeja E, Gonzalez-Gay MA. Localized vasculitis of the gastrointestinal tract. Semin Arthritis Rheum. 2006;35(6):403–6.
31. Uzoigwe CE, Dewsbery S, Bitra K, Iqbal R, Ali F, May JC, et al. A surgical solution for vasculitis? Lancet. 2007;369(9566):1054.
32. Muller-Ladner U. Vasculitides of the gastrointestinal tract. Best Pract Res Clin Gastroenterol. 2001;15(1):59–82.
33. Chetty R, Serra S. A pragmatic approach to vasculitis in the gastrointestinal tract. J Clin Pathol. 2017;70(6):470–5.
34. Gornik HL, Persu A, Adlam D, Aparicio LS, Azizi M, Boulanger M, et al. First international consensus on the diagnosis and management of fibromuscular dysplasia. J Hypertens. 2019;37(2):229–52.
35. Persu A, Giavarini A, Touze E, Januszewicz A, Sapoval M, Azizi M, et al. European consensus on the diagnosis and management of fibromuscular dysplasia. J Hypertens. 2014;32(7):1367–78.
36. Miloslavsky EM, Stone JH, Unizony SH. Challenging mimickers of primary systemic vasculitis. Rheum Dis Clin North Am. 2015;41(1):141–60, ix.
37. Ahn E, Luk A, Chetty R, Butany J. Vasculitides of the gastrointestinal tract. Semin Diagn Pathol. 2009;26(2):77–88.
38. Shenouda M, Riga C, Naji Y, Renton S. Segmental arterial mediolysis: a systematic review of 85 cases. Ann Vasc Surg. 2014;28(1):269–77.
39. Slavin RE. Segmental arterial mediolysis: course, sequelae, prognosis, and pathologic-radiologic correlation. Cardiovasc Pathol. 2009;18(6):352–60.
40. Baker-LePain JC, Stone DH, Mattis AN, Nakamura MC, Fye KH. Clinical diagnosis of segmental arterial mediolysis: differentiation from vasculitis and other mimics. Arthritis Care Res (Hoboken). 2010;62(11):1655–60.

Cutaneous Vasculitis

18

Diana Prieto-Peña, Trinitario Pina,
and Miguel A. González-Gay

Abstract

Cutaneous vasculitis (CV) includes a wide spectrum of entities characterized by predominant skin manifestations and a variable grade of systemic involvement. CV exhibits a variety of cutaneous lesions depending on the size of the involved vessels, with the most common being palpable purpura. CV can be found as part of the clinical spectrum of primary systemic vasculitis, autoimmune diseases, or less commonly as presenting manifestation of mimicking conditions such as infections and neoplastic diseases. In this regard, an adequate clinical approach is required to establish optimal management of this condition. CV limited to the skin usually respond to bed-rest and low-dose glucocorticosteroid therapy. However, when systemic involvement exists, immunosuppressive drugs such as azathioprine, intravenous cyclophosphamide, or rituximab may be considered.

Keywords

Cutaneous vasculitis · Leukocytoclastic vasculitis · Palpable purpura · Cutaneous single-organ vasculitis · Classification · Etiology · Epidemiology · Diagnostic approach · Management

D. Prieto-Peña · T. Pina · M. A. González-Gay (✉)
Rheumatology Division, Hospital Universitario Marqués de Valdecilla, IDIVAL,
University of Cantabria, Santander, Spain
e-mail: trinitario.pina@scsalud.es

© Springer Nature Switzerland AG 2021
C. Salvarani et al. (eds.), *Large and Medium Size Vessel and Single Organ Vasculitis*, Rare Diseases of the Immune System,
https://doi.org/10.1007/978-3-030-67175-4_18

Abbreviations

AAV	ANCA-associated vasculitis
ACR	American College of Rheumatology
ANCA	Anti-neutrophil cytoplasmic antibody
CHCC	Chapel Hill Consensus Conference
CV	Cutaneous vasculitis
EGPA	Eosinophilic granulomatosis with polyangiitis
EULAR	European League Against Rheumatism
GPA	Granulomatosis with polyangiitis
HBV	Hepatitis B virus
HCV	Hepatitis C virus
HV	Hypersensitivity vasculitis
IgAV	IgA vasculitis
MPA	Microscopic polyangiitis
PAN	Polyarteritis nodosa
PRES	Paediatric Rheumatology European Society
PRINTO	Paediatric Rheumatology International Trials Organization
PSS	Primary Sjögren syndrome
RA	Rheumatoid arthritis
SLE	Systemic lupus erythematosus

18.1 Introduction

The term cutaneous vasculitis (CV) encloses a heterogeneous group of vasculitic syndromes characterized by predominant cutaneous involvement [1]. In the absence of an underlying disease, we refer to them as primary or idiopathic systemic vasculitides. However, they are usually related to other conditions such as infections, drug-exposure, malignancies, or connective tissue diseases. CV exhibit a wide spectrum of manifestations depending on the localization and size of the involved vessels, and often have overlapping clinical and pathologic manifestations representing a challenge for the clinician [2]. In the same way, CV may be a process limited to the skin or be a manifestation of a more widespread entity associated with a variable grade of visceral involvement.

18.2 Nomenclature and Classification of Cutaneous Vasculitis

Nowadays, the classification of some CV remains to be controversial. The 2012 Revised Chapel Hill Consensus (2012 CHCC) classified vasculitis according to the size of the affected vessels [3]. However, no special reference to the classification of cutaneous vasculitis was made. In this regard, a consensus group was recently formed to propose an addendum to the 2012 CHCC in order to provide a standardization of names and definitions for CV. They established three forms of CV: (1) a cutaneous component of systemic vasculitis; (2) a skin-limited or skin-dominant expression or variant of systemic vasculitis; (3) a single-organ vasculitis (SOV) of the skin that differs from recognized systemic vasculitides with regard to clinical, laboratory, and pathologic features. In this latter group, they included the following entities: cutaneous IgM/IgG immune complex vasculitis, nodular cutaneous vasculitis (erythema induratum of Bazin), erythema elevatum et diutinum, recurrent macular vasculitis in hypergammaglobulinemia and normocomplementemic urticarial vasculitis [4].

18.3   Clinical Spectrum of Cutaneous Vasculitis

Cutaneous manifestations will depend on the size of the affected vessel. Small-sized blood vessels include capillaries, postcapillary venules, and nonmuscular arterioles (diameter <50 μm) mainly located within the superficial papillary dermis. Cutaneous involvement of small-sized vessels usually manifests as a maculopapular rash followed by palpable purpura, resulting from extravasation of erythrocytes through damaged blood vessel walls into the dermis. These lesions do not blanch when pressure is applied upon the skin, which distinguishes it from simple purpura. Other skin lesions such as nonpalpable macules and patches, urticaria, bullous lesions, vesicles, pustules, splinter hemorrhages, and ulcerations may also be observed. In fact, a combination of different lesions is common [5, 6]. In contrast, medium-sized blood vessels (diameter between 50 and 150 μm) have muscular walls and are particularly found in the deep reticular dermis, near the junction of the dermis and subcutaneous tissues. Its affection is characterized by the presence of subcutaneous nodules, ulcers, livedo reticularis, digital infarctions, and papulonecrotic lesions (Fig. 18.1). Larger vessels are not found within the skin.

Clinicians should keep in mind that palpable purpura is the most common type of cutaneous lesion seen in patients with CV being observed in up to 70% of cases, mainly located in the lower extremities due to the increased hydrostatic pressure [7–11]. Nodules, ulcers, and nonpalpable purpura are probably the next more common lesions observed. However, it is important to take into account that different conditions such as pigmented purpuric eruptions, severe thrombocytopenic purpura or scurvy, may mimic CV [12, 13]. For this reason, a skin biopsy is recommended to confirm the presence of vasculitis and distinguish it from other conditions.

Table 18.1 summarizes the clinical manifestations and histological findings of the main entities that can present with cutaneous vasculitis.

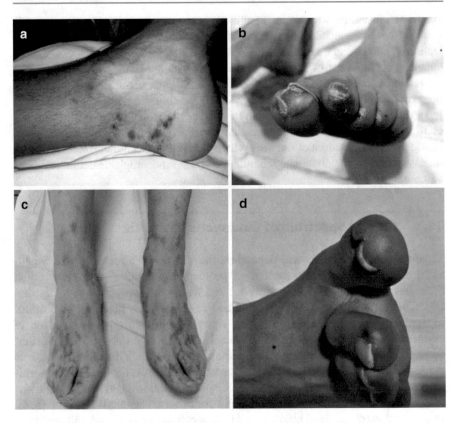

Fig. 18.1 (**a**) Palpable purpuric papules. (**b**) Ulcerative periungual digital lesions (**c**) livedo racemosa. (**d**) Periungual digital nodular lesions

Table 18.1 Clinical manifestations and histological findings of the main entities which can present with cutaneous vasculitis

Main entities which can present with cutaneous vasculitis	Systemic involvement	Main cutaneous manifestations	Histological findings
Medium-vessel vasculitis			
Polyarteritis nodosa	Yes	Palpable purpura, nodules with ulcers	Fibrinoid necrosis with infiltration of arterioles in deep dermis and subcutis
Cutaneous polyarteritis nodosa[a]	Exceptional	Livedo, macules, nodules	Vasculitis of small arteries and arterioles in the panniculus and dermosubcutaneous junction
Small-vessel vasculitis			
Microscopic polyangiitis	Yes	Palpable purpura, nodules, urticaria	Leukocytoclastic vasculitis

Table 18.1 (continued)

Main entities which can present with cutaneous vasculitis	Systemic involvement	Main cutaneous manifestations	Histological findings
Granulomatosis with polyangiitis	Yes	Palpable purpura, nodules, urticaria	Leukocytoclastic vasculitis with extravascular granulomas
Eosinophilic granulomatosis with polyangiitis	Yes	Palpable purpura, nodules, urticaria	Leukocytoclastic vasculitis + eosinophilic infiltrates with extravascular granulomas
IgA vasculitis	Yes	Palpable purpura in buttocks and lower extremities	Leukocytoclastic vasculitis with IgA1-dominant deposits
Cryoglobulinemic vasculitis	Yes	Small petechial palpable lesions in lower extremities	Leukocytoclastic vasculitis with vascular deposits of immunoglobulins
Hypocomplementemic urticarial vasculitis	Yes	Urticarial lesions lasting >48 h	Leukocytoclastic vasculitis with vascular deposits of immunoglobulins
Vasculitis associated with systemic disease			
Rheumatoid arthritis	Yes	Rheumatoid nodules, rheumatoid vasculitis, skin ulcers in unusual locations	Leukocytoclastic vasculitis Necrobiotic granulomas (rheumatoid nodules)
Systemic lupus erythematosus	Yes	Punctate lesions in fingertips, palpable purpura, papules/nodules, urticarial lesions	Leukocytoclastic vasculitis
Primary Sjögren syndrome	Yes	Palpable purpura, urticarial lesions	Leukocytoclastic vasculitis
Cutaneous SOV (according to the addendum 2012 CHCC)			
IgM/IgG vasculitis	No	Palpable purpura	Leukocytoclastic vasculitis with IgM/IgG dominant deposits
Erythema elevatum et diutinum	No	Nonpurpuric edematous erythematous papules on the extensor surface of extremities	Leukocytoclastic vasculitis, vessel occlusion, and fibrosis
Nodular vasculitis	No	Nodules in extremities	Leukocytoclastic vasculitis of small vessels with lobular panniculitis
Hypergammaglobulinemic macular vasculitis	No	Relapsing lived hemorrhagic macules on legs	Leukocytoclastic vasculitis with perivascular deposits of immunoglobulins
Normocomplementemic urticarial vasculitis	No	Urticarial lesions lasting >48 h	Leukocytoclastic vasculitis with vascular deposits of immunoglobulins

[a]Considered by some authors as a different entity from systemic polyarteritis nodosa

18.4   Cutaneous Vasculitic Manifestations in Systemic Vasculitides with Predominant Organ Involvement Different from the Skin

Large vessel vasculitis rarely present with CV because of the absence of large vessels in the skin. In contrast, cutaneous affection is relatively common in vasculitides that involve medium and small vessels including polyarteritis nodosa (PAN), granulomatosis with polyangiitis (GPA), eosinophilic granulomatosis with polyangiitis (EGPA), and microscopic polyangiitis (MPA). CV are frequently found in immune complex small-vessel vasculitis, such as IgA vasculitis, cryoglobulinemic vasculitis, and hypocomplementemic urticarial vasculitis.

18.4.1 Polyarteritis Nodosa

Fiorentino et al. [14] described CV in 49.7% of patients being more frequent in non-HBV-related PAN (57.8% versus 35%). Purpura was the most common lesion regardless HBV infection association (17.9% and 24.4%, respectively), followed by nodules (23.6%) and livedo (20%) in non-HBV-associated PAN. Interestingly, the presence of cutaneous manifestations at diagnosis, especially nodules, was associated with a higher risk of relapse. Another entity to concern about is cutaneous PAN (also named cutaneous arteritis) characterized by the affection of small arteries and arterioles in the panniculus and derma-subcutaneous junction [15]. Livedo, macules, and subcutaneous nodules with or without ulceration are the most frequently observed lesions, usually limited to the extremities [16]. When compared to other similar entities, cutaneous PAN differs from nodular vasculitis because it does not extend beyond the adventitia of the arterial vessels [17]. According to some authors, cutaneous PAN can be considered a different entity from systemic PAN due to a more chronic benign nature and its rare evolution into a systemic vasculitis [18, 19].

18.4.2 Anti-neutrophil Cytoplasmic Antibody (ANCA)-Associated Vasculitis

Cutaneous manifestations in ANCA-associated vasculitis (AAV) enclose both vasculitic and non-vasculitic skin lesions, with a complex clinical and histopathological spectrum. Palpable purpura in the lower extremities is the most common presentation. Nevertheless, other rarer lesions have also been reported, such as livedo racemosa, nodular erythema, or subcutaneous nodules [20]. The most common histopathologic pattern observed in the cutaneous lesions of patients with MPA and GPA is a neutrophilic vasculitis (a leukocytoclastic vasculitis characterized by a predominant infiltrate of neutrophils mixed with nuclear dust). In patients with EGPA, neutrophilic vasculitis may also be observed but extravascular necrotizing granuloma and eosinophilic infiltrates are more common [21–23]. Another characteristic feature is that small-vessel vasculitis involvement and subcutaneous arteritis or phlebitis may be observed at the same time [20].

18.4.2.1 MPA

In a retrospective study of 85 patients with MPA classified according to the 1994 CHCC, Guillevin et al. [21] observed cutaneous involvement in 62.4% of patients. Purpura was the commonest manifestation, accounting for 41:2% of cases, followed by livedo and nodules (12.9% each), and urticaria (3.5%).

18.4.2.2 GPA

The frequency of CV in patients with GPA varies between less than 15 and 46% depending on different series [24, 25], being the presenting manifestations in 10–21% of cases [26, 27]. Several studies have assessed the correlation between CV and the activity and course of the disease. Frances et al. [24] and Barksdale et al. [28] found that patients with CV presented an earlier onset of GPA with a more rapidly progressive and widespread vasculitis and a higher frequency of kidney and joint involvement.

18.4.2.3 EGPA

Bosco et al. observed CV in a range of 40–81% patients with EGPA, being the presenting sign of the disease in 14% of cases. The most common manifestations were palpable purpura of the lower extremities (up to 50% patients) and urticarial lesions (12–31%) [22]. Other reported lesions were papular/nodular lesions, livedo reticularis, ulcerations, bullous lesions, cutaneous infarcts, Raynaud's phenomenon, and vesicles and sterile pustules.

18.4.3 Immune Complex Small-Vessel Vasculitis

18.4.3.1 IgA Vasculitis (IgAV)

Cutaneous involvement is a mandatory criterion in 2010 EULAR/PRINTO/PRES classification criteria for IgAV characterized by a rash of symmetric erythematous papules of the buttocks and lower extremities, which progresses to palpable purpura [29]. Other skin lesions, generally macular, papular, or more rarely urticarial or vesicular, are observed in up to 44% of children [30]. The typical histological pattern is a small-vessel leukocytoclastic vasculitis along with IgA 1-predominant immune deposits in the walls of arterioles, capillaries, and venules. IgAV is classically a childhood disease, generally considered a benign and self-limited entity. Conversely, it is a less common condition in adults in whom it may be associated with a worse outcome due to an increased frequency of severe renal affection [31, 32]. Recent studies addressed the role of the genetic factors in the susceptibility and severity of IgAV. Lopez-Mejías et al. showed that there is a strong association with HLA class II region, which in Europeans is mainly related to HLA-DRB1*01 allele [33–35]. Several authors have reported that cutaneous affection could be correlated with the development of renal affection and relapse in IgAV. Shin et al. [36] and Rigante et al. [37] found that recurrent purpura lasting more than 1 month was an important independent predictive factor for the development of nephritis and relapse in children. In keeping with this report, a recent study suggested that the distribution of the cutaneous lesions on the extremities could also be a predictor of long-term renal involvement in adults with IgAV [38]. Byun et al. [39] observed that relapsing disease was also associated with the presence of severe leukocytoclastic vasculitis with a significant deposition of IgA but not of IgM on direct immunofluorescence.

A new entity named IgM/IgG immune complex vasculitis has been proposed to be considered as a cutaneous SOV. This term is meant for those CV confined to the skin, clinically indistinguishable from IgA cutaneous lesions, characterized by IgM/IgG deposits that do not belong to other defined vasculitis [4].

18.4.3.2   Cryoglobulinemic Vasculitis

Cryoglobulinemic vasculitis is another vasculitis affecting small vessels (predominantly capillaries, venules, or arterioles) with cryoglobulin immune deposits and the presence of cryoglobulins in serum [3]. CV is the most common presenting symptom entailing intermittent episodes of small petechial palpable lesions predominantly localized in the lower extremities [40, 41]. In a series of 443 patients with cryoglobulinemia, Trejo et al. [42] found that patients with a cryocrit >5%, low C4, and positive rheumatoid factor had a higher frequency of palpable purpura. CV are more commonly found in type II cryoglobulinemia, less frequently in type III and rare in type I cryoglobulinemia in which most cutaneous lesions are related to a hyperviscosity-related vasculopathy [43].

18.4.3.3   Urticarial Vasculitis

In contrast to common urticaria, cutaneous lesions of urticarial vasculitis persist for more than 48 h and resolve with purpura and hyperpigmentation. In most cases, it is an idiopathic condition, but it can also occur in the setting of viral infections, serum sickness, drug reactions, or as a paraneoplastic syndrome (usually hematologic disorders) [44]. Normocomplementemic patients usually have minimal or no systemic involvement and often have better outcome. This is the reason why normocomplementemic urticaria has been proposed by the addendum to 2012 CHCC to be part of the group of cutaneous SOV [4]. On the other hand, patients with hypocomplementemic urticaria (also named anti-C1q vasculitis) are more likely to develop severe multi-systemic manifestations (mainly pulmonary) [44]. It has been associated with systemic lupus erythematosus due to some overlapping manifestations and the reported presence of C1q autoantibodies in both conditions [45].

18.5   Cutaneous Vasculitis Associated with Autoimmune Systemic Diseases

Vasculitis may occur in many autoimmune diseases, usually affecting small-sized vessels.

18.5.1 Rheumatoid Arthritis (RA)

Cutaneous involvement is the most common extra-articular manifestation in RA, being rheumatoid nodules the most frequent lesions [46]. Rheumatoid vasculitis has been reported in 15–31% patients according to autopsy data. However, it appears to be far less common in the clinical setting [47]. Rheumatoid vasculitis typically affects middle-aged patients with severe RA with an average of 14 years after the onset of the disease [48]. Palpable purpura in the lower extremities is the most common cutaneous presentation and cannot be distinguished from those occurring in other conditions. Other reported cutaneous lesions are skin ulcers characteristically found in unusual locations of the lower extremities (mainly in the dorsum of the foot or the upper calf), ischemic focal digital lesions, maculopapular erythema, hemorrhagic blisters, erythema elevatum diutinum, livedo reticularis, subcutaneous nodules, and atrophie blanche [47, 48].

18.5.2 Systemic Lupus Erythematous (SLE)

Lopez-Longo et al. [49] reported the presence of CV in 68 patients in a series of 670 patients with SLE. The spectrum of cutaneous manifestations was as follows: erythematous punctate lesions of the fingertips and palms (36%), palpable purpura (25%), ischemic/ulcerated lesions (14%), erythematous papules/macules (14%), urticarial lesions (11%), and nodular lesions (5%). The vast majority showed a pattern of leukocytoclastic vasculitis in the histology. Fukuda et al. [50] found that SLE patients with anti-Ro antibodies seem to have a higher risk of developing CV. Some studies have addressed the correlation between vasculitic skin lesions and the onset and severity of SLE. Lopez-Longo et al. [51] observed that patients with CV had a longer disease duration from SLE onset. In this line, Shinjo et al. [52] showed that CV was associated with a higher frequency of Raynaud phenomenon and ribosomal P protein antibodies, but not with a higher frequency of kidney or nervous system involvement.

18.5.3 Primary Sjögren Syndrome (PSS)

The frequency of CV in PSS varies from 4 to 10% depending on different series [53, 54]. In a series of 588 patients with PSS reported by Ramos-Casals et al. [54], 14 presented with cryoglobulinemic vasculitis, 11 with urticarial vasculitis, and 26 with cutaneous purpura not associated with cryoglobulins. Most patients had small-vessel leukocytoclastic vasculitis with a higher prevalence of extraglandular and immunologic features. Also, 5% of the biopsied patients had medium-sized vessel vasculitis.

18.6 Cutaneous Single-Organ Vasculitis (SOV)

According to 2012 CHCC, the term SOV encloses skin-limited vasculitis that does not share enough clinical, laboratory, and/or pathologic features with a systemic vasculitis [3]. Some of the entities proposed by the addendum to 2012 CHCC to be included in this group have been already mentioned, such as IgM/IgG vasculitis and normocomplementemic urticarial vasculitis. Other proposed conditions are:

18.6.1 Erythema Elevatum et Diutinum (EED)

EED is an uncommon disease characterized by nonpurpuric prominent and persistent edematous erythematous papules and plaques on the extensor surface of the extremities (backs of hands, elbows, or knees) that heal over a period of months or years with fibrosis [55]. EED can be associated with monoclonal gammopathy, infections, and IgG4-related disease [56]. Treatment with dapsone has yielded good results [55].

18.6.2 Nodular Vasculitis (Erythema Induratum of Bazin)

It is a lobular panniculitis with vasculitis of vessels in the panniculus, often related to tuberculosis (erythema induratum of Bazin). Lobular panniculitis distinguishes nodular vasculitis from cutaneous PAN and differs from GPA and EGPA because of the primary localization of vasculitis in the panniculus [4].

18.6.3 Hypergammaglobulinemic Macular Vasculitis (Hypergammaglobulinemic Purpura of Waldenström)

It is characterized by the presence of relapsing lived hemorrhagic macules on the lower extremities associated with elevated erythrocyte rate and the presence of non-IgM rheumatoid factor. It is usually found in the setting of a polyclonal hypergammaglobulinemia, but it can also be associated to autoimmune diseases, specially Sjogren's syndrome and SLE, but not with systemic vasculitis [57, 58].

18.7 Diagnostic Approach in a Patient Presenting with Cutaneous Vasculitis

The first step to be carried out in the study of a patient presenting with palpable purpura or other cutaneous lesions suggestive of vasculitis is to perform a skin biopsy to obtain specimens for routine microscopy and direct immunofluorescence.

Some important considerations about biopsy process should be considered. With respect to this, it is recommended to take a punch or excisional biopsy extending to subcutis from the most tender, reddish, or purpuric lesion. The optimal time for skin biopsy is less than 48 h after the appearance of a vasculitic lesion in an attempt to ensure the accuracy of histology and direct immunofluorescence analysis results. After 24 h neutrophilic infiltration of wall vessels is progressively replaced by lymphocytes and macrophages. As a result, lesions older than 48 h may show a predominant lymphocyte infiltrate regardless of the underlying form of vasculitis. The same concern applies to direct immunofluorescence analysis, the possibility to find immunoglobulins decrease as time goes on. After 72 h only C3 is detected [59, 60].

A complete clinical history should be performed searching for data regarding drug-exposure, recent infections, and the presence of preexisting symptoms suggestive of autoimmune and neoplastic diseases. Careful physical examination, laboratory, electrocardiography, and chest radiograph should also bring about in all patients in order to exclude systemic involvement. Routine laboratory testing should include red blood cell count, erythrocyte sedimentation rate, C-reactive protein, liver, and kidney function test, urinalysis, rheumatoid factor, antinuclear antibodies, ANCA, serum IgA, cryoglobulins, complement levels (C3, C4, CH50), determinations for hepatitis B and C virus. Figure 18.2 shows a work-up in a patient with CV in whom a skin biopsy discloses the presence of a leukocytoclastic vasculitis.

18.8 Treatment of Cutaneous Vasculitis

CV limited to the skin usually has a rapid and complete response after bed-rest and in some cases treatment with low-dose prednisone therapy. The therapeutic efficacy of non-steroidal anti-inflammatory drugs, dapsone, or colchicine remains controversial. In those patients in whom CV is not limited to skin, therapy must be individualized, and it must be focused on the appropriate management of the systemic vasculitis, especially if lung and/or renal involvement exist. In this case, immunosuppressive drugs such as azathioprine, intravenous cyclophosphamide, or rituximab may be considered. When the CV occurs in the setting of a malignancy or an infection, treatment of the underlying disease leads to improvement of the cutaneous manifestations in most cases [2, 12, 13].

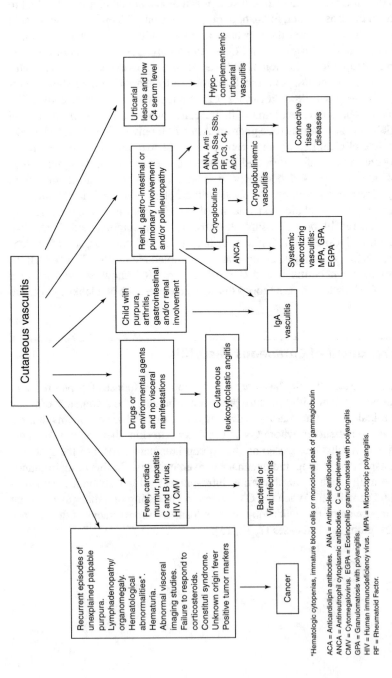

Fig. 18.2 Work-up in a patient with CV in whom a skin biopsy disclosed the presence of a leukocytoclastic vasculitis. *Hematologic cytopenias, immature blood cells or monoclonal peak of gammaglobulin. *ACA* Anticardiolipin antibodies, *ANA* Antinuclear antibodies, *ANCA* antineutrophil cytoplasmic antibodies, *C* Complement, *CMV* Cytomegalovirus, *EGPA* eosinophilic granulomatosis with polyangiitis, *GPA* granulomatosis with polyangiitis, *HIV* Human immunode-ficiency virus, *MPA* Microscopic polyangiitis, *RF* Rheumatoid factor

*Hematologic cytopenias, immature blood cells or monoclonal peak of gammaglobulin

ACA = Anticardiolipin antibodies. ANA = Antinuclear antibodies.
ANCA = Antineutrophil cytoplasmic antibodies. C = Complement
CMV = Cytomegalovirus. EGPA = Eosinophilic granulomatosis with polyangiitis
GPA = Granulomatosis with polyangiitis.
HIV = Human immunodeficiency virus. MPA = Microscopic polyangiitis.
RF = Rheumatoid Factor.

References

1. Gonzalez-Gay MA, Garcia-Porrua C. Epidemiology of the vasculitides. Rheum Dis Clin North Am. 2001;27:729–49.
2. Hunder GG. Vasculitis: diagnosis and therapy. Am J Med. 1996;100(Suppl 2A):37S–45.
3. Jennette JC, Falk RJ, Bacon PA, et al. 2012 revised international Chapel Hill consensus conference nomenclature of vasculitides. Arthritis Rheum. 2013;65(1):1–11.
4. Sunderkötter CH, Zelger B, Chen KR, et al. Nomenclature of cutaneous vasculitis. Arthritis Rheum. 2018;70:171–84.
5. Blanco R, Martinez-Taboada VM, Rodriguez-Valverde V, García-Fuentes M. Cutaneous vasculitis in children and adults. Associated diseases and etiologic factors in 303 patients. Medicine. 1998;77:403–18.
6. Stone JH, Nousari HC. "Essential" cutaneous vasculitis: what every rheumatologist should know about vasculitis of the skin. Curr Opin Rheumatol. 2001;13:23–34.
7. Khetan P, Sethuraman G, Khaitan BK, et al. An aetiological and clinicopathological study on cutaneous vasculitis. Indian J Med Res. 2012;135:107–13.
8. García-Porrúa C, Gonzalez-Gay MA. Comparative clinical and epidemiological study of hypersensitivity vasculitis versus Henoch-Schönlein purpura in adults. Semin Arthritis Rheum. 1999;28:404–12.
9. Leelavathi M, Aziz SA, Gangaram HB, Hussein SH. Cutaneous vasculitis: a review of aetiology and clinical manifestations in 85 patients in Malaysia. Med J Malaysia. 2009;64:210–2.
10. Al-Mutairi N. Spectrum of cutaneous vasculitis in adult patients from the Farwaniya region of Kuwait. Med Princ Pract. 2008;17:43–8.
11. Chua SH, Lim JT, Ang CB. Cutaneous vasculitis seen at a skin referral centre in Singapore. Singap Med J. 1999;40:147–50.
12. Gonzalez-Gay MA, García-Porrua C, Pujol RM. Clinical approach to cutaneous vasculitis. Curr Opin Rheumatol. 2005;17:56–61.
13. Pina T, Blanco R, González-Gay MA. Cutaneous vasculitis: a rheumatologist perspective. Curr Allergy Asthma Rep. 2013;13:545–54.
14. Fiorentino D. Cutaneous vasculitis. J Am Acad Dermatol. 2003;48:311–40.
15. Requena L, Yus ES. Panniculitis. Part I. Mostly septal panniculitis. J Am Acad Dermatol. 2001;45:163–83; quiz 84–6.
16. Criado PR, Marques GF, Morita TC, de Carvalho JF. Epidemiological, clinical and laboratory profiles of cutaneous polyarteritis nodosa patients: report of 22 cases and literature review. Autoimmun Rev. 2016;15:558–63.
17. Carlson JA, Chen KR. Cutaneous vasculitis update: neutrophilic muscular vessel and eosinophilic, granulomatous, and lymphocytic vasculitis syndromes. Am J Dermatopathol. 2007;29:32–43.
18. Daoud MS, Hutton KP, Gibson LE. Cutaneous periarteritis nodosa: a clinicopathological study of 79 cases. Br J Dermatol. 1997;136:706–13.
19. Alibaz-Oner F, Koster MJ, Crowson CS, et al. Clinical spectrum of medium-sized vessel vasculitis. Arthritis Care Res (Hoboken). 2017;69:884–91.
20. Chen KR. Skin involvement in ANCA-associated vasculitis. Clin Exp Nephrol. 2013;17:676–82.
21. Guillevin L, Durand-Gasselin B, Cevallos R, et al. Microscopic polyangiitis. Clinical and laboratory findings in eighty-five patients. Arthritis Rheum. 1999;42:421–30.
22. Bosco L, Peroni A, Schena D, et al. Cutaneous manifestations of Churg-Strauss syndrome: report of two cases and review of the literature. Clin Rheumatol. 2011;30:573–80.
23. Davis MD, Daoud MS, Mcevoy MT, Su WP. Cutaneous manifestations of Churg-Strauss syndrome: a clinicopathologic correlation. J Am Acad Dermatol. 1997;37:199–203.
24. Frances C, Du LT, Piette JC, et al. Wegener's granulomatosis. Dermatological manifestations in 75 cases with clinicopathologic correlation. Arch Dermatol. 1994;130:861–7.
25. Lie JT. Wegener's granulomatosis: histological documentation of common and uncommon manifestations in 216 patients. Vasa. 1997;26:261–70.

26. Patten SE, Tomecki KJ. Wegener's granulomatosis: cutaneous and oral mucosal disease. J Am Acad Dermatol. 1993;28:710–8.
27. Zycinska K, Wardyn K, Zielonka TM, et al. Cutaneous changes: an initial manifestation of pulmonary Wegener's granulomatosis. Adv Exp Med Biol. 2013;755:307–10.
28. Barksdale SK, Hallahan CW, Kerr GS, et al. Cutaneous pathology in Wegener's granulomatosis. A clinicopathologic study of 75 biopsies in 46 patients. Am J Surg Pathol. 1995;19:161–72.
29. Ozen S, Pistorio A, Iusan SM, et al. EULAR/PRINTO/PRES criteria for Henoch-Schonlein purpura, childhood polyarteritis nodosa, childhood Wegener granulomatosis and childhood Takayasu arteritis: Ankara 2008. Part II: final classification criteria. Ann Rheum Dis. 2010;69:798–806.
30. Calviño MC, Llorca J, Garcia-Porrua C, et al. Henoch-Schönlein purpura in children from northwestern Spain: a 20 year epidemiologic and clinical study. Medicine (Baltimore). 2001;80:279–90.
31. Calviño MC, Llorca J, García-Porrúa C, Fernández-Iglesias JL, Rodríguez-Ledo P, Gonzalez-Gay MA. Henoch-Schönlein purpura in children from northwestern Spain: a 20-year epidemiologic and clinical study. Medicine (Baltimore). 2001;80:279–90.
32. García-Porrúa C, Calviño MC, Llorca J, Couselo JM, González-Gay MA. Henoch-Schönlein purpura in children and adults: clinical differences in a defined population. Semin Arthritis Rheum. 2002;32:149–56.
33. González-Gay M, López-Mejías R, Pina T, Blanco R, Castañeda S. IgA vasculitis: genetics and clinical and therapeutical management. Curr Rheumatol Rep. 2018;20:24.
34. López-Mejías R, Genre F, Pérez BS, et al. HLA-DRB1 association with Henoch-Schonlein purpura. Arthritis Rheumatol. 2015;67:823–7.
35. López-Mejías R, Castañeda S, Genre F, et al. Genetics of immunoglobulin-A vasculitis (Henoch-Schönlein purpura): an updated review. Autoimmun Rev. 2018;S1568–9972(18):30012–0.
36. Shin JI, Park JM, Shin YH, et al. Predictive factors for nephritis, relapse, and significant proteinuria in childhood Henoch-Schönlein purpura. Scand J Rheumatol. 2006;35:56–60.
37. Rigante D, Candelli M, Federico G, et al. Predictive factors of renal involvement or relapsing disease in children with Henoch-Schönlein purpura. Rheumatol Int. 2005;25:45–8.
38. St John J, Vedak P, Garza-Mayers AC, Hoang MP, Nigwekar SU, Kroshinsky D. Location of skin lesions in Henoch-Schönlein purpura and its association with significant renal involvement. J Am Acad Dermatol. 2018;78:115–20.
39. Byun JW, Song HJ, Kim L, et al. Predictive factors of relapse in adult with Henoch-Schönlein purpura. Am J Dermatopathol. 2012;34:139–44.
40. Ramos-Casals M, Stone JH, Cid MC, Bosch X. The cryoglobulinaemias. Lancet. 2012;379:348–60.
41. Ferri C, Sebastiani M, Giuggioli D, et al. Mixed cryoglobulinemia: demographic, clinical, and serologic features and survival in 231 patients. Semin Arthritis Rheum. 2004;33:355–74.
42. Trejo O, Ramos-Casals M, Garcia-Carrasco M, et al. Cryoglobulinemia. Study of etiologic factors and clinical and immunologic features in 443 patients from a single center. Medicine (Baltimore). 2001;80:252–62.
43. Terrier B, Karras A, Kahn JE, et al. The spectrum of type I cryoglobulinemia vasculitis. New insights based on 64 cases. Medicine (Baltimore). 2013;92:61–8.
44. Venzor J, Lee WL, Huston DP. Urticarial vasculitis. Clin Rev Allergy Immunol. 2002;23:201–16.
45. Saigal K, Valencia IC, Cohen J, et al. Hypocomplementemic urticarial vasculitis with angioedema, a rare presentation of systemic lupus erythematosus: rapid response to rituximab. J Am Acad Dermatol. 2003;49:S283–5.
46. Turesson C, O'Fallon WM, Crowson CS, et al. Extra-articular disease manifestations in rheumatoid arthritis: incidence trends and risk factors over 46 years. Ann Rheum Dis. 2003;62:722–7.
47. Genta MS, Genta RM, Gabay C. Systemic rheumatoid vasculitis: a review. Semin Arthritis Rheum. 2006;36:88–98.
48. Chen KR, Toyohara A, Suzuki A, Miyakawa S. Clinical and histopathological spectrum of cutaneous vasculitis in rheumatoid arthritis. Br J Dermatol. 2002;147:905–13.

49. Lopez-Longo FJ, Gonzalez-Fernandez CM, Rodriguez-Mahou M, et al. Vasculitis in systemic lupus erithematosus. Prevalence and clinical characteristic in 670 patients. Medicine (Baltimore). 2006;85:95–104.
50. Fukuda MV, Lo SC, Almeida CS, Shinjo SK. Anti-Ro antibody and cutaneous vasculitis in systemic lupus erythematosus. Clin Rheumatol. 2009;28:301–4.
51. Lopez-Longo FJ, Gonzalez-Fernandez CM, Rodriguez-Mahou M, et al. Clinical expression of systemic lupus erythematosus with anti-U1-RNP and anti-Sm antibodies. Rev Clin Esp. 1997;197:329–35.
52. Shinjo SK, Bonfa E. Cutaneous vasculitis in systemic lupus erythematosus: association with anti-ribosomal P protein antibody and Raynaud phenomenon. Clin Rheumatol. 2011;30:173–7.
53. Malladi AS, Sack KE, Shiboski SC, et al. Primary Sjögren syndrome as a systemic disease: a study of participants enrolled in an international Sjögren's syndrome registry. Arthritis Care Res. 2012;64:911–8.
54. Ramos-Casals M, Anaya JM, Garcia-Carrasco M, et al. Cutaneous vasculitis in primary Sjögren syndrome: classification and clinical significance of 52 patients. Medicine (Baltimore). 2004;83:96–106.
55. Wahl CE, Bouldin MB, Gibson LE. Erythema elevatum diutinum: clinical, histopathologic, and immunohistochemical characteristics of six patients. Am J Dermatopathol. 2005;27:397–400.
56. Kavand S, Lehman JS, Gibson LE. Granuloma faciale and erythema elevatum diutinum in relation to immunoglobulin G4-related disease: an appraisal of 32 cases. Am J Clin Pathol. 2016;145:401–6.
57. Malaviya AN, Kaushik P, Budhiraja S, al-Mutairi M, Nampoory MR, Hussein A, et al. Hypergammaglobulinemic purpura of Waldenstr€om: report of 3 cases with a short review. Clin Exp Rheumatol. 2000;18:518–22.
58. Capra JD, Winchester RJ, Kunkel HG. Hypergammaglobulinemic purpura: studies on the unusual anti-globulins characteristic of the sera of these patients. Medicine (Baltimore). 1971;50:125–38.
59. Carlson JA. The histological assessment of cutaneous vasculitis. Histopathology. 2010;56:3–23.
60. Kluger N, Frances C. Cutaneous vasculitis and their differential diagnosis. Clin Exp Rheumatol. 2009;27(Suppl 52):S124–38.

Single-Organ Genitourinary Vasculitis

José Hernández-Rodríguez and Gary S. Hoffman

Abstract

Single-organ vasculitis (SOV) comprises a group of diseases in which vasculitic involvement is confined to a specific organ, system, or territory. SOV may be divided into focal and diffuse forms. Gynecologic, testicular, prostate, and urinary structures may be involved in different systemic vasculitides. In addition, these organs may be occasionally affected in an isolated manner as focal SOV. The discovery of SOV involving genital and urinary structures is usually incidental in evaluations for malignant or infectious conditions. To achieve an accurate diagnosis of SOV, a comprehensive evaluation ruling-out systemic vasculitis is warranted since a systemic involvement will always require immunosuppressive therapy. Once the diagnosis of genitourinary SOV is confirmed, the resection of the affected tissue may lead to the resolution of the vasculitic process. With regard to SOV or systemic vasculitis affecting the prostate and urinary structures (ureter, bladder, and urethra), vasculitis lesions may cause urinary tract obstruction at any level, often requiring additional urologic surgical management.

Keywords

Vasculitis · Single-organ vasculitis · Genitourinary vasculitis · Genital · Prostate · Ureter · Bladder · Urethra

J. Hernández-Rodríguez (✉)
Vasculitis Research Unit, Department of Autoimmune Diseases, Hospital Clínic of Barcelona, IDIBAPS, University of Barcelona, Barcelona, Spain
e-mail: jhernan@clinic.cat

G. S. Hoffman
Department of Rheumatic and Immunologic Diseases, Cleveland Clinic, Center for Vasculitis Care and Research, Cleveland, OH, USA

© Springer Nature Switzerland AG 2021
C. Salvarani et al. (eds.), *Large and Medium Size Vessel and Single Organ Vasculitis*, Rare Diseases of the Immune System,
https://doi.org/10.1007/978-3-030-67175-4_19

19.1   Introduction

Single-organ vasculitis (SOV), also known as isolated or localized vasculitis, comprises a group of diseases in which vasculitic involvement is confined to a specific organ, system, or territory [1, 2]. SOV may be divided into focal and diffuse forms [1, 2].

Focal SOV has been described involving the aorta, breast, gallbladder, gastrointestinal tract, and genitourinary structures [2–8]. Focal forms of SOV tend to be incidentally discovered after surgical resection of lesions that were initially suspected to be due to infectious or malignant processes. In most cases, the resection of the lesion satisfactorily eliminates vasculitis and systemic therapy is usually not required [2–8]. However, these patients may require a thorough evaluation to ensure that such focal lesions are not the first manifestation of an underlying systemic disease.

Diffuse or multifocal SOV may affect a single organ in multiple sites, such as the skin [9], central nervous system [10], retina [11], kidneys [12], peripheral nerves [13], calf muscles [14, 15], or coronary and pulmonary vessels [16]. The diffuse nature of the lesions makes surgical resection not feasible. This form of SOV may be chronic and relapsing (e.g., cutaneous vasculitis) or associated with severe morbidity or fatal consequences (e.g., retinal vasculitis, primary central nervous system vasculitis). Thus, diffuse forms of SOV usually require systemic therapy [2, 11].

The names reserved for systemic vasculitides [e.g., polyarteritis nodosa (PAN), giant-cell arteritis (GCA), or granulomatosis with polyangiitis (GPA) (Wegener)] should not be used for isolated vasculitis. Instead, the names for SOV should be descriptive and include the involved organ, vessel type, and histopathology findings. Several examples of this nomenclature include the terms cutaneous arteritis or cutaneous small-vessel vasculitis, ovarian arteritis, or urinary bladder small-vessel vasculitis; with the addition of granulomatous or non-granulomatous to describe the inflammatory pattern [1, 2].

Female and male genital organs and the urinary tract may be involved in systemic vasculitides. However, these structures have also been reported to be affected as SOV. This chapter reviews the main clinical and histological characteristics of SOV involving genitourinary structures (Fig. 19.1).

19.2   Gynecologic Single-Organ Vasculitis

Female genital structures encompass ovaries, fallopian tubes, uterus, vagina, and vulva (Fig. 19.1). These territories may be affected by vasculitis in an isolated manner. The incidence of unanticipated findings of vasculitis among gynecologic surgeries performed for different indications in two large studies ranged from 0.04 to 0.15% [7, 17]. The unexpected finding of vasculitis affecting gynecologic structures is not generally associated with progression to systemic disease [7, 18]. However, very rarely, systemic vasculitides such as GCA may initially present as asymptomatic or painful pelvic masses in the absence of evidence of a systemic disease [7].

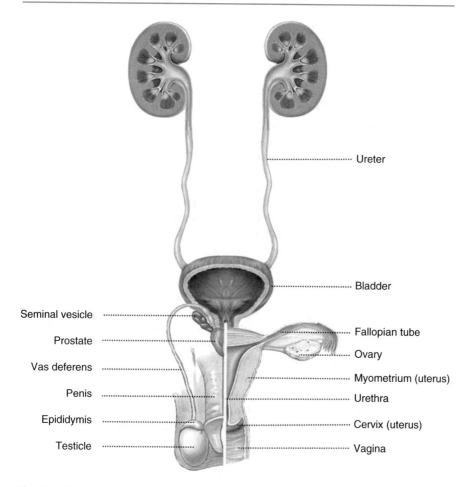

Fig. 19.1 Genitourinary organs involved in systemic and single-organ vasculitis

A retrospective literature review analyzing 163 patients with gynecologic vasculitis (115 with SOV and 48 with systemic vasculitis) provided useful information in characterizing gynecologic SOV [7]. In descending order of frequency, clinical manifestations leading to a diagnosis of gynecologic vasculitis included vaginal bleeding, followed by asymptomatic abdominal masses, uterine prolapse, atypical cervical smear, and pelvic pain [7]. While vasculitis was the only lesion in about a third of the resected specimens, the remaining two third of patients presented with a wide range of concomitant benign and malignant lesions [7]. Some of these adjacent (non-vasculitic) lesions have been histopathologically identified as leiomyomas, myometrial adenomyosis, endometriosis, endometrial carcinoma, chronic salpingitis, cystadenofibroma of fallopian tubes, adenofibroma and carcinoma affecting the ovaries, chronic cervicitis, Nabothian cysts, and cervical squamous metaplasia and carcinoma [7, 18]. While the most common non-vasculitic concomitant benign lesion was leiomyoma, the most prevalent malignant lesion was endometrial carcinoma [7, 18]. Except for benign ovarian abnormalities, which were observed more frequently in systemic vasculitis than in SOV, all the remaining benign and malignant non-vasculitic lesions appear to be similarly present in patients with gynecologic SOV and systemic vasculitis [7].

Several clinical, laboratory, and histopathologic characteristics may contribute in distinguishing isolated from the systemic disease in patients with gynecologic vasculitis [7]. Although patients with gynecologic SOV tend to be younger than those with systemic vasculitis (median age 51 years; range 18–80 years vs. 68 years; 32–83 years), the age range of both groups clearly overlaps and make age not a useful distinction in clinical practice. Compared to patients with systemic involvement, patients with gynecologic SOV are less likely to have fever, constitutional and musculoskeletal symptoms (75% vs. 7%), abnormal erythrocyte sedimentation rates (ESR) (97% vs. 26%), and anemia (80% vs. 17%). Regarding local manifestations, patients with SOV present more often with vaginal bleeding (57% vs. 25%) than patients with a systemic disease. Conversely, asymptomatic pelvic masses appear to be more frequent in systemic vasculitis patients (6% vs. 35%) [7]. The areas of the genital tract affected by vasculitis tend to differ between systemic and SOV forms. While in SOV, the uterus and particularly the cervix are more frequently affected as focal lesions, in systemic diseases, multifocal lesions tend to be present in different territories, mostly ovaries, fallopian tubes, and myometrium [7].

Histopathology of female genital SOV is characterized by a non-granulomatous pattern in the majority (>90%) of patients [7, 18]. However, granulomatous vasculitis has been observed in about two thirds of patients with systemic vasculitis (Fig. 19.2) [7]. With regard to the size of the inflamed vessel, medium and small vessels have been similarly involved in systemic and SOV forms [7].

Patients with gynecologic SOV do not require any treatment beyond the excisional surgical procedure [7, 18]. In this regard, in patients with cervix SOV diagnosed by incisional biopsy (without resection of the whole lesion) and not receiving any systemic therapy, local vasculitis does not tend to evolve to a systemic form [7, 18]. Conversely, almost all patients with a systemic gynecologic vasculitis require glucocorticoid therapy and about one third may receive additional immunosuppressive agents [7].

Among systemic vasculitides, the most frequently reported with gynecologic involvement is GCA, followed by PAN and GPA, and less often, microscopic polyangiitis, cryoglobulinemic vasculitis, and vasculitis associated with rheumatoid arthritis and systemic lupus erythematosus [7]. Of note, up to a third of the reported patients with GCA and gynecologic involvement presented as a silent form, without classic symptoms or signs of GCA, such as craniofacial features, large-vessel involvement, or polymyalgia rheumatica [7, 19]. Therefore, the unexpected finding of a pelvic mass showing granulomatous vasculitis in genital structures in women older than 50 years always warrants to rule out a systemic disease, especially GCA [7].

With regard to vaginal and vulvar vasculitis, vaginal involvement has been sporadically reported as SOV [20] and vasculitis affecting the vulva has been associated with Epstein–Barr virus infection [21], Behçet disease [22], GPA [23], and rheumatoid vasculitis [24].

Fig. 19.2 Histological features in two patients with gynecologic vasculitis. (**a**) Granulomatous vasculitis affecting medium-sized vessels of the ovary with muscular layer destruction (short arrows) and giant cells (long arrow) from a patient with giant cell arteritis. (**b**) Non-granulomatous vasculitis of medium-sized arteries of the cervix, with lymphocytes infiltrating muscular wall (long arrows) and fibrinoid necrosis (short arrow) from a patient with single-organ vasculitis. All samples were stained with hematoxylin-eosin, original magnification ×400

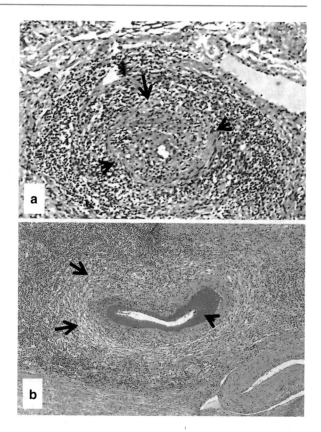

19.3   Male Genital Tract Single-Organ Vasculitis

Structures of the male genital tract include testicles, epididymis, vas deferens, spermatic cords, seminal vesicles, prostate, and penis (Fig. 19.1). Each structure may be affected by vasculitis, either as focal SOV or as part of a systemic vasculitis [8].

19.3.1 Testicles, Epididymis, and Spermatic Cords

The clinical presentation of vasculitis involving the testicles and surrounding structures mostly resembles that of a testicular tumor, local infection, or torsion of the spermatic cord. The incidental finding of vasculitis in testicular surgery is lower than in gynecologic surgery, as illustrated by a large study that found an incidence of 0.003% of unexpected vasculitis in all testicular surgeries [8].

In a review of 72 patients with testicular vasculitis (37 with SOV and 35 with systemic vasculitis), a painful testicular mass or enlarged testicle was the most frequent manifestation, present in about 75% of individuals [8]. Less common symptoms included a painless mass or swelling affecting the testicle or epididymis.

Bilateral involvement has been reported in 15% of patients, and sequential presentation may also occur. Testicular vasculitis has also been discovered after surgical interventions for prostate adenocarcinoma or incomplete testicular descent, or at autopsy [8]. Vasculitic lesions, either in SOV or systemic forms, may occur alone or affect different testicular parts in a multifocal fashion. Among genital structures, the testicle is the territory more frequently affected (80%) by vasculitis, followed by epididymis (45%) and vas deferens/spermatic cord (31%) [8]. Orchiectomy is the most frequent confirmatory procedure for testicular vasculitis, followed by testicular biopsy, and epididymis and spermatic cord resection or biopsy [8].

Patients' age, testicular manifestations, and their duration appear to be similar in patients with SOV and systemic vasculitis. However, compared with systemic vasculitis, patients with SOV presented less often with fever, constitutional and/or musculoskeletal symptoms (74% vs. 8%), elevated ESR (95% vs. 16%), and anemia (50% vs. 0%). The proportion of testicular, epididymis, and vas deferens/spermatic cord vasculitis involvement, and the extent as focal or multifocal vasculitis did not differ between the two groups [8].

Testicular ultrasound with or without Doppler is the imaging technique of choice in most cases of genital abnormalities and commonly detects vasculitic lesions as heterogeneous masses and hypoechoic areas (or both) with normal or decreased vascular flow [8]. Unfortunately, this technique is not able to accurately distinguish vasculitis lesions from testicular neoplasms, infections, or torsion. In addition, vascular signal and ultrasound features do not discriminate between systemic vasculitis and SOV [8].

Non-granulomatous vasculitis involving medium-sized vessels is the predominant histopathologic feature in the majority of patients with either isolated or systemic testicular vasculitis (Fig. 19.3) [8]. With regard to coexistent lesions, testicular carcinoma has been found only in less than 2% of SOV patients [8]. As in gynecologic SOV, concomitant lesions that might trigger isolated vasculitis in the testicular structures have not been identified to be associated to testicular SOV [8].

Compared to patients with systemic vasculitis, those with testicular SOV are most often diagnosed by orchiectomy (43% vs. 81%) and less often by testicular biopsy (29% vs. 3%). These differences may be explained because a malignant lesion has been shown to be more frequently suspected in SOV than in systemic vasculitis patients (74% vs. 32%) [8]. Patients with testicular SOV do not require treatment apart from surgery. By contrast, patients with systemic disease usually require glucocorticoid treatment and more than a half are also treated with additional immunosuppressive drugs [8].

PAN is the systemic condition most frequently associated with testicular vasculitis as PAN accounts for about two thirds of all the reported patients with systemic vasculitis and testicular involvement [8]. Since the initial description of testicular involvement in PAN, in the early 1900s and afterward, testicular vasculitis and PAN have shown a close relationship [8]. Although testicular vasculitis becomes clinically apparent in less than 20% of PAN patients [25, 26], vasculitic lesions in genital structures have been demonstrated in almost all cases at necropsy examination [25]. In 1990, American College of Rheumatology (ACR) classification criteria for PAN, the presence of testicular vasculitis was included as a clinical criterion [27]. However, these criteria have been infrequently used after the 1994 and 2012 Chapel

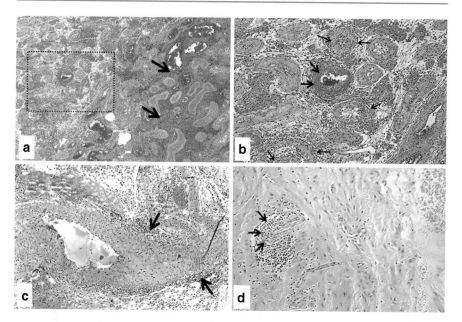

Fig. 19.3 Histological findings in four patients with isolated testicular vasculitis. (**a**) Non-granulomatous (necrotizing) vasculitis involving medium and small vessels in the testicle (square) with infarcted and hemorrhagic testicular tissue (arrows). (**b**) Profuse vasculitic changes with lymphocytic infiltrates (tiny arrows) and a medium-sized artery showing fibrinoid necrosis (thick arrows) from the previous marked area. (**c**) Medium-sized artery with lymphocytic adventitial infiltrates (arrows). (**d**) Small vessel vasculitis with lymphocytes surrounding and infiltrating the vessel wall (arrows). All samples were stained with hematoxylin-eosin, magnification (**a**) ×100, (**b, c**) ×200; and (**d**) ×400

Hill Consensus Conference (CHCC) on the nomenclature and classification of vasculitides. The CHCC nomenclature scheme differentiated hepatitis-B virus (HBV)-associated vasculitis as a secondary form of systemic vasculitis that may also present with testicular vasculitis [1, 28].

Apart from PAN and HBV-associated vasculitis, other systemic vasculitides in which testicular vasculitis may occur include GPA, and less frequently, immunoglobulin A (IgA) vasculitis (Henoch-Schönlein), microscopic polyangiitis, cryoglobulinemic vasculitis, GCA, eosinophilic granulomatosis with polyangiitis (EGPA) (Churg–Strauss) and anti-glomerular basement membrane (anti-GBM) disease (Goodpasture) [8]. Recently, testicular vasculitis has also been described in a patient with deficiency of adenosine deaminase 2 (DADA2), a monogenic autoinflammatory disease that can mimic PAN [29].

19.3.2 Prostate, Seminal Vesicles, and Penis

Prostate SOV has been reported in several patients with symptoms suggestive of urinary obstruction or prostatitis, and biopsies revealed granulomatous vasculitis with eosinophilic infiltrates or necrotizing vasculitis involving prostatic arteries

without apparent disease beyond the prostate [30–32]. In these cases, local abnormalities resolved after glucocorticoid treatment [30–32]. However, a large surgical
study evaluating prostatic specimens from 540 patients with benign prostatic hyperplasia showed lymphocytic vasculitis affecting small to medium-sized arteries in
12.4% of cases. The presence of prostatic infarction was found to be a risk factor
clearly associated with lymphocytic vasculitis. A benign clinical course confirmed
the isolated nature of vasculitis in all cases since surgical excision was the only
therapeutic intervention [33].

Among the systemic vasculitides that may involve the prostate, GPA is the most
common (Fig. 19.4) [34, 35], followed by microscopic polyangiitis [36], EGPA

Fig. 19.4 Prostate
vasculitis in a patient with
granulomatosis with
polyangiitis. (**a**)
Granulomatous infiltrate
with predominance of
histiocytes and plasma
cells. (**b**, **c**) Inflammatory
area with lymphocytic
vasculitis. Lymphocytes
infiltrating the vessel wall
of a small artery in detail
(**c**). All samples were
stained with hematoxylin-
eosin, magnification (**a**, **b**)
×200; and (**c**) ×400

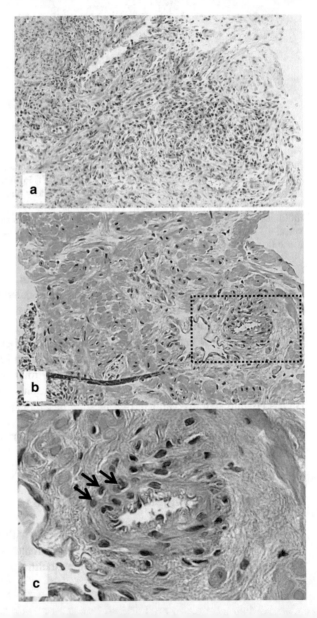

[37], PAN [38], and HBV-associated vasculitis [39]. Local symptoms usually improve after systemic immunosuppressive therapy, but some cases, mainly those with GPA, may require of additional prostate surgery [35–39].

SOV of the seminal vesicles has been described in prostate specimens after radical prostatectomy in two patients who had an associated prostate adenocarcinoma [40]. No cases of seminal vesicle involvement as part of a systemic vasculitis have been reported.

Penile vasculitis has occurred as ulcerations and ischemic lesions of the glans, for which a malignant lesion is frequently suspected. In addition, it has also been described as periurethral aseptic abscesses developing urethral-cutaneous fistula. While only one clear case of penis SOV has been reported [41], most penile vasculitis have been associated with systemic vasculitides, in particular with GPA [34, 35, 42, 43], but also with PAN [44, 45], IgA vasculitis [46], lupus-associated vasculitis [47], Behçet disease [48], and Buerger's disease [49]. Systemic treatment is warranted in all patients with systemic vasculitis [34, 35, 42–48], and penile resection has been required in some cases [35, 49].

19.4 Urinary Tract Single-Organ Vasculitis

Ureter, urinary bladder, and urethra are the three segments of the urinary tract (Fig. 19.1), which can be infrequently involved in systemic vasculitides. The unexpected discovery of SOV in the urinary tract has been anecdotal. Vasculitic lesions affecting urinary structures, either isolated or as part of a systemic vasculitis, may be associated with a significant risk of obstruction and secondary renal failure.

19.4.1 Ureters

Vasculitis involving the ureter is usually found after the development of obstructive hydronephrosis secondary to ureter stricture or blockade caused by an inflammatory thickening of the ureteral wall. Endoscopic surgical procedures are often required to restore urine flow. SOV involving the ureter in the absence of a systemic disease has been seldom reported [50–52]. Systemic vasculitides involving the ureter include GPA [34, 35], PAN [53–55], EGPA [53], and IgA vasculitis [56, 57].

19.4.2 Urinary Bladder

Urinary bladder vasculitis has been rarely reported in both SOV and systemic vasculitis. The risk of bladder cancer is the primary concern in patients with prior exposure to cyclophosphamide [58].

A clear case of isolated bladder vasculitis was described in a patient who was apparently cured after a partial resection of the lesion without receiving any medical treatment [59]. Other cases reported as bladder SOV should be considered as nonconsistent SOV since they were additionally treated with prednisone alone [60] or in combination with cytotoxic drugs [61, 62]. Systemic vasculitides in which bladder involvement has been occasionally diagnosed include GPA [34, 42], EGPA [63], PAN [64, 65], HBV-associated vasculitis [62], IgA vasculitis [57], and Behçet disease [66].

Clinical manifestations of urinary bladder vasculitis, either systemic or SOV, are diverse and include macroscopic hematuria [57, 59–62], obstructive manifestations [62, 65], and cystitis [60, 63]. The development of vesico-vaginal fistula has been described in GPA [42] and neurogenic bladder may be caused by a necrotizing vasculitis involving medium-sized arteries of the perivesicular fat in patients with PAN [64].

Imaging techniques or cystoscopy may reveal abnormalities of the bladder wall or mucosa, including a thickened or irregular wall or vesical mass [34, 59–62, 65] and a diffuse erythematous mucosa suggesting transitional cell carcinoma in situ [60, 62]. All patients reported with bladder involvement and systemic vasculitis were treated with glucocorticoids and additional immunosuppressive drugs [34, 42, 57, 62–66].

19.4.3 Urethra

The urethra has been very rarely associated with a localized form of granulomatous vasculitis. On the one hand, in cases reported as urethral SOV, GPA was considered as the possible diagnosis and systemic immunosuppressive therapy was administered with control of local disease [20, 67]. On the other hand, GPA has been reported as the most common cause of urethral vasculitis [20, 42, 43, 68], followed by sporadic cases associated with EGPA [69], PAN [70], Kawasaki disease [71], and Behçet disease [48]. In all cases, urethral vasculitis was manifested as urethral obstruction, and systemic and surgical therapy were always provided [20, 42, 43, 48, 68–71].

19.5   Conclusions

Gynecologic, testicular, prostate, and urinary structures may be involved in different systemic vasculitides. In addition, these organs may be occasionally affected in an isolated manner as focal SOV. The discovery of SOV involving genital and urinary structures is usually incidental in evaluations for malignant or infectious conditions. To achieve an accurate diagnosis of SOV, a comprehensive evaluation ruling-out systemic vasculitis is warranted since a systemic involvement will always require systemic immunosuppressive therapy. Once the diagnosis of genitourinary SOV is confirmed, the resection of the affected tissue may lead to the resolution of the vasculitic process. With regard to SOV or systemic vasculitis affecting the prostate and urinary structures (ureter, bladder, and urethra), vasculitis lesions may cause urinary tract obstruction at any level, often requiring additional urologic surgical management.

References

1. Jennette JC, Falk RJ, Bacon PA, et al. 2012 revised International Chapel Hill Consensus Conference Nomenclature of Vasculitides. Arthritis Rheum. 2013;65:1–11.
2. Hernández-Rodríguez J, Hoffman GS. Updating single-organ vasculitis. Curr Opin Rheumatol. 2012;24:38–45.
3. Rojo-Leyva F, Ratliff NB, Cosgrove DM 3rd, Hoffman GS. Study of 52 patients with idiopathic aortitis from a cohort of 1,204 surgical cases. Arthritis Rheum. 2000;43:901–7.
4. Hernández-Rodríguez J, Tan CD, Molloy ES, Khasnis A, Rodríguez ER, Hoffman GS. Vasculitis involving the breast: a clinical and histopathologic analysis of 34 patients. Medicine (Baltimore). 2008;87:61–9.
5. Hernández-Rodríguez J, Tan CD, Rodriguez ER, Hoffman GS. Single-organ gallbladder vasculitis: characterization and distinction from systemic vasculitis involving the gallbladder. An analysis of 61 patients. Medicine (Baltimore). 2014;93:405–13.
6. Salvarani C, Calamia KT, Crowson CS, et al. Localized vasculitis of the gastrointestinal tract: a case series. Rheumatology (Oxford). 2010;49:1326–35.
7. Hernández-Rodríguez J, Tan CD, Rodríguez ER, Hoffman GS. Gynecologic vasculitis: an analysis of 163 patients. Medicine (Baltimore). 2009;88:169–81.
8. Hernández-Rodríguez J, Tan CD, Koening CL, Khasnis A, Rodríguez ER, Hoffman GS. Testicular vasculitis: findings differentiating isolated from systemic disease in 72 patients. Medicine (Baltimore). 2012;91(2):75–85.
9. Diaz-Perez JL, De Lagran ZM, Diaz-Ramon JL, Winkelmann RK. Cutaneous polyarteritis nodosa. Semin Cutan Med Surg. 2007;26:77–86.
10. Calabrese LH, Mallek JA. Primary angiitis of the central nervous system. Report of 8 new cases, review of the literature, and proposal for diagnostic criteria. Medicine (Baltimore). 1988;67:20–39.
11. Pelegrín L, Hernández-Rodríguez J, Espinosa G, et al. Characterization of isolated retinal vasculitis. Analysis of a cohort from a single center and literature review. Autoimmun Rev. 2017;16:237–43.
12. Weidner S, Geuss S, Hafezi-Rachti S, Wonka A, Rupprecht HD. ANCA-associated vasculitis with renal involvement: an outcome analysis. Nephrol Dial Transplant. 2004;19:1403–11.
13. Puechal X, Said G. Necrotizing vasculitis of the peripheral nervous system: nonsystemic or clinically undetectable? Arthritis Rheum. 1999;42:824–5.
14. García F, Pedrol E, Casademont J, et al. Polyarteritis nodosa confined to calf muscles. J Rheumatol. 1992;19:303–5.
15. Khellaf M, Hamidou M, Pagnoux C, et al. Vasculitis restricted to the lower limbs: a clinical and histopathological study. Ann Rheum Dis. 2007;66:554–6.
16. Lie JT. Pathology of isolated nonclassical and catastrophic manifestations of Takayasu arteritis. Int J Cardiol. 1998;66(Suppl 1):S11–21.
17. Ganesan R, Ferryman SR, Meier L, Rollason TP. Vasculitis of the female genital tract with clinicopathologic correlation: a study of 46 cases with follow-up. Int J Gynecol Pathol. 2000;19:258–65.
18. Roma AA, Amador-Ortiz C, Liapis H. Significance of isolated vasculitis in the gynecological tract: what clinicians do with the pathologic diagnosis of vasculitis? Ann Diagn Pathol. 2014;18:199–202.
19. Besse MC, Collercandy N, Diot E. Gynecologic vasculitis: positron emission tomography-computed tomography contribution in a rare localization of giant cell arteritis. J Rheumatol. 2019;46:439.
20. Soro Marin S, Judez Navarro E, Sianes Fernandez M, Sanchez Nievas G, Romero JG. An unusual presentation of limited granulomatosis with polyangiitis involving vagina and urethra. Case Rep Rheumatol. 2017;2017:9407675.
21. Barrett MM, Sangueza M, Werner B, Kutzner H, Carlson JA. Lymphocytic arteritis in Epstein-Barr virus vulvar ulceration (Lipschutz disease): a report of 7 cases. Am J Dermatopathol. 2015;37:691–8.

22. Chun SI, Su WP, Lee S. Histopathologic study of cutaneous lesions in Behcet's syndrome. J Dermatol. 1990;17:333–41.
23. Lewis FM. Vulvar involvement in Wegener's granulomatosis. A case report. J Reprod Med. 2002;47:725–7.
24. Appleton MA, Ismail SM. Ulcerating rheumatoid nodule of the vulva. J Clin Pathol. 1996;49:85–7.
25. Dahl EV, Baggenstoss AH, Deweerd JH. Testicular lesions of periarteritis nodosa, with special reference to diagnosis. Am J Med. 1960;28:222–8.
26. Pagnoux C, Seror R, Henegar C, et al. Clinical features and outcomes in 348 patients with polyarteritis nodosa: a systematic retrospective study of patients diagnosed between 1963 and 2005 and entered into the French Vasculitis Study Group Database. Arthritis Rheum. 2010;62:616–26.
27. Lightfoot RW Jr, Michel BA, Bloch DA, et al. The American College of Rheumatology 1990 criteria for the classification of polyarteritis nodosa. Arthritis Rheum. 1990;33:1088–93.
28. Jennette JC, Falk RJ, Andrassy K, et al. Nomenclature of systemic vasculitides. Proposal of an international consensus conference. Arthritis Rheum. 1994;37:187–92.
29. Clarke K, Campbell C, Omoyinmi E, et al. Testicular ischemia in deficiency of adenosine deaminase 2 (DADA2). Pediatr Rheumatol Online J. 2019;17:39.
30. Bretal-Laranga M, Insua-Vilarino S, Blanco-Rodriguez J, Caamano-Freire M, Mera-Varela A, Lamas-Cedron P. Giant cell arteritis limited to the prostate. J Rheumatol. 1995;22:566–8.
31. Yonker RA, Katz P. Necrotizing granulomatous vasculitis with eosinophilic infiltrates limited to the prostate. Case report and review of the literature. Am J Med. 1984;77:362–4.
32. Kopolovic J, Rivkind A, Sherman Y. Granulomatous prostatitis with vasculitis. A sequel to transurethral prostatic resection. Arch Pathol Lab Med. 1984;108:732–3.
33. Lopez-Beltran A, Vidal A, Montironi R, et al. Lymphocytic vasculitis of the prostate transition zone. BJU Int. 2012;110:1775–80.
34. Huong DL, Papo T, Piette JC, et al. Urogenital manifestations of Wegener granulomatosis. Medicine (Baltimore). 1995;74:152–61.
35. Dufour JF, Le Gallou T, Cordier JF, et al. Urogenital manifestations in Wegener granulomatosis: a study of 11 cases and review of the literature. Medicine (Baltimore). 2012;91:67–74.
36. Lamarche JA, Peguero AM, Rosario JO, Patel A, Courville C. Anti-MPO small-vessel vasculitis causing prostatis and nephritis. Clin Exp Nephrol. 2007;11:180–3.
37. Kiyokawa H, Koyama M, Kato H. Churg-Strauss syndrome presenting with eosinophilic prostatitis. Int J Urol. 2006;13:838–40.
38. Gonzalez-La Riviere O, de la Torre-Rendon F, Hernandez-Vasquez R, Arce-Salinas CA. Polyarteritis nodosa mimicking prostatic cancer. J Rheumatol. 2000;27:2504–6.
39. Cheatum DE, Sowell DS 3rd, Dulany RB. Hepatitis B antigen-associated periarteritis nodosa with prostatic vasculitis. Diagnosis by needle biopsy. Arch Intern Med. 1981;141:107–8.
40. Argani P, Carter HB, Epstein JI. Isolated vasculitis of the seminal vesicle. Urology. 1998;52:131–3.
41. Rubio FA, Robayna G, Herranz P, De Lucas R, Garcia-Jimenez JA, Casado M. Necrotizing vasculitis of the glans penis. Br J Dermatol. 1999;140:756–7.
42. Davenport A, Downey SE, Goel S, Maciver AG. Wegener's granulomatosis involving the urogenital tract. Br J Urol. 1996;78:354–7.
43. Ebo DG, Mertens AV, De Clerck LS, Gentens P, Daelemans R. Relapse of Wegener's granulomatosis presenting as a destructive urethritis and penile ulceration. Clin Rheumatol. 1998;17:239–41.
44. Watanabe K, Nanki T, Sugihara T, Miyasaka N. A case of polyarteritis nodosa with periurethralaseptic abscesses and testicular lesions. Clin Exp Rheumatol. 2008;26:1113–5.
45. Karademir K, Senkul T, Atasoyu E, Yildirim S, Nalbant S. Ulcerative necrosis of the glans penis resulting from polyarteritis nodosa. J Clin Rheumatol. 2005;11:167–9.
46. Sandell J, Ramanan R, Shah D. Penile involvement in Henoch-Schonlein purpura. Indian J Pediatr. 2002;69:529–30.
47. Tripp BM, Chu F, Halwani F, Hassouna MM. Necrotizing vasculitis of the penis in systemic lupus erythematosus. J Urol. 1995;154:528–9.

48. Ghosh S, Kumar M, Kumari P, Gadpayle AK. Acquired urethral meatal stenosis: a rare sequel of an aggressive form of Behcet's disease. BMJ Case Rep. 2013;2013:bcr2013009344.
49. Pham KN, Sokoloff MH, Steiger CA. Severe gangrene at the glans penis requiring penectomy as the first major complication of Buerger's disease. Am J Clin Exp Urol. 2016;4:9–11.
50. Duclos JM, Bensadoun H, Herreman G, Baviera E. [Pseudotumor of the ureter manifesting periarteritis nodosa]. Ann Urol (Paris). 1984;18:418–9.
51. Goodman GR, Woodside JR, Slichenmyer WJ. Chronic vasculitis causing unilateral ureteral stenosis. Urology. 1988;32:354–6.
52. Kamar N, Malavaud B, Alric L, et al. Ureteral stenosis as the sole manifestation of Wegener's granulomatosis. Urology. 2003;62:352.
53. Azar N, Guillevin L, Huong Du LT, Herreman G, Meyrier A, Godeau P. Symptomatic uro-genital manifestations of polyarteritis nodosa and Churg-Strauss angiitis: analysis of 8 of 165 patients. J Urol. 1989;142:136–8.
54. Bolat D, Zumrutbas AE, Baser A, Tuncay L. Spontaneous ureteral rupture in a patient with polyarteritis nodosa. Int Urol Nephrol. 2016;48:223–4.
55. Bulbuloglu E, Kantarceken B, Yuksel M, Ciralik H, Sahinkanat T, Kale IT. An unusual presentation of polyarteritis nodosa: a case report. West Indian Med J. 2006;55:56–9.
56. Dalpiaz A, Schwamb R, Miao Y, Gonka J, Walzter W, Khan SA. Urological manifestations of Henoch-Schonlein purpura: a review. Curr Urol. 2015;8:66–73.
57. Siegenthaler GM, Rizzi M, Bettinelli A, Simonetti GD, Ferrarini A, Bianchetti MG. Ureteral or vesical involvement in Henoch-Schonlein syndrome: a systematic review of the literature. Pediatr Nephrol. 2014;29:235–9.
58. Hellmich B, Kausch I, Doehn C, Jocham D, Holl-Ulrich K, Gross WL. Urinary bladder cancer in Wegener's granulomatosis: is it more than cyclophosphamide? Ann Rheum Dis. 2004;63:1183–5.
59. Kassir R, Mouracade P, Barabino G, Peoc'h M, Cuilleron M, Gigante M. Vasculitis of the bladder: an extremely rare case report. Int J Surg Case Rep. 2013;4:782–4.
60. Katz DJ, Sengupta S, Snow RM. Isolated vasculitis of the bladder. Urology. 2005;65:797.
61. Fall M, Hoper L, Kabjorn-Gustafsson C, Trysberg E. Isolated vasculitis of the urinary bladder: a note on diagnosis and prognosis. Scand J Urol. 2018;52:230–1.
62. Fischer AH, Wallace VL, Keane TE, Clarke HS. Two cases of vasculitis of the urinary bladder: diagnostic and pathogenetic considerations. Arch Pathol Lab Med. 1998;122:903–6.
63. Heers H, Ramaswamy A, Hofmann R. A case of Churg-Strauss syndrome (eosinophilic granulomatosis with polyangiitis) of the urinary bladder. Urology. 2017;108:7–10.
64. Amarenco P, Amarenco G, Baudrimont M, Roullet E, Marteau R. Bladder neuropathy in periarteritis nodosa. Ann Intern Med. 1989;110:411–2.
65. Borkum M, Abdelrahman HY, Roberts R, Kalla AA, Okpechi IG. Polyarteritis nodosa presenting as a bladder outlet obstruction. S Afr Med J. 2016;106:1086–7.
66. Cetinel B, Akpinar H, Tufek I, Uygun N, Solok V, Yazici H. Bladder involvement in Behcet's syndrome. J Urol. 1999;161:52–6.
67. Dore B, Duriez P, Grange P, Aubert J. [Wegener's granulomatosis with urethral-penile location. Apropos of a case]. Ann Urol (Paris). 1990;24:256–8.
68. Anderson PT, Gottheil S, Gabril M, Barra L, Power N. Acute urinary retention secondary to urethral involvement of granulomatosis with polyangiitis. Can Urol Assoc J. 2017;11:E38–40.
69. Walsh I, Loughridge WG, Keane PF. Eosinophilic vasculitis (Churg-Strauss syndrome) involving the urethra. Br J Urol. 1994;74:255–6.
70. Giannarini G, Pomara G, Moro U, et al. Isolated polyarteritis nodosa of the genitourinary tract presenting with severe erectile dysfunction: a case report with long-term follow-up. J Sex Med. 2009;6:1189–93.
71. Watanabe T, Abe Y, Sato S, Uehara Y, Ikeno K, Abe T. Sterile pyuria in patients with Kawasaki disease originates from both the urethra and the kidney. Pediatr Nephrol. 2007;22:987–91.

Arterial and Venous Involvement in Behçet's Disease

20

Fatma Alibaz-Oner and Haner Direskeneli

Abstract

Behçet's disease (BD) is a chronic, multisystemic, inflammatory disease characterized by recurrent attacks of mucocutaneous, ocular, musculoskeletal, vascular, central nervous system and gastrointestinal manifestations. Vascular involvement is observed in up to 40% of the patients with BD, especially in young males and is one of the major causes of mortality and morbidity. Both venous and arterial disease is observed. Glucocorticoids, azathioprine and cyclophosphamide are recommended as the first-line treatments in vascular BD (VBD). But increasing data with TNF inhibitors and interferons suggest that these agents may also be acceptable options for the management of refractory cases. Anticoagulant usage is still controversial with limited data coming from retrospective studies. There is a clear need for randomized, controlled studies for the management of VBD.

Keywords

Arterial thrombosis · Aneursyms · Venous thrombosis

Behçet's disease (BD) is a systemic inflammatory disease characterized by oral and genital ulcers, ocular manifestations, and systemic involvement including gastrointestinal, musculoskeletal, neurological systems, and major vessels. Vasculitis is one of the main pathological findings in BD. Vessels of all sizes can be involved both in the arterial and venous systems [1, 2].

F. Alibaz-Oner · H. Direskeneli (✉)
Division of Rheumatology, Department of Internal Medicine, Marmara University, School of Medicine, Istanbul, Turkey

© Springer Nature Switzerland AG 2021
C. Salvarani et al. (eds.), *Large and Medium Size Vessel and Single Organ Vasculitis*, Rare Diseases of the Immune System,
https://doi.org/10.1007/978-3-030-67175-4_20

20.1 Epidemiology

Vascular involvement is seen in the range of 15–50% in BD [3]. It is more commonly observed in Middle-Eastern and Northern African countries such as Turkey, Jordan, Israel, Iran, Morocco, Algeria, and South European countries with immigrant populations such as France, whereas observed quite rare in East Asia such as Japan (<10%) [4] and Korea (<5%) [5]. While venous involvement consists of 67–84% of all vascular manifestations [6, 7], arterial involvement rate is below 15% in all series [8]. Lower extremity deep vein thrombosis (DVT) is the most frequent form of vascular involvement. Although venous thrombosis is seen primarily in the lower extremities, it may affect many different sites including the inferior and superior vena cava, pulmonary artery, suprahepatic vessels, and cardiac cavities. In BD patients, vascular involvement is one of the major causes of mortality and morbidity, up to 17% of the mortality in BD is reported to be associated with vascular involvement such as pulmonary embolism or Budd-Chiari syndrome (BCS) [9]. More than 80% of patients with vascular Behçet disease (VBD) are males [10]. Males also had more severe disease course [6, 7].

Vascular involvement can develop before fulfilling International Study Group (ISG) Criteria for BD in up to 10% of the patients. In this group, the most frequent type of involvement is DVT (86.8%). In about 20% of the patients, vascular involvement develops at disease-onset. After the diagnosis, median time to first vascular event was found to be 1.4 years in a large VBD cohort from Turkey. In majority of the patients (74.6%), first vascular event developed within 5 years after disease-onset. While DVT and cerebral sinus thrombosis develop earlier within median 1 year after disease-onset, pulmonary artery involvement, vena cava thrombosis, and BCS develop within a few years of disease-onset. Non-pulmonary arterial involvement seems to develop at later ages within a median of 5 years during the disease course [6].

20.2 Pathology

BD is a unique systemic vasculitis involving both arterial and venous vessels of all sizes. It is defined as *"variable vessel vasculitis"* in CHCC in 2012 due to atypical histological and clinical features of BD [11]. It mainly affects venous rather than arterial vessels in contrast to other systemic vasculitides. Inflammation in venous vessels leads significant thrombotic tendency which appears to be unrelated to thrombophilic factors [8]. On the other hand, arterial vessel inflammation leads the tendency for aneurysm formation in especially pulmonary arteries having less elastic and thinner vessel wall and lower intraluminal pressure similar to venous vessels. Arterial disease can also rarely manifest with thrombotic occlusions. Features of arterial involvement are also quite different from other large-vessel vasculitis leading to homogenous, concentric wall thickness [12]. The entire aorta is macroscopically rough and wrinkled indicating scattered aortitis. Loss or interruption of medial elastic fibers are present together with the perivascular lymphocytic infiltration and proliferation of vasa vasorum [13]. There is irregular fibrous thickening in all layers and focal aneurysmal dilatation in aortic involvement [14]. Aneurysms were seen mostly in abdominal aorta, but may also be present in arcus aorta and the other large arteries. Aneurysms mostly had saccular or fusiform shape and are filled with a thick thrombus with lamellar structure [15]. While fibrous thickening of adventitia and the proliferation of the vasa vasorum are seen in chronic large-vessel involvement, occlusion, and stenosis are mostly observed in medium or smaller arteries not having prominent changes in vasa vasorum. When inflamed vessel is not thrombosed, inflammation leads to the weakening in the arterial wall, resulting in pseudoaneurysms [16]. As cardiac involvement, histopathology shows an organizing intracardiac thrombus formation with mononuclear inflammatory cell infiltration with or without involvement of the underlying cardiac tissue [17].

Sticky and organized thrombi in the inflamed vessel wall is the main pathologic feature of venous involvement. The mechanisms underlying the thrombotic tendency in BD is still unknown. In the inflamed vessel wall, there is an occlusive inflammatory thrombus development, strictly adherent to vessel wall. This thrombus formation is typically not complicated by thromboembolism [14, 18, 19]. The other pathological change is leukocytoclastic vasculitis in veins, venules, capillaries, and arterioles. Vessel wall is invaded by neutrophils and fibrinoid necrosis, leukocytoclasis, endothelial swelling, and erythrocyte extravasation is present. Lymphocytic vasculitis may also be less commonly seen in BD [20].

20.3 Pathophysiology

There is no specific defect in the coagulation cascade in BD pateints with thrombosis [21]. But increased levels of thrombin-antithrombin III complex and prothrombin fragments 1 + 2 support intravascular thrombin generation in these patients as a result of the activation of the coagulation cascade. Various procoagulant conditions associated with an increased risk of thrombosis such as deficiencies of protein C, protein S and antithrombin III, factor V Leiden, and prothrombin 20210A mutations, may contribute to the prothrombotic state of BD. Several fold increases in the risk of thrombosis was reported in carriers of factor V Leiden and prothrombin gene mutations in patients with BD, especially in series from Turkey [22]. A meta-analysis suggested that increased homocysteine levels are also more prominent in BD patients with thrombosis and may be considered to be associated with thrombosis in BD [23]. Anticardiolipin antibodies do not seem to be important in the thrombotic tendency of BD [24]. In a small study from Turkey, combined thrombophilias were higher in BD patients with recurrent thrombotic events compared to patients with only one thrombotic event [25]. The cumulative evidence suggests that the pathogenesis of thrombosis in BD is probably not due to a hypercoagulable state but rather to the vascular damage induced by inflammation or intrinsic endothelial dysfunction. The vascular damage may serve as a source of thrombogenic stimuli [26–28].

Neutrophils and lymphocytes are the dominant inflammatory cells in histopathologic samples of BD. These cells are mainly localized around the vessel wall rather than inside the wall. Mainly neutrophilic perivascular inflammation pattern was demonstrated in vascular manifestations similar to cutaneous manifestations [29–31]. The role of neutrophils was first suggested by Matsumura et al. in 1975. This study showed a prominent high chemotactic activity of neutrophils in BD [32]. It was suggested that HLA-B*51 probably contributes to the neutrophil hyperactivation in BD [33]. Cytokine levels, such as CXCL8 and G-CSF having important role in neutrophil recruitment and activation, were found higher in active BD [34, 35]. In another study from Turkey, testosterone is shown to activate neutrophils in male BD patients, suggesting the role of gender in severe manifestations [36].

Neutrophils generate neutrophil extracellular traps (NETs) by a distinct process of cell death termed "NETosis" during inflammatory or infectious conditions. NETs consist of extruded cell-free DNA with histones and granular components and also contain antimicrobial peptides and proteases [37]. NETs were found in many autoimmune diseases including rheumatoid arthritis, systemic lupus erythematosus, and anti-neutrophil cytoplasmic antibodies-associated vasculitis [38]. NETs are also suggested as a key trigger of thrombus initiation and progression in deep vein thrombosis [39]. In a recent study, it was shown that neutrophils of BD patients are prone to undergo NETosis in vitro even without stimulation. The level of NETs were found significantly increased in active BD compared to inactives and were also higher in vascular BD, suggesting that NETs may contribute to the vascular disease pathogenesis and thrombosis in VBD [40].

Mechanisms other than NETosis are also implicated for the role of neutrophils during thrombosis in BD. Increased leukocyte oxidative stress and reactive oxygen species (ROS) generation from neutrophils lead to reduced fibrin susceptibility to plasmin lysis and post-translational modifications (carbonylation) of fibrinogen [41]. It is well known that there is a strict relationship among inflammation, endothelial dysfunction, and oxidative stress [42]. It was also shown that neutrophils activation has important roles in inducing platelet activation, affecting the anti-thrombotic function of the endothelium and inhibiting response to fibrinolytic agents and tissue factor carriage [43, 44]. Moreover, neutrophil ROS via NADPH oxidase modify fibrinogen structure promoting changes in fibrinogen function and lead to a clot with tight fibrin network and resistant to plasmin-induced lysis [45]. All these findings explain why the thrombus in BD is responsive to immunosuppressive treatment rather than anticoagulants.

Microparticles (MPs) are sub-micronic vesicles forming during budding from the cell membrane of any cell type in response to cellular activity or apoptosis. They can be formed as circulating MPs or MPs generated within tissues. They can participate in the maintenance of organ or vascular homeostasis as well as inducing dysfunction according to the their cellular origin. MPs are suggested to have procoagulant properties [46]. Increased MPs are shown in BD [47, 48] Khan E et al. also observed that BD patients had increased MPs expressing tissue factor compared to healthy controls. Furthermore, BD patients with thrombosis history had higher MPs expressing tissue factor in BD. These findings may add additional association between inflammation and thrombosis in BS [49].

20.4 Clinical Features and Prognosis of Venous Involvement

20.4.1 Deep Vein Thrombosis of Lower Extremities

DVT in lower extremity is the most common manifestation of vascular involvement in BD, observed in approximately 70% [7]. Femoral (superficial, deep, and common) and popliteal veins are the most frequently involved veins and are followed by crural, external iliac, and common iliac veins. When compared to DVT associated with non-BD reasons, bilateral involvement, less complete recanalization, and more collateral development are more frequent in VBD [50, 51]. Despite immunosuppressive (IS) treatment, about one third of patients relapse during follow-up [6, 7]. In a prospective follow-up of 33 patients with DVT in lower extremities, relapse rates were 29%, 37%, and 45% at 6, 12, and 24 months, respectively. In this study, poor recanalization was the only predictor factor for relapse [52]. Post-thrombotic syndrome (PTS) is the most frequent complication of DVT and is associated with varying combinations of leg pain, heaviness, swelling, edema, hyperpigmentation, and varicose collateral veins. In severe cases, lipodermatosclerosis and venous ulcers may also occur [53]. Presence of PTS effects quality of life (QoL) negatively [54]. PTS is observed in up to 64% of BD with DVT. Severe PTS rate is 10%. Venous disease-associated QoL is also impaired in BD when assessed with Venous Insufficiency Epidemiological and Economic Study Quality of Life/Symptom (VEINES-QoL/Sym) questionnaire [55]. Successful control of BD activity might decrease the development of PTS, improve venous disease-specific QoL, and prevent relapses in VBD [49]. As majority of VBD patients are young males who are an active population both in work and daily life, prevention of PTS should be a key target in the management of VBD patients. In another study, severe PTS was found significantly higher in BD compared to DVT associated with non-BD reasons. However, majority of BD patients were male (71 vs 7) in this study, whereas half of DVT associated with non-BD reasons group was female (29 vs 27), and this gender difference might have influenced the results [48].

Leg ulcers are the sign of severe PTS, and they should be differentiated from pyoderma gangrenosum and vasculitic lesions in BD [56]. A recent survey reported that half of the leg ulcers in BD were refractory to standard treatments [57].

20.4.2 Venous Wall Thickness in Behçet's Disease

Despite the dominance of veins in vascular involvement, limited data is present for the assessment of veins in BD. In a magnetic resonance imaging study, Ambrose N et al. first demonstrated increased vein wall thickness (VWT) in popliteal veins of BD patients [58]. Boulon C. et al. later published the findings of a vascular BD case presenting with acute calf pain (without thrombosis) by venous Doppler ultrasound (US). Increased VWT in right great saphenous vein was reported in this case which decreased after corticosteroid (CS) treatment [59]. Our group recently published the first controlled Doppler US study showing increased VWT of lower extremity veins in male BD patients. When common femoral vein (CFV), the largest of lower extremity veins, was chosen as the primary site of US assessment, cut-off values for right and left CFV ≥0.5 mm had high area under the receiver operating characteristic (ROC) curves (>0.8) with sensitivities of 81–82.8% and specificities of 78.4–81.1%. Positive (PPV) and negative predictive values (NPV) in our tertiary clinical setting were also acceptable (PPV: 85.7–87.5%, NPV: 72.5–75%) [60, 61]. Our observations were also confirmed in another study by Seyahi E et al. from Turkey [62]. We recently investigated further the *diagnostic performance* of CFV thickness using Doppler US as an easy and fast method in BD, compared to multiple disease controls. Increased CFV thickness was observed as a distinctive feature of BD which is rarely present in healthy and other inflammatory or vascular diseased controls such as ankylosing spondylitis, systemic vasculitides, venous insufficiency, and non-inflammatory DVT, with the exception of APS. The cut-off value of ≥0.5 mm, determined in our first study, performed quite well against all control groups with a sensitivity >90%. The specificities were also found >80% compared to all control groups, except APS. Values especially higher than 0.75 mm seem to indicate a very high probability of BD. (Alibaz-Oner F, et al. Rheumatology (Oxford), in press).

20.4.3 Thrombosis of Superior and Inferior Vena Cava

Thrombosis of vena cava (VC) superior and inferior consists of 9% and 8% of major vessel manifestations in BD, respectively [6, 7]. They are generally associated with other vascular involvements such as BCS, pulmonary artery involvement, and cerebral sinus thrombosis [6, 63, 64]. Thrombosis in VC superior can cause VC superior syndrome (VCSS) which presents with swelling and cyanosis of the face, neck, and upper extremities and prominent venous collaterals in the area drained by the VC superior. VCSS in BD has generally a benign course due to venous collateral development [8]. It may rarely be complicated with pleural effusion, chylothorax, and mediastinal fibrosis [65]. Thrombosis in VC inferior is divided into three anatomical sites as infrahepatic, hepatic, and suprahepatic. Hepatic and suprahepatic VC inferior thrombosis cause BCS. Infrahepatic part is most commonly involved due to the extension of the lower extremity DVT. If there is bilateral common femoral vein thrombosis in BD, iliac vein thrombosis was seen in 50% and VC inferior thrombosis was seen in 20% of these patients. Lower back or abdominal pain may be seen during the acute presentation. Collateral presentation of abdominal veins is a typical sign. Swelling and ulcers in legs and scrotum may also be seen. VC inferior thrombosis often develops insidiously except in the presence of BCS [8].

20.4.4 Budd-Chiari Syndrome

Budd-Chiari syndrome is a rare manifestation of BD. The frequency is below 5% among all vascular manifestations; however, it is the most lethal complication among all vascular manifestations [8]. In a retrospective survey of 43 BCS with BD, two different clinical presentations were reported as "symptomatic" and "silent" presentations. In symptomatic presentation, patients may present with abdominal pain, ascites, collaterals on the abdominal wall, edema on the scrotum, and diffuse swelling in the lower extremities—together with the signs of hepatic failure such as jaundice, encephalopathy, splenomegaly, hypersplenism, and bleeding from esophageal varices. In patients presenting with ascites, the mortality rate is up to 60% within a median of 10 months after the diagnosis. In silent presentation, BCS develops insidiously without ascites or any other symptoms associated with liver failure. The patient is usually diagnosed with efficient collateral formation. The mortality rate is expected to be <10% in patients with silent presentation. When compared to BCS with non-BD reasons, younger age, male predominance, and occlusion of the VC inferior are more frequent in BCS with BD. No effect of anticoagulation or thrombolytic therapy is observed on mortality [66]. In two other case series, mortality was reported below 20% during follow-up [67, 68].

20.4.5 Cerebral Sinus Thrombosis

Cerebral sinus thrombosis (CST) consists of approximately one third of neurologic involvement of BD, again mainly seen in males [69]. In a large CST cohort from Turkey, BD as an etiological factor was present in 108 (9.4%) of 1144 patients. Transverse sinuses were the most common sites of thrombosis, followed by the superior sagittal sinuses [70]. It generally presents signs and symptoms of intracranial hypertension such as headache and papilledema. Fever and nausea/vomiting can be seen in about one fifth of patients. Seizure and confusion can rarely be seen. CST is strongly associated with peripheral vascular involvement in BD [71]. Prognosis is good in CST with BD. In a retrospective study, 90% of patients responded well to the treatment within 1 month [72]. In a systematic review including 290 cases of CST, a good response was achieved in more than half of the patients whereas a sequelae developed in 20%. Most frequent sequelae were optic nerve atrophy and blindness/reduced visual acuity. There was no mortality except one case due to suicide [73].

20.5 Clinical Features and Prognosis of Arterial Involvement

20.5.1 Pulmonary Arterial Involvement

Despite being the most frequent form of arterial involvement, pulmonary arterial involvement (PAI) rate is only 5–10% among all vascular manifestations. It affects mainly males [7, 74]. PAI can manifest as aneurysm formation, thrombosis, or both [29], but aneurysm formation is more frequent. Isolated "in situ" pulmonary artery thrombosis (PAT) is seen in up to 28% of PAI. In about one third of isolated pulmonary thrombosis, aneurysm formation develops during follow-up [75, 76]. Aneurysms are usually multiple and bilateral. Most frequent localization is lobar arteries [77, 78]. Hemoptysis is the most frequent symptom of pulmonary arterial aneurysm (up to 90%) and is usually the presenting symptom. Life-threatening massive hemoptysis is seen in half of the patients. Hemoptysis, especially massive hemoptysis is seen less frequent in PAT. Constitutional symptoms, fever, dyspnea, cough, and chest pain may also be seen in patients with PAI [10, 27]. An association between PAI and venous involvement was previously shown [6]. In PAT, thromboembolism is not expected due to tightly adherent thrombi to the vessel wall [8]. Mortality rate was around 25% during the follow-up in patients with pulmonary aneurysm. The risk was higher in patients with larger aneurysms and higher systolic pulmonary artery pressure levels [10, 72]. Chronic thromboembolic pulmonary hypertension (CTEPH) may be seen as a rare complication of PAI. In a case series from Turkey with nine patients undergone pulmonary endarterectomy, one patient was deceased due to postoperative complications 1 month after surgery. After a median follow-up of 24 months, eight patients were alive with improvements in pulmonary symptoms [79].

20.5.2 Peripheral Arterial Involvement

The frequency of peripheral arterial involvement is around 5% among all vascular manifestations. It develops late compared to other vascular manifestations, generally mean 5–10 years after the disease-onset. Male predominance is present similar to other vascular manifestations [6]. Peripheral arterial involvement mainly manifests with aneurysms rather than thrombosis [80]. Abdominal aorta, femoral, popliteal, and carotid arteries are the most frequent involvement sites of aneurysm formation. Aneurysm may be seen also in visceral and cerebral arteries. Constitutional symptoms and elevated acute-phase response may be seen in early stages of peripheral arterial involvement [8, 81]. Aneurysms present with painful and pulsatile masses. These pulsatile aneurysms have the risk of rupture or leakage. Abdominal aortic aneurysms usually present with nonspecific symptoms such as back or flank pain, abdominal discomfort and constipation. The rupture of abdominal aorta has a risk of mortality [82]. In a retrospective study of 12 patients with abdominal aneurysms, overall recurrence rate after surgical intervention was 50% [83].

Tüzün H. et al. reported the prognosis of 25 (24 M/1 F) BD patients with non-pulmonary arterial involvement. Twenty-three of the patients had aneurysms while the remaining had arterial occlusions. There was one mortality and 23 patients (92%) were under follow-up after a mean of 7.4 ± 2.9 years. Recurrence rate in this series was 20% [78]. Saadoun et al. reported outcome of 101 patients with arterial involvement among a cohort of 820 patients. Involved arteries were mainly aorta ($n = 25$), femoral ($n = 23$), and pulmonary ($n = 21$) arteries. After a median follow-up of 7.6 years, complete remission was achieved in 39% of the patients, while 28% experienced a relapsing course. Mortality developed in 14%. The 20-year survival rate was found significantly lower in patients with arterial involvement than in those without arterial lesions (73% vs. 89%, respectively) [84].

20.5.3 Cardiac Involvement

Cardiac involvement is a very rare form of vascular involvement in BD (<5%) [7]. Most fequent forms of cardiac involvement is intracardiac thrombosis. Coronary arteritis, pericarditis, myocarditis, endocarditis with valvular regurgitation, endo-myocardial fibrosis, and sinus of valsalva aneurysms were also rarely reported. Intracardiac thrombus is mainly seen in males, and the majority of lesions are located at the right side of the heart. Cardiac valves may rarely be affected. Most frequent symptom is fever, seen in >80% of patients with intracardiac thrombus. Dyspnea, chest pain, and hemoptysis are seen in one third of patients. There is limited data for the prognosis of cardiac involvement. During follow-up of 22 BD patients with intra-cardiac thrombosis, thrombus disappeared in 13 cases and thrombus size was reduced in 7 cases [85]. Valvular regurgitation is seen mostly in the aortic valve and less commonly in the mitral and tricuspid valves. Heart failure may rarely be the first presentation of patients before BD diagnosis. Embolism from these valvular lesions is unexpected due to the tightly attachment to endocardium or myocardium [86]. In a French series of 52 patients, mortality rate was 15% during a median follow-up of 3 (IQR: 1.75–4.2) years. A relapsing disease course was seen in eight (15%) patients. The 5-year survival rates were 83.6% and 95.8% in BD patients with and without cardiac involvement, respectively [87]. Intracardiac thrombosis is strongly associated with PAI [6]. Thus, evaluation of pulmonary arteries with CT angiography is strongly recommended, when intracardiac thrombosis is observed [17].

Coronary artery involvement is an extremely rare form of vascular involvement in BD. It was reported to be 0.5% among all vascular manifestations [88]. Coronary involvement can cause aneurysms or occlusion of coronary artery and may be presented with myocardial infarction or aneurysm rupture [89].

20.6   Imaging in Vascular Involvement of Behçet's Disease

Venous Doppler ultrasound (US) is the mostly used imaging tool to detect venous thrombosis in BD in especially lower extremities, but also for the diagnosis of BCS. A Turkish study compared the diagnostic value of magnetic resonance (MR) venography and Doppler US in 28 BD patients with chronic DVT. While Doppler US detected chronic findings in all patients, MR venography detected in 93%. Collateral veins were detected in 19 patients with MR venography, whereas they were present in only seven patients with US. MR venography might be an alternative or additional method to detect chronic thrombosis in the lower extremities [90]. Contrast-enhanced computerized tomograpraphy (CT) scan and MR angiography (MRA) as noninvasive radiological interventions are the preferred imaging methods to diagnose vena cava thrombosis [91]. For cerebral sinus thrombosis, both CT and MRA may be used for diagnosis, but MR is superior to CT for detecting a clot in the cortical or deep veins. MR also easily shows the ischemic damage (even hemor-rhagic ones) in the cerebral parenchyma in cases of CVT [92].

Invasive procedures are not preferred in vascular BD for imaging of arterial sys-tem due to the risk of aneursym formation at the insertion site [93]. Therefore, conventional angiography should be avoided unless endovascular interventions are planned. For the diagnosis of pulmonary arterial involvement, contrast-enhanced CT is the best option. MRA may be another option, but CT is better to show small aneurysms [29, 94, 95].

For the imaging of peripheral arterial involvement in BD, both CT and MR angiography can be used. The development of multidetector CT has enabled reconstructions of three-dimensional, high-resolution images within very short time. This also allowed the assessment PET is the widely used imaging tool for LVV in recent years. It can be an option in suspicion of isolated aortic involvement in BD of the vessel wall thickening and mural thrombus. There is limited data with PET-CT imaging to show inflammatory activity in pulmonary arteries [96, 97].

20.7   Diagnosis

There is no spesific diagnostic test for BD and the diagnosis depends on clinical features. International Study Group (ISG) for Behçet's disease developed a set of classification criteria in 1990. ISG criteria was validated and is widely used for BD, with a sensitivity and specificity >90%. The diagnosis requires recurrent oral ulcers plus at least two of genital ulcers, erythema-nodosum-like lesions, folliculitis, uveitis (anterior or pan-uveitis) and pathergy test [98]. This criteria set does not include major organ involvement except ocular involvement. The 2014 International Criteria for Behçet's Disease seems to be more sensitive especially in early disease due to including scores for major organ involvement. However, it may cause overdiagnosis and patients especially with spondyloarthropathic features can be mislabeled as BD [99].

Diagnosing BD can be a clinical challenge, especially in patients presenting with major manifestations such as vascular, ocular, or neurologic involvement with or without oral aphthous lesions. These patients not meeting diagnostic criteria, had BD diagnosis with "expert opinion" in countries with high prevalence of BD. Incomplete BD was also reported as increased in recent years in Far-East countries such as Japan and Korea [100]. Furthermore, early diagnosis is of utmost importance especially in severe cases with venous thrombosis as their management differ from non-inflammatory DVT, necessitating immunosuppressive use rather than anticoagulant therapy. Our recent studies previously mentioned showed that measurement of CFV thickness with Doppler ultrasound (US) can be a diagnostic test for BD with sensitivity and the specificities higher than 80% for the cut-off value of ≥ 0.5 mm (Alibaz-Oner et al., Rheum(Oxford) in press).

20.8   Treatment

20.8.1 Medical Treatment

The primary pathology leading to thrombosis in BD is the inflammation of the vessel wall and systemic ISs are used to reduce this inflammation. However, there are no controlled studies of ISs for the management of major vessel disease in

BD. According to the EULAR 2018 recommendations, glucocorticoids (GC) and ISs such as azathioprine, cyclophosphamide, or cyclosporine-A are recommended for the management of acute DVT in BD, monoclonal tumor necrosis factor (TNF) inhibitors could be considered in refractory patients [101]. Hamuryudan et al. reported the follow-up results of patients included in an RCT of azathioprine for ocular involvement. In this study, vascular and neurological involvement was less present among patients who had been treated with azathioprine [102]. Retrospective case series also showed the beneficial effects of azathioprine in vascular involvement [6]. A recent prospective study from Turkey showed that 45% of the 29 patients with DVT relapsed under azathioprine treatment during a mean follow-up of 40.7 ± 13.4 months. In this study, 13 of 14 patients treated with interferon-alpha had good recanalization, and only 2 (11%) had a relapse during a mean follow-up of 29 ± 20 months. Interferon-alpha seems as promising agent for the treatment of VBD [52].

In a recent retrospective study including 70 patients with DVT or superficial thrombophlebitis, biologic treatments, and conventional IS therapies including azathioprine, cyclosporine-A, and cyclophosphamide were compared. Vascular response rate was higher in adalimumab-based regimens (34/35, 97%) compared to conventional IS therapies (23/35, 66%) during a mean follow-up of 25.7 ± 23.2 months. Relapse rate was also found lower in patients treated with adalimumab-based regimens compared to patients treated with conventional therapies (9% vs 40%) [103]. As a general approach, life-threatening conditions such as pulmonary arterial aneurysm (PAA) and BCS are managed with more aggressive medical treatment including cyclophosphamide and glucocorticoid pulses [8]. Monoclonal TNF inhibitors should be considered in refractory cases.

There is now increasing data of TNF inhibitors for the treatment of all types of refractory VBD [104–106]. *Desbois* et al. reported 18 VBD patients treated with TNF inhibitors and refractory to conventional immunosuppressants. Clinical remission was achieved in about 90% of patients. Relapse developed in two (11%) patients after discontinuation of TNF inhibitors [107]. In a series of 27 refractory VBD patients treated with TNFα inhibitor agents, complete clinical remission was achieved in 22 (80%) patients within 3 months. The median daily dose of GCs significantly decreased at 3 months. Infliximab was the first choice of TNFα inhibitor in 24 and adalimumab in three patients. A trend toward a higher rate of complete remission was observed with concomitant IS use compared to monotherapy of TNFα inhibitors (93% vs 67%, $p = 0.09$) [108].

There are limited data with other biological agents showing the efficacy of anakinra [109], alemtuzumab [110], and tociluzumab [111] in refractory VBD.

20.9   Anticoagulation

IS treatment is the mainstay of VBD. But there is no concensus for anticoagulation. Data for anticoagulation in the treatment of VBD comes from only retrospective studies. *Desbois AC* et al. analyzed their retrospective cohort of 807 BD patients. All BD patients with deep vein thrombosis ($n = 296$) received anticoagulation therapy despite a high number of associated arterial aneurysms ($n = 44$), eight of which were pulmonary. Hemorrhagic complications were seen in only 2% of the patients. The rate of immunosuppressive usage was only 46.8% in patients having deep venous thrombosis in this study; however, IS agents significantly reduced venous thrombosis relapses [112]. In a multicenter retrospective study from Turkey evaluating different treatment modalities in VBD, the relapse rate was found similar between patients using only ISs and those using anticoagulants together with ISs (29.1% vs 22.4%, $p = 0.08$). In multivariate analysis, development of vascular relapse negatively correlated with only IS treatments, adding anticoagulants on ISs had no additional positive effect [7]. In a retrospective study, any positive effect of anticoagulants on development of post-thrombotic syndrome after DVT is also not shown [51]. A meta-analysis of three retrospective studies showed that ISs and anticoagulants are superior to anticoagulants alone (RR 0.17, 95% CI 0.08–0.35), and adding anticoagulants to ISs provides no benefit (RR 0.75, 95% CI 0.48–1.17). According to EULAR Recommendations, anticoagulants may be added, provided the risk of bleeding in general is low and coexistent pulmonary artery aneurysms are ruled out [113].

20.10 Surgical Treatment

As indications for surgical interventions in venous disease is rare, surgery is an option for mainly arterial involvement in VBD [8]. In a recent case series and systematic review, the results of initial endovascular or surgical interventions were unfavorable in 22 (53.6%) of 41 BD patients with venous thrombosis [114]. In case of need for surgical interventions, there is no consensus for optimal intervention modality or optimal graft type in VBD. But, peri- and postoperative IS treatment were suggested to reduce surgical complications and relapses [115]. For PAAs, surgical treatment without IS treatment is not a successful option due to multiple location of aneurysms in different parts of lungs. Nevertheless, lobectomy may be an option together with peri- and postopperative IS treatment in selected cases. Endovascular embolization may be effective in PAA in patients refractory to medical treatments [75, 116]. Endovascular embolization should also be preferred to open surgery in patients with a high risk of major bleeding [113]. Recently, in refractory cases, pulmonary endarterectomy was reported to be well tolerated and effective in VBD with pulmonary hypertension due to thrombi [79].

Peripheral arterial aneurysms should be treated surgically [80]. For both pulmonary and peripheral artery aneurysms, the choice of surgical intervention between graft insertion, ligation, and bypass surgery should be made according to the size and location of the aneurysm and the surgeon's experience. Synthetic grafts should be preferred since venous grafts have a higher risk of thrombosis in patients with BS [113].

20.11 Conclusion

Vascular BD is a complex vasculitis involving all size veins and arteries. It is one of the major causes of mortality and morbidity, especially in males. While vein involvement presents with thrombosis, arterial involvement present with both aneurysm and thrombosis. DVT in lower extremity is the most frequent vascular involvement type. Current evidence suggests that the pathogenesis of thrombosis in BD is probably not due to a hypercoagulable state but rather to the vascular damage induced by inflammation or intrinsic endothelial dysfunction. Recent studies showed that neutrophils have critical role in inflammation-associated thrombosis in BD. There is no specific diagnostic test for BD and the diagnosis depends on clinical features. For the cases presenting with oral ulcers and especially recurrent vascular involvement, measurement of common femoral vein thickness can be used as a diagnostic test. Glucocorticoids, azathioprine, and cyclophosphamide are still recommended as the first-line treatments in VBD. However, TNF inhibitors and interferon-alpha can be used in refractory patients. Anticoagulant usage for VBD is still controversial due to limited data coming from only retrospective studies. There is a clear need for randomized controlled studies for the management of VBD.

References

1. Calamia KT, Schirmer M, Melikoglu M. Major vessel involvement in Behcçet's disease: an update. Curr Opin Rheumatol. 2011;23:24–31.
2. Yazici H, Yurdakul S, Hamuryudan V. Behcçet disease. Curr Opin Rheumatol. 2001;13:18–22.
3. Ozguler Y, Esatoglu SN, Seyahi E, Melikoglu M. Vascular and cardiac involvement. In: Yazici Y, et al., editors. Behçet syndrome. 2nd ed. Springer Nature Switzerland AG; 2020. p. 83–103.
4. Ishido T, Horita N, Takeuchi M, Kawagoe T, Shibuya E, Yamane T, et al. Clinical manifestations of Behçet's disease depending on sex and age: results from Japanese Nationwide Registration. Rheumatology (Oxford). 2017;56(11):1918–27.
5. Ryu HJ, Seo MR, Choi HJ, Baek HJ. Clinical phenotypes of Korean patients with Behcet disease according to gender, age at onset, and HLA-B51. Korean J Intern Med. 2018;33(5):1025–31.
6. Tascilar K, Melikoglu M, Ugurlu S, Sut N, Caglar E, Yazici H. Vascular involvement in Behcet's syndrome: a retrospective analysis of associations and the time course. Rheumatology (Oxford). 2014;53(11):2018–22.
7. Alibaz-Oner F, Karadeniz A, Yılmaz S, Balkarlı A, Kimyon G, Yazıcı A. Behçet disease with vascular involvement: effects of different therapeutic regimens on the incidence of new relapses. Medicine (Baltimore). 2015;94(6):e494.
8. Seyahi E. Behcet's disease: how to diagnose and treat vascular involvement. Best Pract Res Clin Rheumatol. 2016;30(2):279–95.
9. Saadoun D, Wechsler B, Desseaux K, Le Thi Huong D, Amoura Z, Resche-Rigon M, et al. Mortality in Behçet's disease. Arthritis Rheum. 2010;62:2806–12.
10. Kural-Seyahi E, Fresko I, Seyahi N, Ozyazgan Y, Mat C, Hamuryudan V, et al. The long-term mortality and morbidity of Behcet syndrome: a 2-decade outcome survey of 387 patients followed at a dedicated center. Medicine (Baltimore). 2003;82:60–76.

11. Jennette JC, Falk RJ, Bacon PA, Basu N, Cid MC, Ferrario F, et al. 2012 revised international chapel hill consensus conference nomenclature of vasculitides. Arthritis Rheum. 2013;65:1–11.
12. Yazici H, Seyahi E, Hatemi G, Yazici Y. Behcet syndrome: a contemporary view. Nat Rev Rheumatol. 2018;14(2):119.
13. Yazawa S, Ishihara A, Kawasaki S. Fatal thoracic aortic aneurysm in a patient with childhood-onset vasculo-Behçet's disease: an autopsy report. Intern Med. 2001;40(11):1154–7.
14. Fukuda Y, Watanabe I, Hayashi H, Kuwabara N. Pathological studies on Behçet's disease. Ryumachi. 1980;20(4):268–75.
15. Lakhanpal S, Tani K, Lie JT, Katoh K, Ishigatsubo Y, Ohokubo T. Pathologic features of Behçet's syndrome: a review of Japanese autopsy registry data. Hum Pathol. 1985;16(8):790–5.
16. Ko GY, Byun JY, Choi BG, Cho SH. The vascular manifestations of Behçet's disease: angiographic and CT findings. Br J Radiol. 2000;73(876):1270–4.
17. Mogulkoc N, Burgess MI, Bishop PW. Intracardiac thrombus in Behçet's disease: a systematic review. Chest. 2000;118(2):479–87.
18. Kobayashi M, Ito M, Nakagawa A, Matsushita M, Nishikimi N, Sakurai T, et al. Neutrophil and endothelial cell activation in the vasa vasorum in vasculo-Behcet disease. Histopathology. 2000;36(4):362–71.
19. Matsumoto T, Uekusa T, Fukuda Y. Vasculo-Behçet's disease: a pathologic study of eight cases. Hum Pathol. 1991;22(1):45–51.
20. Kim B, LeBoit PE. Histopathologic features of erythema nodosum—like lesions in Behçet disease: a comparison with erythema nodosum focusing on the role of vasculitis. Am J Dermatopathol. 2000;22(5):379–90.
21. Kiraz S, Ertenli I, Ozturk MA, Haznedaroglu IC, Celik I, Calguneri M. Pathological haemostasis and "prothrombotic state" in Behcet's disease. Thromb Res. 2002;105(2):125–33.
22. Chamorro AJ, Marcos M, Hernandez-Garcia I, Calvo A, Mejia JC, Cervera R, et al. Association of allelic variants of factor V Leiden, prothrombin and methylenetetrahydrofolate reductase with thrombosis or ocular involvement in Behcet's disease: a systematic review and meta-analysis. Autoimmun Rev. 2013;12(5):607–16.
23. La Regina M, Orlandini F, Prisco D, Dentali F. Homocysteine in vascular Behcet disease: a meta-analysis. Arterioscler Thromb Vasc Biol. 2010;30(10):2067–74.
24. Tokay S, Direskeneli H, Yurdakul S, Akoglu T. Anticardiolipin antibodies in Behçet's disease: a reassessment. Rheumatology (Oxford). 2001;40(2):192–5.
25. Yaşar NŞ, Salgür F, Cansu DÜ, Kaşifoğlu T, Korkmaz C. Combined thrombophilic factors increase the risk of recurrent thrombotic events in Behcet's disease. Clin Rheumatol. 2010;29(12):1367–72.
26. Espinosa G, Font J, Tassies D, Vidaller A, Deulofeu R, Lopez-Soto A, et al. Vascular involvement in Behcet's disease: relation with thrombophilic factors, coagulation activation, and thrombomodulin. Am J Med. 2002;112(1):37–43.
27. Leiba M, Seligsohn U, Sidi Y, Harats D, Sela BA, Griffin JH, et al. Thrombophilic factors are not the leading cause of thrombosis in Behcet's disease. Ann Rheum Dis. 2004;63(11):1445–9.
28. Chambers JC, Haskard DO, Kooner JS. Vascular endothelial function and oxidative stress mechanisms in patients with Behçet's syndrome. J Am Coll Cardiol. 2001;37(2):517–20.
29. Erkan F, Gül A, Tasali E. Pulmonary manifestations of Behçet's disease. Thorax. 2001;56:572–8.
30. Hirohata S, Kikuchi H. Histopathology of the ruptured pulmonary artery aneurysm in a patient with Behçet's disease. Clin Exp Rheumatol. 2009;27:S91–5.
31. Ergun T, Gürbüz O, Harvell J, et al. The histopathology of pathergy: a chronologic study of skin hyperreactivity in Behçet's disease. Int J Dermatol. 1998;37:929–93.
32. Matsumura N, Mizushima Y. Leucocyte movement and colchicine treatment in Behçet's disease. Lancet. 1975;2:813.

33. Eksioglu-Demiralp E, Direskeneli H, Kibaroglu A, Yavuz S, Ergun T, Akoglu T. Neutrophil activation in Behçet's disease. Clin Exp Rheumatol. 2001;19:S19–24.
34. Saruhan-Direskeneli G, Yentur SP, Akman-Demir G, Isik N, Serdaroglu P. Cytokines and chemokines in neuro-Behcet's disease compared to multiple sclerosis and other neurological diseases. J Neuroimmunol. 2003;145:127–34.
35. Kawakami T, Ohashi S, Kawa Y, Takahama H, Ito M, Soma Y, et al. Elevated serum granulocyte colony stimulating factor levels in patients with active phase of sweet syndrome and patients with active behcet disease: implication in neutrophil apoptosis dysfunction. Arch Dermatol. 2004;140:570–4.
36. Yavuz S, Akdeniz T, Hancer V, Bicakcigil M, Can M, Yanikkaya-Demirel G. Dual effect of testosterone in Behcet's disease: implications for a role in disease pathogenesis. Genes Immun. 2016;17(6):335–41.
37. Ørensen OE, Borregaard N. Neutrophil extracellular traps—the dark side of neutrophils. J Clin Invest. 2016;126:1612–20.
38. Lee KH, Kronbichler A, Park DD, Park Y, Moon H, Kim H, et al. Neutrophil extracellular traps (NETs) in autoimmune diseases: a comprehensive review. Autoimmun Rev. 2017;16(11):1160–73.
39. Martinod K, Wagner DD. Thrombosis: tangled up in nets. Blood. 2014;123:2768–76.
40. Le Joncour A, Martos R, Loyau S, Lelay N, Dossier A, Cazes A, et al. Critical role of neutrophil extracellular traps (NETs) in patients with Behcet's disease. Ann Rheum Dis. 2019;78(9):1274–82.
41. Becatti M, Emmi G, Silvestri E, Bruschi G, Ciucciarelli L, Squatrito D, et al. Neutrophil activation promotes fibrinogen oxidation and thrombus formation in Behcet disease. Circulation. 2016;133:302–11.
42. Mittal M, Siddiqui MR, Tran K, Reddy SP, Malik AB. Reactive oxygen species in inflammation and tissue injury. Antioxid Redox Signal. 2014;20:1126–67.
43. Soehnlein O. Multiple roles for neutrophils in atherosclerosis. Circ Res. 2012;110:875–88.
44. van Montfoort ML, Stephan F, Lauw MN, Hutten BA, Van Mierlo GJ, Solati S, et al. Circulating nucleosomes and neutrophil activation as risk factors for deep vein thrombosis. Arterioscler Thromb Vasc Biol. 2013;33:147–51.
45. Emmi G, Becatti M, Bettiol A, Hatemi G, Prisco D, Fiorillo C. Behçet's syndrome as a model of thrombo-inflammation: the role of neutrophils. Front Immunol. 2019;10:1085.
46. Vallier L, Cointe S, Lacroix R, Bonifay A, Judicone C, Dignat-George F, Kwaan HC. Microparticles and fibrinolysis. Semin Thromb Hemost. 2017;43(2):129–34.
47. Mejía JC, Ortiz T, Tàssies D, Solanich X, Vidaller A, Cervera R, et al. Procoagulant microparticles are increased in patients with Behçet's disease but do not define a specific subset of clinical manifestations. Clin Rheumatol. 2016;35(3):695–9.
48. Macey M, Hagi-Pavli E, Stewart J, Wallace GR, Stanford M, Shirlaw P, et al. Age, gender and disease-related platelet and neutrophil activation ex vivo in whole blood samples from patients with Behçet's disease. Rheumatology (Oxford). 2011;50(10):1849–59.
49. Khan E, Ambrose NL, Ahnström J, Kiprianos AP, Stanford MR, Eleftheriou D, et al. A low balance between microparticles expressing tissue factor pathway inhibitor and tissue factor is associated with thrombosis in Behçet's Syndrome. Sci Rep. 2016;6:38104.
50. Seyahi E, Cakmak OS, Tutar B, Arslan C, Dikici AS, Sut N, et al. Clinical and Ultrasonographic evaluation of lower-extremity vein thrombosis in Behcet syndrome: an observational study. Medicine (Baltimore). 2015;94(44):e1899.
51. Alibaz-Oner F, Aldag B, Aldag M, Unal AU, Mutiş A, Toptas T, Ergun T, Direskeneli H. Post-thrombotic syndrome and venous disease-specific quality of life in patients with vascular Behçet's disease. J Vasc Surg Venous Lymphat Disord. 2016;4(3):301–6.
52. Ozguler Y, Hatemi G, Cetinkaya F, Tascilar K, Hamuryudan V, Ugurlu S, Seyahi E, Yazici H, Melikoglu M. Clinical course of acute deep vein thrombosis of the legs in Behçet's syndrome. Rheumatology (Oxford). 2020;59(4):799–806.

53. Kahn SR, Ginsberg JS. Relationship between deep venous thrombosis and the postthrombotic syndrome. Arch Intern Med. 2004;164:17–26.
54. Kahn SR, Hirsch A, Shrier I. Effect of post-thrombotic syndrome on health-related quality of life after deep venous thrombosis. Arch Intern Med. 2002;162:1144–8.
55. Kahn SR, Lamping DL, Ducruet T, Arsenault L, Miron MJ, Roussin A, et al. VEINES-QOL/Sym questionnaire was a reliable and valid disease-specific quality of life measure for deep venous thrombosis. J Clin Epidemiol. 2006;59:1049–56.
56. Jung JY, Kim DY, Bang D. Leg ulcers in Behcet's disease. Br J Dermatol. 2008;158(1):178–9.
57. Ozguler Y, Kutlubay Z, Dikici AS, Melikoglu M, Mat C, Yazici H, et al. Leg ulcers in Behçet's syndrome: an observational survey in 24 patients. Arthritis Rheumatol. 2018;70(Suppl 10):9.
58. Ambrose N, Pierce IT, Gatehouse PD, Haskard DO, Firmin DN. Magnetic resonance imaging of vein wall thickness in patients with Behçet's syndrome. Clin Exp Rheumatol. 2014;32:S99–102.
59. Boulon C, Skopinski S, Constans J. Vein inflammation and ultrasound in Behçet's syndrome. Rheumatology (Oxford). 2016;55:1750.
60. Alibaz-Oner F, Mutis A, Ergelen R, Erturk Z, Ergun E, Direskeneli D. Venous vessel wall thickness in lower extremity is increased in male Behcet's disease patients without vascular involvement. Rheumatology (Oxford). 2017;56(Suppl 3).
61. Alibaz-Oner F, Ergelen R, Mutis A, Erturk Z, Asadov R, Mumcu G, et al. Venous vessel wall thickness in lower extremity is increased in male patients with Behçet's disease. Clin Rheumatol. 2019;38(5):1447–51.
62. Seyahi E, Gjoni M, Durmaz ES, Durmaz EŞ, Akbaş S, Sut N, et al. Increased vein wall thickness in Behçet disease. J Vasc Surg Venous Lymphat Disord. 2019;7(5):677–684.e2.
63. Kansu E, Ozer FL, Akalin E, Guler Y, Zileli T, Tanman E, et al. Behcet's syndrome with obstruction of the venae cavae. A report of seven cases. Q J Med. 1972;41(162):151–68.
64. Houman H, Lamloum M, Ben Ghorbel I, Khiari-Ben Salah I, Miled M. Vena cava thrombosis in Behcet's disease. Analysis of a series of 10 cases. Ann Med Interne (Paris). 1999;150(8):587–90.
65. Benjilali L, Harmouche H, Alaoui-Bennesser H, Mezalek ZT, Adnaoui M, Aouni M, et al. Chylothorax and chylopericardium in a young man with Behcet's disease. Joint Bone Spine. 2008;75(6):743–5.
66. Seyahi E, Caglar E, Ugurlu S, Kantarci F, Hamuryudan V, Sonsuz A, Melikoglu M, Yurdakul S, Yazici H. An outcome survey of 43 patients with Budd-Chiari syndrome due to Behçet's syndrome followed up at a single, dedicated center. Semin Arthritis Rheum. 2015;44(5):602–9.
67. Desbois AC, Rautou PE, Biard L, Belmatoug N, Wechsler B, Resche-Rigon M, et al. Behcet's disease in Budd-Chiari syndrome. Orphanet J Rare Dis. 2014;9:104.
68. Sakr MA, Reda MA, Ebada HE, Abdelmoaty AS, Hefny ZM, Ibrahim ZH, et al. Characteristics and outcome of primary Budd-Chiari syndrome due to Behçet's syndrome. Clin Res Hepatol Gastroenterol. 2019. pii: S2210-7401(19)30249-9.
69. Akman-Demir G, Serdaroglu P, Tasçi B. Clinical patterns of neurological involvement in Behçet's disease: evaluation of 200 patients. The Neuro-Behçet Study Group. Brain. 1999;122(Pt 11):2171–82.
70. Uluduz D, Midi I, Duman T, Colakoglu S, Tüfekci A, Bakar M, et al. Behçet's disease as a causative factor of cerebral venous sinus thrombosis: subgroup analysis of data from the VENOST study. Rheumatology (Oxford). 2019;58(4):600–8.
71. Saadoun D, Wechsler B, Resche-Rigon M, Trad S, Le Thi Huong D, Sbai A, et al. Cerebral venous thrombosis in Behçet's disease. Arthritis Rheum. 2009;61(4):518–26.
72. Yesilot N, Bahar S, Yilmazer S, Mutlu M, Kurtuncu M, Tuncay R, Coban O, Akman-Demir G. Cerebral venous thrombosis in Behçet's disease compared to those associated with other etiologies. J Neurol. 2009;256(7):1134–42.
73. Aguiar de Sousa D, Mestre T, Ferro JM. Cerebral venous thrombosis in Behçet's disease: a systematic review. J Neurol. 2011;258(5):719–27.

74. Hamuryudan V, Er T, Seyahi E, Akman C, Tüzün H, Fresko I, et al. Pulmonary artery aneurysms in Behçet syndrome. Am J Med. 2004;117:867–70.
75. Seyahi E, Melikoglu M, Akman C, Hamuryudan V, Ozer H, Hatemi G, et al. Pulmonary artery involvement and associated lung disease in Behcet disease: a series of 47 patients. Medicine (Baltimore). 2012;91(1):35–48.
76. Uzun O, Akpolat T, Erkan L. Pulmonary vasculitis in behcet disease: a cumulative analysis. Chest. 2005;127(6):2243–53.
77. Yuan S. Pulmonary artery aneurysms in Behçet disease. J Vasc Bras. 2014;13(3):217–28.
78. Tunaci M, Ozkorkmaz B, Tunaci A, Gul A, Engin G, Acunas B. CT findings of pulmonary artery aneurysms during treatment for Behcet's disease. AJR Am J Roentgenol. 1999;172(3):729–33.
79. Yildizeli SO, Yanartas M, Tas S, Direskeneli H, Mutlu B, Ceyhan B, et al. Outcomes of patients with Behçet's syndrome after pulmonary endarterectomy. Thorac Cardiovasc Surg. 2018;66(2):187–92.
80. Tuzun H, Seyahi E, Arslan C, Hamuryudan V, Besirli K, Yazici H. Management and prognosis of nonpulmonary large arterial disease in patients with Behçet disease. J Vasc Surg. 2012;55:157–63.
81. Chae EJ, Do KH, Seo JB, Park SH, Kang JW, Jang YM, et al. Radiologic and clinical findings of Behcet disease: comprehensive review of multisystemic involvement. Radiographics. 2008;28(5):e31.
82. Tuzun H, Besirli K, Sayin A, Vural FS, Hamuryudan V, Hizli N, et al. Management of aneurysms in Behcet's syndrome: an analysis of 24 patients. Surgery. 1997;121(2):150–6.
83. Kwon TW, Park SJ, Kim HK, Yoon HK, Kim GE, Yu B. Surgical treatment result of abdominal aortic aneurysm in Behçet's disease. Eur J Vasc Endovasc Surg. 2008;35:173–80.
84. Saadoun D, Asli B, Wechsler B, Houman H, Geri G, Desseaux K, et al. Long-term outcome of arterial lesions in Behçet disease: a series of 101 patients. Medicine (Baltimore). 2012;91(1):18–24.
85. Emmungil H, Yaşar Bilge NŞ, Küçükşahin O, Kılıç L, Okutucu S, Gücenmez S, et al. A rare but serious manifestation of Behçet's disease: intracardiac thrombus in 22 patients. Clin Exp Rheumatol. 2014;32(4 Suppl 84):S87–92. Epub 2014 Jul 28.
86. Lee I, Park S, Hwang I, Kim MJ, Nah SS, Yoo B, et al. Cardiac Behcet disease presenting as aortic valvulitis/aortitis or right heart inflammatory mass: a clinicopathologic study of 12 cases. Am J Surg Pathol. 2008;32(3):390–8.
87. Geri G, Wechsler B, Thi Huong DL, Isnard R, Piette JC, Amoura Z, et al. Spectrum of cardiac lesions in Behcet disease: a series of 52 patients and review of the literature. Medicine (Baltimore). 2012;91(1):25–34.
88. Fei Y, Li X, Lin S, Song X, Wu Q, Zhu Y, et al. Major vascular involvement in Behçet's disease: a retrospective study of 796 patients. Clin Rheumatol. 2013;32(6):845–52.
89. Farouk H, Zayed HS, El-Chilali K. Cardiac findings in patients with Behcet's disease: facts and controversies. Anatol J Cardiol. 2016;16(7):529–33.
90. Tutar B, Kantarci F, Cakmak OS, Yazici H, Seyahi E. Assessment of deep venous thrombosis in the lower extremity in Behçet's syndrome: MR venography versus Doppler ultrasonography. Intern Emerg Med. 2019;14(5):705–11.
91. Tunaci A, Berkmen YM, Gokmen E. Thoracic involvement in Behçet's disease: pathologic, clinical, and imaging features. AJR Am J Roentgenol. 1995;164(1):51–6.
92. Bonneville F. Imaging of cerebral venous thrombosis. Diagn Interv Imaging. 2014;95(12):1145–50.
93. Bradbury AW, Milne AA, Murie JA. Surgical aspects of Behçet's disease. Br J Surg. 1994;81:1712–21.
94. Esatoglu SN, Seyahi E, Ugurlu S, Gulsen F, Akman C, Cantasdemir M, et al. Bronchial artery enlargement may be the cause of recurrent haemoptysis in Behçet's syndrome patients with pulmonary artery involvement during follow-up. Clin Exp Rheumatol. 2016;34(6 Suppl 102):92–6.

95. Mehdipoor G, Davatchi F, Ghoreishian H, Arjmand Shabestari A. Imaging manifestations of Behcet's disease: key considerations and major features. Eur J Radiol. 2018;98:214–25.

96. Cho SB, Yun M, Lee JH, Kim J, Shim WH, Bang D. Detection of cardiovascular system involvement in Behcet's disease using fluorodeoxyglucose positron emission tomography. Semin Arthritis Rheum. 2011;40(5):461–6.

97. Trad S, Bensimhon L, El Hajjam M, Chinet T, Wechsler B, Saadoun D. 18F-fluorodeoxy-glucose-positron emission tomography scanning is a useful tool for therapy evaluation of arterial aneurysm in Behcet's disease. Joint Bone Spine. 2013;80(4):420–3.

98. International Study Group for Behçet's Disease. Criteria for diagnosis of Behçet's disease. Lancet. 1990;335:1078–80.

99. The International Criteria for Behçet's Disease (ICBD): a collaborative study of 27 countries on the sensitivity and specificity of the new criteria. International Team for the Revision of the International Criteria for Behçet's Disease (ITR-ICBD). J Eur Acad Dermatol Venereol. 2014;28(3):338–47.

100. Kirino Y, Ideguchi H, Takeno M, Suda A, Higashitani K, Kunishita Y, et al. Continuous evolution of clinical phenotype in 578 Japanese patients with Behcet's disease: a retrospective observational study. Arthritis Res Ther. 2016;18:217.

101. Hatemi G, Christensen R, Bang D, Bodaghi B, Celik AF, Fortune F, et al. 2018 update of the EULAR recommendations for the management of Behcet's syndrome. Ann Rheum Dis. 2018;77(6):808–18.

102. Hamuryudan V, Ozyazgan Y, Hizli N, et al. Azathioprine in Behcet's syndrome: effects on long-term prognosis. Arthritis Rheum. 1997;40:769–74.

103. Emmi G, Vitale A, Silvestri E, Boddi M, Becatti M, Fiorillo C, et al. Adalimumab-based treatment versus disease-modifying antirheumatic drugs for venous thrombosis in Behcet's syndrome: a retrospective study of seventy patients with vascular involvement. Arthritis Rheumatol. 2018;70(9):1500–7.

104. Adler S, Baumgartner I, Villiger PM. Behcet's disease: successful treatment with infliximab in 7 patients with severe vascular manifestations. A retrospective analysis. Arthritis Care Res (Hoboken). 2012;64:607–11.

105. Vitale A, Emmi G, Lopalco G, Gentileschi S, Silvestri E, Fabiani C, et al. Adalimumab effectiveness in Behcet's disease: short and long-term data from a multicenter retrospective observational study. Clin Rheumatol. 2017;36(2):451–5.

106. Chan E, Sangle SR, Coghlan JG, D'Cruz DD. Pulmonary artery aneurysms in Behcet's disease treated with anti-TNFα: a case series and review of the literature. Autoimmun Rev. 2016;15(4):375–8.

107. Desbois AC, Biard L, Addimanda O, Lambert M, Hachulla E, Launay D, et al. Efficacy of anti-TNF alpha in severe and refractory major vessel involvement of Behcet's disease: a multicenter observational study of 18 patients. Clin Immunol. 2018;197:54–9.

108. Aksoy A, Yazici A, Omma A, Cefle A, Onen F, Tasdemir U, et al. Efficacy of TNFα inhibitors for refractory vascular Behcet's disease: a multicenter observational study of 27 patients and a review of the literature. Int J Rheum Dis. 2020;23(2):256–61.

109. Cantarini L, Vitale A, Scalini P, Dinarello CA, Rigante D, Franceschini R, et al. Anakinra treatment in drug-resistant Behcet's disease: a case series. Clin Rheumatol. 2015;34:1293–301.

110. Mohammad AJ, Smith RM, Chow YW, Chaudhry AN, Jayne DR. Alemtuzumab as remission induction therapy in Behçet disease: a 20-year experience. J Rheumatol. 2015;42(10):1906–13.

111. Ding Y, Li C, Liu J, Yu X, Wang Y, Shi J, et al. Tocilizumab in the treatment of severe and/or refractory vasculo-Behcet's disease: a single-centre experience in China. Rheumatology (Oxford). 2018;57(11):2057–9.

112. Desbois AC, Wechsler B, Resche-Rigon M, Piette JC, Huong Dle T, Amoura Z, et al. Immunosuppressants reduce venous thrombosis relapse in Behcet's disease. Arthritis Rheum. 2012;64(8):2753–60.

113. Hatemi G, Christensen R, Bang D, Bodaghi B, Celik AF, Fortune F, et al. 2018 update of the EULAR recommendations for the management of Behçet's syndrome. Ann Rheum Dis. 2018;77(6):808–18.
114. Dincses E, Esatoglu SN, Fresko I, Melikoglu M, Seyahi E. Outcome of invasive procedures for venous thrombosis in Behçet's syndrome: case series and systematic literature review. Clin Exp Rheumatol. 2019;37 Suppl 121(6):125–31.
115. Ozguler Y, Hatemi G. Management of Behçet's syndrome. Curr Opin Rheumatol. 2016;28(1):45–50.
116. Alpay-Kanitez N, Çelik S, Baltacioğlu F, Içaçan OC, Bes C, Yildizeli B. Endovascular embolisation with Amplatzer vascular plug of ruptured pulmonary artery aneurism in Behçet's disease. Clin Exp Rheumatol. 2019;37 Suppl 121(6):152–3.

Correction to: Isolated Gastrointestinal Vasculitis

Thomas D. Garvey and Kenneth J. Warrington

Correction to: C. Salvarani et al. (eds.), *Large and Medium Size Vessel and Single Organ Vasculitis, Rare Diseases of the Immune System*, https://doi.org/10.1007/978-3-030-67175-4_17

Owing to an oversight on the part of the production, this chapter was initially published with incorrect authorship. The chapter was published with Kenneth J. Warrington name alone, and co-author Thomas D. Garvey details were inadvertently missed. The authorship has now been updated with this erratum.

The updated online version of the chapter can be found at https://doi.org/10.1007/978-3-030-67175-4_17

© Springer Nature Switzerland AG 2021
C. Salvarani et al. (eds.), *Large and Medium Size Vessel and Single Organ Vasculitis*, Rare Diseases of the Immune System,
https://doi.org/10.1007/978-3-030-67175-4_21

Index

© Springer Nature Switzerland AG 2021   277
C. Salvarani et al. (eds.), *Large and Medium Size Vessel and Single Organ*
Vasculitis, Rare Diseases of the Immune System,
https://doi.org/10.1007/978-3-030-67175-4

Printed in the United States
by Baker & Taylor Publisher Services